Lasers in Proctology

Kamal Gupta

Lasers in Proctology

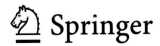 Springer

Kamal Gupta
Department of Surgery
Karan Hospital
Jalandhar, India

ISBN 978-981-19-5824-3   ISBN 978-981-19-5825-0   (eBook)
https://doi.org/10.1007/978-981-19-5825-0

This Springer imprint is published by the registered company Springer Nature Singapore Pte Ltd.
The registered company address is: 152 Beach Road, #21-01/04 Gateway East, Singapore
189721, Singapore

Dedicated to

A few good women

My mother, Mrs. Ved Gupta; my wife, Dr. Ruby; and my daughters Ankita and Nikita

and

A few good men

My father, Dr. Sat Paul Gupta; my mentor, Guru, and teacher, Dr. Kushal Mital; and my friend and critic, Dr. Niranjan Agarwal

Foreword

In the last decade, there has been a surge in publications on *Lasers in Proctology*. Many surgeons own laser equipment, yet there is no in-depth narrative on using lasers in proctology. A considerable variation in results, the wavelength used, type of laser machines, and amount of energy used has been mentioned in the literature, leaving a surgeon dazed. The missing piece is how exactly the procedure is done, how to select patients, how much energy is safe, and what steps are to be taken to avoid potential complications. The book *Lasers in Proctology* arrives when there is a surge in patients opting for lasers for anorectal diseases.

Lasers in Proctology is a comprehensive book with 19 chapters spread over 200 pages with more than 200 professional illustrations, giving in-depth knowledge of the "Art of Application of Laser Technology in Proctology." If a surgeon is practicing proctology, this book should be read cover to cover, over and over again. After reading it, practice it. You would notice a difference in the outcome of the results.

The book came out on the demand of surgeons using LASERS in practice. I met Dr. Kamal Gupta for the first time in the Minimal Invasive Benign Proctology course at CeMAST, Mumbai, in 2017. He was a student seeking knowledge, and I was the Director and one of the course faculty. As a student, he was seeking answers to never-ending questions. At the time, he was far ahead of us in lasers but not quite getting the desired results. After thoroughly understanding the anatomy taught in the course, he focused on improving outcomes in patients undergoing laser surgery. After he proved that lasers were safe and the techniques reproducible, he was offered a faculty position to teach lasers in proctology at CeMAST.

Over the next 6 months, he sent me over 300 articles from PubMed on lasers in proctology and videos of his procedures. Impressed, I invited him to train me in lasers for all anorectal diseases. In three sessions, one each month, I did 30 cases with him hovering over me. The next step was to promote safe laser surgery among surgeons across India. Because of the repeatable techniques, safety, and good results, soon he was a guest speaker at all surgical conferences in India. He started demonstrating live surgeries in the conferences, and surgeons started following his surgical techniques.

As the tale goes, he has been faculty at IMMAST (formerly known as CEMAST), Mumbai, India, and MASST, Chennai, India, since 2018 and 2022, respectively. I was his strongest critic. Newer techniques were designed, lower wattage was used, different sites of entry points were devised, and safety points were created. Above all, everything was documented. Several papers have been published on the laser in proctology in the past 4 years.

However, one issue was left, how do we train surgeons worldwide? It is just not laser surgery; he needed surgeons to understand why a particular method was used. The book *Laser in Proctology* answers all the queries.

Lasers in Proctology book has been built from the base up. The text is written in a simple format as if the author is speaking to the reader. The author offers time-tested techniques based on evidence-based practices to improve patient management outcomes.

I wish the best for Dr. Kamal Gupta. The readers are in for a surgical feast.

Kushal Mital
Hon. Secretary
Association of Colon and Rectal
Surgeons of India
Medicare Hospital
Thane, Maharashtra, India

Foreword

It is a proud privilege to write this foreword for this book authored by Dr. Kamal Gupta. Having witnessed his journey in the field of proctology for the last 5–6 years, I have no reservations in acclaiming that I am yet to see a more dedicated person in the field. His yearning to know the minutest details of the anal canal anatomy, the various principle behind each surgery, and the reasons for their failures based on anatomy physiology have made him a perfectionist, if I could call it so. He is never tired of learning, de-learning, relearning, and readopting anything in proctology. His indent knowledge in the field of laser proctology is unmatched, and his desire to teach the intricacies of the same to all has persuaded him to write this book.

Having him as a co-author for the chapter on hemorrhoids, I can tell he can improvize on anything he writes within a day. This is because he reads and studies the topic repeatedly and has something new to add every time.

Though he describes me as his strongest critic, I know how impressed I am with this personality. His penchant for learning and teaching has resulted in developing clear concepts in this field.

This book of his on lasers in proctology reflects his hard work. It will act as a ready reckoner for the readers to understand the various aspects of anorectal disorders as well as their surgical management, especially the laser-based procedure. He has explained each aspect in simple language and helps develop a clear understanding of the subject. The opinions of surgeons with extensive training who, in some or other way, are experts in their respective fields speak volumes about the book. His innovative ideas of hybridizing minimally invasive procedures in proctology have shown great results. If duplicated by others may lead to change in gold standard managements of some of these disorders.

In addition to general surgeons, surgery residents, and medical students interested in laser surgery, the book will hopefully be a source of helpful knowledge and perhaps even a guide for surgeons who want to develop expertise in the field of lasers in colorectal surgery. Kamal has put a lot of work into the book, taking time out of his hectic schedule to put his frequently original perspectives on paper.

I commend Kamal on his superb work in publishing this textbook. I'm expecting that after reading this book, readers will have new insights into the concept of employing lasers in anorectal surgery, especially in fistula surgery, where it's crucial to know when to use lasers and when not to.

To conclude, I must say everything may be accomplished by taking small steps, one at a time: overcoming anxieties and apprehensions, realizing aspirations, or becoming someone you want to be different from the mass.

The journey of a thousand miles begins with one step.—Lao Tzu.

Niranjan Agarwal
Consultant Colorectal Surgeon
Bombay Hospital
Mumbai, India

Foreword

My first reaction to Kamal's request for a foreword was a surprise mixed with great satisfaction of his achievements in such a short time over a decade. I vividly remember an inquisitive young surgeon asking me for a few minutes to discuss various aspects of anorectal problems, predominantly DGHAL AND RAR. I always enjoyed expressing tricks and tips for success in these procedures. Shortly, I started seeing him as a faculty performing surgeries at state, national, and international conferences. This was soul-satisfying to me as he addressed me as his GURU. He focused more and more on *Lasers in Proctology*, soon becoming famous as the LASER MAN OF INDIA. Now was the turn of Guru, making students learn laser procedures in anorectal surgeries. He has trained over 400 surgeons in laser in anorectal procedures through regular workshops.

I saw an excellent teacher in him, inspiring, talented, precise, revealing tricks and tips, and encouraging full audience participation. Thus, teacher in him evolved to a level to research, study, get peers' views, discuss, express, and write a comprehensive book. Right from anatomy, physiology, physiopathology, and functional disturbances, he has written so well that with the academic experience of decades, I feel this book will be a boon in understanding, practicing, managing complications, and improving their skills by practical demonstrations and live operating workshops to young surgeons and experienced to refresh the standard to latest advances in knowledge. Kamal has solicited a galaxy of authors of repute to contribute and share their less-known secrets of success in this broad specialty.

It is a great pleasure to see a student and my teacher in laser proctology progressing so fast and so well with a down-to-earth attitude and exemplary humility.

I wish him all success in life.

NEVER MISTAKE KNOWLEDGE FOR WISDOM. ONE HELPS YOU MAKE A LIVING, AND THE OTHER HELPS MAKE A LIFE.

Prof. (Dr.) Rama Kant
Former Head of Department of Surgery
King George Medical University
Lucknow, India

Foreword

Education is never as expensive as ignorance.—Anon

It gives me great joy to write a foreword for this outstanding multidisciplinary book on anorectal disorders authored by Dr. Kamal Gupta, popularly known as the "laser man" of India. So little is known about these hugely common conditions that often one can only share his/her ignorance in the field; this book stands out in terms of the latest information brought out with clarity and brevity. The author has covered all aspects of these disorders ranging from applied surgical anatomy and physiology to the latest management modalities available. The surgical anatomy has been covered tastefully with surgical aspects and relevance optimally addressed. Having known the author for a long time as a very passionate student of medicine and a dedicated teacher of the science and art of it, one can vouch for this masterpiece as being among the best available in the field.

Each chapter is oozing with information and instructions on the do's and don'ts in the field. The diagrams, sketches, and photographs have been tastefully done to complement the rich text. A must-have book for all practicing surgeons, residents, and other students training to be surgeons, especially the budding colo-proctologists. I would recommend the book for all trainees appearing for MS, MRCS, FRCS, and similar examinations. I would like to congratulate the author for an outstanding effort and wish this masterpiece great success.

Prof. (Dr.) Chintamani
Former Head of Department of Surgery
Safdarjang Hospital and VMMC
New Delhi, India

Foreword

Traditionally, perianal region is a poorly understood region. Modern advancements in the area are gradually taking the place of conventional surgical procedures. Numerous novel techniques have replaced traditional invasive surgery, including band ligations, hemorrhoid artery ligations, foam sclerotherapy, and stapled hemorrhoidectomy. As a result, some severe complications are reported in centers of excellence from peripheral hospitals, which underlines the requirement for postgraduates to have proper training.

Every good surgical textbook aims to convey concept clarity while teaching expertise in surgery. This book primarily aims to bring together all current threads of pertinent knowledge. The book contains a very explicatory explained anatomical features of the anal and perianal region.

The book *Lasers in Proctology* well explains laser hemorrhoidoplasty. Laser hemorrhoidoplasty is a laser-based technique that is minimally invasive and has the least number of complications. More comprehensive laser applications have been described in the treatment of fistula-in-ano, pilonidal sinus, and all the complications of hemorrhoids in this book. The hybrid technique of combining video-assisted laser ablation of the fistulous tract has been very nicely explained.

Another valuable procedure in the book is laser lateral internal sphincterotomy, a minimally invasive technique for anal fissures. The chapters are thorough without adding extraneous details. All the complicated procedures have been very aptly described. Frequent queries, as well as some unusual ones that present an intriguing method of treating individuals with anorectal issues, have been addressed in this book. Once one begins reading the book, one will discover new concepts of hybrid procedures that will enable one to handle issues that may have previously been very difficult for one to handle. With time, the widespread availability of these new procedures will add to the armamentarium of training for young surgeons. However, I feel in years to come, the forbidding costs of the equipment should also come down to make these procedures more cost-effective.

To be precise, I strongly recommend this book as a must-read for young and aspiring surgeons.

Abdul Majeed Chaudhary
Professor and Chairman, Department of Surgery
Lahore Medical and Dental College
Lahore, Pakistan

Preface

No teaching hospital will be considered complete unless it includes a proctologist on its staff.—Lockhart Mummery, 1914

Lockhart Mummery's statement accurately emphasizes the importance of proctology, a field generally regarded as one of the neglected branches of general surgery.

During my years in private practice, I was particularly intrigued and moved by the reluctance patients with anorectal problems exhibit when approaching a specialist. My desire to alleviate their suffering drew my attention to this field and consequently drove me to relentlessly work in and pursue the field of proctology.

In my experience, surgeons typically receive a significant part of their surgical training during residency. Later, in practice, they encounter situations where the formal classroom training seems inadequate. Then, they realize the importance of thinking outside the box and coming up with innovative solutions for the problems they encounter. The use of laser in surgery is one such innovative element that has successfully provided better and more accessible treatment. I am particularly reminded of a quote penned by Christian Lous Lange: "Technology is a useful servant but a dangerous master." This leads me to conclude that technology can successfully present a solution when appropriately applied. That is precisely what this book attempts to achieve.

I have constantly been asked why I decided to write this book. To my mind, authors may write books for various reasons: Few may want to be known as distinguished book authors; some may want to leave a legacy behind; for others, writing and publishing may be the preferred method to gain fame while imparting knowledge at the same time. While my humble self cannot determine what truly motivates others, the reason I felt compelled to write this book is that I wanted to share the concepts that had matured from my pertinacious tiny mind, the myths behind laser surgery in proctology, and my desire to dispel certain misconceptions about the use of lasers in surgery. By striving to write this book, I have had the opportunity to pen down my operative techniques as procedure protocols. I quote the famous quotation by Toni Morrison that I fondly remember:

If there's a book you want to read, but it hasn't been written yet, then you must write it.

The book 'Lasers in proctology!' aims to provide a one-stop guide to the basics of laser surgery for common anorectal disorders and provides information for aspiring surgeons who aim to build their reputation as specialists in proctology. While writing this book, I have not only tried to find answers to my questions but also explored this from the perspective of what I would have liked to learn or, more pertinently, what I would have liked to be taught during my residency days. I hope this book provides a practical guide for all those practicing (or desirous of practicing) colorectal surgery.

The book contains 19 chapters that aim to guide surgical aspirants to practice lasers in proctology. The content is attempted to be written in a manner that will hopefully provide practical insight into lasers. The endeavor has been to ensure that the chapters are easy to understand with minimal need for academic supervision. All the chapters have diagrammatic representations of the procedures to understand the surgical approach. I have also shared my experience and opinion with case studies in the various chapters to provide a step-wise guide.

My persistence has yielded favorable results as I have managed to persuade some of the most esteemed and highly experienced anorectal surgeons of national and international repute to review some of the chapters, and they have been gracious to share with me (and you) their knowledge.

Since this book is targeted at and brought into existence for you, dear readers, I welcome suggestions, opinions, and criticism as learning is a continuous process.

Jalandhar, Punjab, India   Kamal Gupta

Acknowledgments

Writing this book seemed daunting, but I was blessed to receive unwavering support from my esteemed colleagues and family, which made this exercise possible.

Foremost, I would like to thank my wife, Dr. Ruby, for demonstrating inexplicable amounts of patience when I was in the middle of writing the book. Reading various versions and providing feedback on every chapter so I could make this book more insightful is, to my mind, one of the more formidable of her many talents. Without her constant support, positive criticism, and encouragement, this book would not have seen the light of the day.

The term "Minimally Invasive Proctology" was first introduced to me during my training in VAAFT at IMMAST, Mumbai, by my mentor and teacher, Dr. Kushal Mital. I visited IMMAST twice as a student and was taught all there is to know about minimally invasive procedures, except for lasers. Dr. Mital asked me to join a faculty for lasers in Proctology at IMMAST (formerly known as CeMAST), and that, accompanied by my thirst for knowledge, is the genesis of this book. For this, I will always remain indebted to him.

The chapter on laser hemorrhoidoplasty was written first and sent for review to Prof. Chintamani, President and Governor of the American College of Surgeons (Indian Chapter). I am deeply thankful to him for providing insight from a reader and an author's perspective. With his constant encouragement and excellent suggestions, I could sail through and finish what I started.

I am also incredibly grateful to Dr. Gulshan Jit Singh and Dr. Jas Kohli for their contribution to the first chapter on the introduction to lasers. Dr. Gulshan Jit is the former head of the department of surgery, Vardhman Medical College and Safdarjung Hospital, Delhi, India, and a well-known laser surgeon for varicose veins. After his post-graduation in general surgery, he did his Ph.D. in Biomedical Engineering from IIT Delhi. Dr. Jas Kohli is an M.Ch. in plastic surgery from Safdarjung Hospital, Delhi, India, and presently practices in Ludhiana. He is a renowned cosmetic surgeon with a keen interest in lasers. He is also a well-known humor writer.

I would like to express my deepest gratitude to Dr. Indru Kubhchandani and Dr. Abdul Majeed Chaudhary for going through the anatomy of the anal canal and the pathophysiology of hemorrhoids chapters and providing insightful comments. Dr. Indru Kubhchandani, a colorectal surgeon, practices in Pennsylvania, USA. He has also served as the president of the

American Society of Colon and Rectal Surgeons. Dr. Abdul Majeed Chaudhary is the principal and chairman of the department of surgery at Lahore Medical College.

To be a co-author of the chapter on hemorrhoids, with my dear friend Dr. Niranjan Agarwal, for the Colon and Rectal surgery textbook, by the Association of Colon and Rectal Surgeons of India was a privilege and an honor. He also reviewed chapters on anal abscesses and fistula. Dr. Niranjan Agarwal served as the president of the association. He is an esteemed academician and a member of the International Society University of Colon and Rectal Surgeons executive board. The credit for individualizing the chapters on conventional procedures from lasers goes to him. I found him to be a very positive critic and a man with a golden heart.

I sincerely appreciate the feedback on the fistulotomy chapter given by Dr. Ajit Naniksingh Kukreja from Ahmedabad, India. He is the author of the book *Anorectal Surgery Made Easy*.

I want to extend my sincere appreciation and gratitude to the surgeons at St. Mark's Hospital and Academic Institute, London, for allowing me to undergo a traveling fellowship in colorectal surgery. This fellowship program was granted to me as a scholarship by the Association of Colon and Rectal Surgeons of India. St. Mark's hospital is revered for surgical management of anorectal disorders. Established in 1835 by Frederick Salmon, this academic institute is known for its clinical excellence worldwide. This hospital stands out as a temple of learning due to the experts who shaped it.

The most outstanding surgeons at St. Mark's Hospital are recognized for their advancements in surgical techniques in bowel diseases. They are E. T. C. Milligan, Morgan, W. B. Gabriel, Park, Goligher, Goodsall, Lockhart-Mummery, H. Graeme Anderson, and F. S. Edwards, to name a few. To reach an unattainable level of competence, these outstanding surgeons have passed on their knowledge from generation to generation. Modern techniques and terminology of some important anatomical landmarks are based on the ground-breaking research these surgeons accomplished.

My knowledge and surgical techniques in anal fistula are primarily drawn from the wealth of St. Mark's literature. I think it was Park who first introduced the idea of minimally invasive surgery for anal fistula. He published an article in 1961 about the importance of excision of the central source of infection and the core out procedure for the distal tract. This article, in my opinion, was years ahead of its time. My surgical methods are based on Park's justification for eliminating the internal opening and sphincter-saving during core out. The degree of the sphincter to be cut during fistulotomy has also been followed as per Park.

I want to thank Dr. Phil Tozer and Dr. G.P Thomas for the valuable knowledge they have provided me during my fellowship at St. Mark's. It was always a pleasure to discuss the surgical procedures with them. During my talk on "Lasers in Proctology," in the grand rounds, it was an honor to have Dr. Tozer as a chairperson.

A father figure whom I would like to thank the most is Prof. Ramakant, former Head of Department of Surgery, King George Medical University, Lucknow, India, and past president of the Association of Surgeons of India.

He taught me the technique of finger-guided hemorrhoidal artery ligation (FGHAL) in a very informal way. Today, FGHAL is a well-accepted technique for the management of hemorrhoids. In 2018, I had the first publication on the FGHAL technique and compared it with Doppler-guided hemorrhoidal artery ligation (DGHAL). Later, different authors published many papers on this technique under different names.

This project would not have been possible without the help of my surgical team. I would like to thank Dr. Neeru Sahni for collecting and compiling the data. She had collected hundreds of publications on each topic before I started to pen down the book. My first surgical assistant, Ms. Harjeet, deserves a special mention for her patience and assistance in modifying most laser procedures, especially fistulas. Ms. Nupur, my office manager, was kind enough to help me prepare rough digital sketches. My sincere thanks to Mr. Partap for creating clear illustrations out of most of my concept diagrams and all other members of my dedicated surgical team for their unwavering support.

I want to extend my gratitude to Dr. Suchitra Bindoria for believing in me and giving me an opportunity to be a faculty at IMMAST, Mumbai. This is the platform from where I have been able to share my knowledge with all the young surgeons who come to learn Minimally Invasive Proctology.

Last but not least, I would like to express my gratitude to Dr. Vistasp H. Edibam from Surat, India, and Dr. Chandan Juneja from Bengaluru, India, for extending me unconditional support during my learning days. Both are my batch mates and very dear friends.

A heartfelt thanks to the editors of Springer for publishing this book and giving me a chance to convey to surgeons the right and safe way of using lasers in proctology.

Kamal Gupta

Contents

1 Lasers in Surgery: From Past to Present 1
  1.1 Introduction 1
  1.2 History of Lasers 2
  1.3 Classification 2
  1.4 Laser Light Characteristics 2
  1.5 Thermal Relaxation Time 4
  1.6 Delivery Systems 4
  1.7 Laser and Tissue Interaction 4
    1.7.1 Photothermal Interactions 4
    1.7.2 Photochemical Interactions 6
    1.7.3 Photodisruption (Photoacoustic) Interactions 6
    1.7.4 Photoablation Interactions 6
    1.7.5 Plasma-Induced Ablation 6
  1.8 Interaction Parameters 6
  1.9 The Optical Fibers: Size, Structure, and Power Density 7
  1.10 Types of Fibers to Be Used in Proctology 7
  1.11 A Comparative Study of the Various Wavelengths
     of Diode Laser 8
  1.12 Tips Before Use of Lasers 8
  1.13 Laser Safety 9
    1.13.1 Safety Measures While Using Laser Fibers 9
    1.13.2 Precautions 9
  1.14 Laser Versus Cautery 9
  1.15 Your Queries! My Answers! 10
  1.16 Discussion 10
  1.17 Terminology 11
  References 11

2 Surgical Anatomy of Anal Canal 13
  2.1 Introduction 13
  2.2 Anatomical Relations of Anal Canal 14
  2.3 Urogenital Triangle 15
  2.4 Interior of Anal Canal 16
  2.5 Upper Columnar Zone: Contents 17
    2.5.1 Morgagni Columns 17
    2.5.2 Anal Valves 17
    2.5.3 Anal Crypts and Anal Glands 17

2.5.4 Dentate Line................................... 17
2.5.5 Anal Papillae 18
2.5.6 Anal Cushions 19
2.5.7 Anal Transitional Zone (ATZ) 20
2.6 Intermediate Zone 21
2.7 Lower Cutaneous Zone 22
2.8 Internal Anal Sphincter (IAS) 23
2.8.1 Origin and Insertion........................... 23
2.8.2 Thickness.................................... 23
2.8.3 Importance................................... 23
2.8.4 Innervation.................................. 23
2.8.5 Blood Supply 23
2.8.6 Functions 24
2.8.7 Features 24
2.9 Conjoined Longitudinal Muscle (CLM) 24
2.9.1 Thickness.................................... 24
2.9.2 Functions 24
2.10 EAS (External Anal Sphincter) 24
2.10.1 Origin and Insertion........................... 25
2.10.2 Thickness.................................... 25
2.10.3 Relations of External Anal Sphincter
with Muscles of Perineum 25
2.10.4 Innervation.................................. 25
2.10.5 Blood Supply 26
2.10.6 Functions 26
2.10.7 Features 26
2.11 Blood Supply to Anal Canal 27
2.11.1 Arterial Supply............................... 27
2.11.2 Venous Supply 27
2.12 Escape Valve Mechanism: A Significant Finding 29
2.13 Anal Canal Lymphatic Drainage 29
2.14 Anal Canal Innervation 30
2.14.1 Above Dentate Line........................... 30
2.14.2 Below Dentate Line 30
2.15 Anal Canal Histology................................. 31
2.16 Pelvic Floor Muscles 31
2.16.1 Levator Ani 31
2.16.2 Blood Supply 32
2.16.3 Innervation.................................. 32
2.16.4 Functions 32
2.16.5 Features 32
2.17 Anorectal Ring..................................... 33
2.18 Anorectal Triangle 33
2.19 Anorectal Angle.................................... 34
2.20 Physiology of Anal Canal and Defecation................ 34
References... 35

3 Anal Cushions and Pathophysiology of Hemorrhoids................ 37
  3.1 Introduction 37
  3.2 Anatomy of Anal Cushions and Hemorrhoids............. 38
      3.2.1 Nonvascular Component of Anal Cushions......... 38
      3.2.2 Vascular Component of Hemorrhoids 38
  3.3 Functions of Anal Cushions........................... 39
  3.4 Superior Hemorrhoidal Artery (SHA) and Formation
      of Corpus Cavernosum Recti (CCR) 39
  3.5 Physiological Significance of Anal Cushions
      and Their Relation to Defecation...................... 42
  3.6 Pathophysiology of Hemorrhoids 43
      3.6.1 Sliding Anal Cushion Theory................... 43
      3.6.2 Hypervascularization Theory................... 43
      3.6.3 Theory of Straining and Constipation 44
  3.7 Correlation Between Anal Tone and Formation
      of Hemorrhoids 44
  3.8 The Fate of Anal Cushions........................... 44
  3.9 Classification of Hemorrhoids 44
      3.9.1 Internal Hemorrhoids........................ 44
      3.9.2 External Hemorrhoids 46
      3.9.3 Mixed Hemorrhoids.......................... 47
  3.10 Rectal Varices and Hemorrhoids 47
  References.. 48

4 Clinical Evaluation of Hemorrhoids 49
  4.1 Introduction 49
  4.2 Clinical Features 49
      4.2.1 Bleeding................................... 49
      4.2.2 Prolapse 49
      4.2.3 Thrombosis 50
      4.2.4 Mucus Discharge 50
      4.2.5 Pain 50
      4.2.6 Pruritus Ani 51
      4.2.7 Feeling of Lump............................ 51
  4.3 History for Evaluation of Hemorrhoids................. 51
  4.4 Physical Examination................................. 51
      4.4.1 Inspection................................. 51
      4.4.2 Palpation 52
      4.4.3 Digital Rectal Examination (DRE) 52
      4.4.4 Proctoscopy 53
      4.4.5 Symptoms, Signs, Examination Findings
            and Differential Diagnosis at a Glance 53
  4.5 Evaluation and Clinical Correlation of Anorectal
      Symptoms 54
      4.5.1 Rectal Bleeding 54
      4.5.2 Pain 54
      4.5.3 Perianal/Rectal Mass 55
      4.5.4 Mucus Discharge 55

4.6 Diagnostic Evaluations 55
  4.6.1 Sigmoidoscopy 55
  4.6.2 Colonoscopy 55
4.7 Indications and Contraindications of Colonoscopy
  and Sigmoidoscopy 56
References 56

5 **Nonsurgical Management of Hemorrhoids** 59
5.1 Introduction 59
5.2 History 59
5.3 Nonsurgical Management of Hemorrhoids 60
  5.3.1 Lifestyle and Dietary Modification 60
  5.3.2 Medical Management 61
  5.3.3 Ambulatory Treatment (Office Procedures) 62
5.4 A Word About Cryotherapy 66
5.5 Discussion 67
5.6 Which Is the Best Office Procedure Out of Sclerotherapy,
  Infrared Coagulation, and Rubber Band Ligation? 67
References 68

6 **Hemorrhoidectomy: The Gold Standard** 71
6.1 Introduction 71
6.2 Historical Background 71
6.3 Indications of Hemorrhoidectomy 72
6.4 Principle of Hemorrhoidectomy 72
6.5 Modifications in Hemorrhoidectomy Over the Years 72
6.6 Evolution of Hemorrhoidectomy 72
  6.6.1 Excision and High Ligation 72
  6.6.2 Miles' Hemorrhoidectomy
       (Excision with Low Ligation) 72
  6.6.3 Milligan-Morgan's Hemorrhoidectomy 73
  6.6.4 Ferguson's Closed Hemorrhoidectomy 73
  6.6.5 Whitehead Hemorrhoidectomy 74
  6.6.6 Submucosal Hemorrhoidectomy (Park's Procedure) .. 75
  6.6.7 Rise and Fall of Lord's Procedure 75
6.7 Thermal Devices in Hemorrhoidectomy 76
  6.7.1 Bipolar Diathermy in Hemorrhoidectomy 76
  6.7.2 Ligasure in Hemorrhoidectomy 76
  6.7.3 Harmonic Scalpel in Hemorrhoidectomy 77
6.8 Carbon Dioxide Laser Hemorrhoidectomy 77
  6.8.1 Principle 77
  6.8.2 Technique 77
  6.8.3 Advantages 77
6.9 Radiofrequency Ablation 77
  6.9.1 Principle 77
  6.9.2 Technique 77
  6.9.3 Advantages of Radiofrequency Ablation 78

6.10 Complications of Excisional Hemorrhoidectomy 78
6.11 Management of Commonest Complications
     After Hemorrhoidectomy. 78
     6.11.1 Bleeding. 78
     6.11.2 Postoperative Pain 78
     6.11.3 Urinary Retention. 79
     6.11.4 Local Infection and Sepsis. 79
     6.11.5 Anal Tags 79
     6.11.6 Anal Stenosis 79
6.12 Comparative Study of Hemorrhoidectomy
     with Minimally Invasive Techniques 80
6.13 Discussion 81
References. 82

7 Minimal Invasive Procedures for Hemorrhoids. 85
   7.1 Introduction 85
   7.2 Doppler-Guided Hemorrhoidal Artery
       Ligation (DGHAL) 86
       7.2.1 Principle. 86
       7.2.2 Indication 86
       7.2.3 Contraindication. 86
       7.2.4 Instrumentation 86
       7.2.5 Technique. 86
       7.2.6 Advantages. 88
       7.2.7 Results 88
   7.3 Stapled Hemorrhoidopexy (Procedure for Prolapsed
       Hemorrhoids: PPH) 88
       7.3.1 Principle. 88
       7.3.2 Indication 88
       7.3.3 Contraindication. 88
       7.3.4 Instrumentation 88
       7.3.5 Technique. 88
       7.3.6 Results 90
       7.3.7 Complications 90
   7.4 Comparison of Excisional Hemorrhoidectomy
       with DGHAL and PPH 91
   7.5 Transanal Suture Rectopexy 92
       7.5.1 Principle. 92
       7.5.2 Indications 92
       7.5.3 Technique. 92
       7.5.4 Results 92
   7.6 Superior Hemorrhoidal Artery Embolization. 93
       7.6.1 Principle. 93
       7.6.2 Indications 93
       7.6.3 Technique. 93
       7.6.4 Results 93
   7.7 Discussion 93
   References. 94

8   Laser Hemorrhoidoplasty 97
  8.1   Introduction 97
  8.2   Principle of Laser Energy 97
  8.3   Laser Hemorrhoidoplasty............................ 98
        8.3.1   Indications 98
        8.3.2   Contraindications.......................... 98
  8.4   Hybrid Procedure: A Combination of Finger-Guided
        Hemorrhoidal Artery Ligation and Laser
        Hemorrhoidoplasty (FGHAL with LHP)................ 98
        8.4.1   Procedure for FGHAL and LHP 98
        8.4.2   Instrument Required........................ 99
        8.4.3   Finger-Guided Hemorrhoidal Artery
                Ligation - An Introduction.................... 99
        8.4.4   Laser Hemorrhoidoplasty..................... 103
  8.5   Hemorrhoids in Patients with Anticoagulants 106
  8.6   Why Recurrence After Surgical Procedures
        for Hemorrhoids?.................................. 107
        8.6.1   Diversion of Blood Flow and Formation
                of Collaterals 107
        8.6.2   Persistence of the Greater Caliber of the
                Superior Hemorrhoidal Artery in
                Hemorrhoidal Disease 107
        8.6.3   Inability to Ligate Posterolateral Branches
                of SHA................................... 107
  8.7   Recurrence After Laser Hemorrhoidoplasty 108
  8.8   Complications Following FGHAL and LHP:
        Why and How to Manage?............................ 108
        8.8.1   Hematoma Formation at the Site of HAL 108
        8.8.2   Bleeding at the Point of Entry of Laser Fiber 109
        8.8.3   Pain: VAS Score of 4–5 Within 24 h 109
        8.8.4   Postoperative Edema: (2.34%)................. 109
        8.8.5   Thrombosis: (0.89%)........................ 109
        8.8.6   Burning and Itching: (10.1%) 109
        8.8.7   Hemorrhage and Abscess: (0.58%) 110
        8.8.8   Skin Tags: (0.2%).......................... 110
  8.9   Your Queries, My Answers!.......................... 110
  8.10 Discussion 112
  8.11 Case Presentations 113
  8.12 Bottom Line...................................... 114
  References... 115

**9   Lasers in External and Complicated Internal
      Hemorrhoids** 117
  9.1   Introduction 117
  9.2   External Hemorrhoids 117
        9.2.1   Thrombosed External Hemorrhoids.............. 118
  9.3   Thrombosed Internal Hemorrhoids 120

        9.3.1   Pathophysiology of Thrombosed Internal
                Hemorrhoids 120
        9.3.2   Management of Thrombosed Internal Hemorrhoids . . 120
    9.4 Strangulated Internal Hemorrhoids 120
        9.4.1   Pathophysiology of Strangulated Hemorrhoids 120
        9.4.2   Management of Strangulated Hemorrhoids 121
    9.5 Discussion 121
    References... 122

10 Anatomy of Para-Anal and Pararectal Spaces................ 125
    10.1   Introduction 125
    10.2   Anatomy of Para-Anal and Pararectal Spaces 125
        10.2.1 Ischioanal/Ischiorectal Space................... 125
        10.2.2 Perianal Space 127
        10.2.3 Intersphincteric Space 127
        10.2.4 Submucosal Space 128
        10.2.5 Superficial Postanal Space.................... 128
        10.2.6 Deep Postanal Space 128
        10.2.7 Supralevator Space.......................... 129
        10.2.8 Retrorectal Space 130
    10.3   Anal Glands...................................... 130
        10.3.1 Location of Anal Glands 131
        10.3.2 The Fate of Anal Glands 131
        10.3.3 Surgical Importance of Anal Glands 132
    10.4   The Relation of Anal Glands with Crohn's Disease,
           Ulcerative Colitis, and Carcinoma Rectum 132
    10.5   Importance of Anatomical Landmarks Related
           to the Conjoined Longitudinal Muscle 133
    10.6   A Word About Milligan's Septum 134
    10.7   Anococcygeal Ligament and Anococcygeal Raphe........ 134
    10.8   A Word About Deep Intersphincteric Space 135
        10.8.1 Boundaries............................... 135
        10.8.2 Surgical Relevance of Deep Intersphincteric
                Space 135
    10.9   A Word About Deep Anterior Anal Space 136
        10.9.1 Surgical Relevance......................... 136
    10.10 A Word About Infralevator Space 137
        10.10.1 Surgical Importance........................ 137
    10.11 Discussion 138
    References... 139

11 Evaluation and Management of Anorectal Abscess........... 141
    11.1   Introduction 141
    11.2   Epidemiology..................................... 141
    11.3   Etiology of Anorectal Abscess....................... 141
    11.4   Pathogenesis of Abscess 142
    11.5   Organisms Responsible for Abscess 142
    11.6   Relation Between Fistulas and Abscess................. 142
    11.7   Fate of Abscess 144

11.8   Types of Abscesses.................................. 144
11.9   Pathway of the Spread of an Abscess.................. 145
        11.9.1   Formation of a Horseshoe Abscess and Fistula.... 145
11.10   Clinical Evaluation................................. 146
11.11   Imaging in Anorectal Abscesses 146
11.12   Perianal Abscess.................................... 146
        11.12.1 Differential Diagnosis 147
11.13   Ischiorectal Abscess................................ 151
        11.13.1 Managing Ischiorectal Abscess 151
        11.13.2 How to Identify Communicating Fistula Tract? ... 151
11.14   Intersphincteric Abscess............................ 156
        11.14.1 Differential Diagnosis 157
        11.14.2 Managing Intersphincteric Abscess 157
11.15   Supralevator Abscess 159
        11.15.1 Managing Supralevator Abscess 159
        11.15.2 Principle of Drainage of Supralevator
                 Abscess: A Paradigm Shift.................... 163
11.16   Deep Postanal Abscess............................... 164
        11.16.1 Managing Deep Postanal Abscess
                 (Hanley's Technique)........................ 165
        11.16.2 Modified Hanley's Technique 165
        11.16.3 Core Tip 165
11.17   Deep Anterior Anal Space Abscess 166
        11.17.1 Management of Deep Anterior Abscess.......... 166
11.18   Superficial Postanal Space Abscess................... 167
11.19   Horseshoe Abscess.................................. 167
        11.19.1 Managing Horseshoe Abscess 168
11.20   A Word About Retrorectal Abscess 170
        11.20.1 Management............................... 170
11.21   Whether to Perform Primary Fistulotomy in Patients
        with Anorectal Abscess! 171
        11.21.1 Absolute Contraindications for Primary
                 Fistulotomy 171
        11.21.2 Tips and Tricks of Doing Primary
                 Fistulotomy 171
11.22   Complications of Anorectal Abscess................... 172
11.23   Postoperative Care 172
11.24   Case Studies....................................... 173
11.25   Discussion 177
References.. 179

12   Clinical Evaluation and Classification of Anal Fistula 181
     12.1   Introduction 181
     12.2   Symptoms 181
     12.3   History 181
     12.4   Clinical Examination 182
            12.4.1   Inspection.............................. 182
            12.4.2   Palpation 182

12.4.3 Digital Rectal Examination (DRE) 182
12.4.4 Proctoscopy 183
12.4.5 Sigmoidoscopy. 183
12.4.6 Fistula Tract Identification. 183
12.5 Goodsall's Rule and Its Clinical Significance 184
12.5.1 Exceptions to the Rule. 184
12.6 Classification of Fistula! Why Do We Classify Them? 184
12.7 Park's Classification. 185
12.7.1 Intersphincteric Fistula. 185
12.7.2 Trans-Sphincteric Fistula. 187
12.7.3 Suprasphincteric Fistula. 189
12.7.4 Extrasphincteric Fistula 189
12.8 Simple and Complex Fistula 190
12.8.1 Simple Fistula 191
12.8.2 Complex Fistula. 191
12.9 Preoperative Evaluation and Imaging in Anal Fistula 191
12.9.1 Anal Endosonography 191
12.9.2 Magnetic Resonance Imaging 192
12.10 Differential Diagnosis 193
12.11 Evaluating Incontinence. 194
12.11.1 Wexner's Score 194
References. 194

13 Fistulotomy: Still a Gold Standard! 197
13.1 Introduction 197
13.2 Fistulotomy 197
13.2.1 Principle. 197
13.2.2 Indications 198
13.2.3 Contraindications. 198
13.3 Management of Intersphincteric Fistula 199
13.3.1 Simple Intersphincteric Fistula (A1) 199
13.3.2 Intersphincteric Fistula with High Blind
Tract (A2). 200
13.3.3 Intersphincteric Fistula with an Opening
in the Lower Rectum (A3) 201
13.3.4 High Intersphincteric Fistula Without an
External Opening (A4). 201
13.3.5 High Intersphincteric Fistula with Pelvic
Extension (A5). 202
13.3.6 Intersphincteric Fistula Extending from
Pelvic Disease (A6) 202
13.4 Management of Trans-sphincteric Fistula 204
13.4.1 B1 Uncomplicated. 204
13.4.2 B2 Complicated 204
13.5 Management of Suprasphincteric Fistula. 207
13.6 Management of Extrasphincteric Fistula. 208
13.7 Simple Fistulotomy Technique 210
13.7.1 Advantages of Marsupialization 211
13.7.2 Results 211

13.8   Discussion 212
     13.8.1   Intersphincteric Fistula....................... 212
     13.8.2   Trans-sphincteric Fistulas 212
     13.8.3   Suprasphincteric Fistula...................... 212
     13.8.4   Extrasphincteric Fistula 213
13.9   Points to Ponder.................................. 213
13.10   Core Tips 214
13.11   Fistulectomy...................................... 215
     13.11.1   Indications 215
     13.11.2   Technique.................................... 215
     13.11.3   Advantages................................... 215
     13.11.4   Disadvantages 215
13.12   Fistulotomy Versus Fistulectomy: A Surgeon's Dilemma! .. 215
13.13   Primary Sphincter Repair........................... 216
     13.13.1   Indications 216
     13.13.2   Advantages................................... 216
     13.13.3   Technique.................................... 216
     13.13.4   Postoperative Care 216
     13.13.5   Core Tips 216
     13.13.6   Discussion 216
     13.13.7   Core Tips 217
13.14   Case Studies...................................... 217
References... 219

14   **Sphincter-Saving Techniques**........................... 221
14.1   Introduction 221
14.2   Principle.. 221
14.3   Endorectal Advancement Flap 221
     14.3.1   Principle..................................... 222
     14.3.2   Indications 222
     14.3.3   Contraindication.............................. 222
     14.3.4   Some Aspects of the Surgical Technique......... 222
     14.3.5   Technique.................................... 223
     14.3.6   Core Tip 223
     14.3.7   Advantage 223
     14.3.8   Results 223
14.4   Fibrin Glue.. 224
     14.4.1   Principle..................................... 224
     14.4.2   Mechanism of Action.......................... 224
     14.4.3   Indications 224
     14.4.4   Technique.................................... 224
     14.4.5   Results 224
     14.4.6   Advantages................................... 225
     14.4.7   Complications with Fibrin Glue 225
14.5   Fistula Plugs....................................... 225
     14.5.1   Principle..................................... 225
     14.5.2   Indications 225

14.5.3   Contraindications. 225
14.5.4   Technique. 226
14.5.5   Core Tips for Fistula Plug Usage. 226
14.5.6   Complications 226
14.5.7   Results 226
14.6   Seton 227
14.6.1   Principle. 227
14.6.2   What All to Include While Placing Seton? 227
14.6.3   Types of Seton 227
14.6.4   Loose Setons 227
14.6.5   Tight Setons 227
14.6.6   Materials Used for Setons 227
14.6.7   Indications 228
14.6.8   Complications 228
14.6.9   Technique. 228
14.6.10   Seton and Staged Fistulotomy 228
14.6.11   Snug Seton Technique 228
14.6.12   Double Seton Technique 228
14.6.13   Kshar Sutra. 229
14.6.14   Results 229
14.6.15   Core Tips 229
14.7   Ligation of Intersphincteric Fistula Tract (LIFT) 229
14.7.1   Principle. 229
14.7.2   Indication 229
14.7.3   Technique. 230
14.7.4   Results 230
14.7.5   Advantages of LIFT. 230
14.7.6   Pitfalls of LIFT 230
14.7.7   Complications After LIFT 230
14.8   Video-Assisted Anal Fistula Treatment (VAAFT). 230
14.8.1   Principle. 230
14.8.2   Indications 231
14.8.3   Contraindications. 231
14.8.4   Equipment 231
14.8.5   Technique. 231
14.8.6   Advantages. 231
14.8.7   Results 231
14.8.8   Pitfalls of VAAFT 232
14.9   Stem Cells 232
14.9.1   Principle. 232
14.9.2   Indications 232
14.9.3   Technique. 232
14.9.4   Results 232
14.9.5   Core Tip 233
14.10   Submucosal Ligation of Fistula Tract (SLOFT) 233
14.10.1   Principle. 233
14.10.2   Indications 233

        14.10.3 Contraindications............................. 233
        14.10.4 Technique.................................. 233
        14.10.5 Results 233
        14.10.6 Comparison with LIFT 234
    14.11 Discussion 234
    References... 235

15 **Role of Lasers in Fistula: Fistula Laser Closure (FiLaC)**...... 239
    15.1   Introduction 239
    15.2   Principle.. 239
    15.3   Indications 239
    15.4   Contraindications.................................. 240
    15.5   Technique... 240
    15.6   Pitfalls 242
    15.7   Results 242
    15.8   Discussion 242
    15.9   Core Tips 244
    15.10 Your Queries! My Answers! 244
    References... 245

16 **Hybrid Procedures-Future of Fistula Surgery!** 247
    16.1   Introduction 247
    16.2   Why Hybrid Procedures! Aims and Objectives! 247
    16.3   Indications 247
    16.4   Contraindications.................................. 247
    16.5   Hybrid Procedures 248
    16.6   Distal Laser Proximal SLOFT (DLPS) 248
        16.6.1   Principle................................... 248
        16.6.2   Indications 248
        16.6.3   Advantages................................ 248
        16.6.4   Technique.................................. 248
        16.6.5   Results 249
        16.6.6   Discussion 250
    16.7   Distal Coring Using FiXcision with Proximal
           SLOFT (DCPS) 250
        16.7.1   Principle................................... 250
        16.7.2   Indications 250
        16.7.3   Contraindications........................... 250
        16.7.4   FiXcision Instrument 250
        16.7.5   Technique.................................. 250
        16.7.6   Pitfalls 251
        16.7.7   Discussion 251
    16.8   Distal Laser with Proximal LIFT (DLPL)............... 252
        16.8.1   Principle................................... 252
        16.8.2   Technique.................................. 252
        16.8.3   Results 252
        16.8.4   Discussion 252

16.9   VAAFT with LIFT with Laser Ablation of the
        Distal Tract (VA-LIFT) 254
        16.9.1   Principle.............................. 254
        16.9.2   Indications 254
        16.9.3   Technique............................. 254
        16.9.4   Results 255
        16.9.5   Discussion 256
16.10   Distal Coring with Proximal Fistulotomy and Laser
        Ablation (DCPF) 256
        16.10.1 Principle.............................. 256
        16.10.2 Indications 256
        16.10.3 Technique............................. 256
        16.10.4 Discussion 256
        16.10.5 Results of Histopathology Examination
                 of Fistula Tracts 258
16.11   Anal Glands: Pathological Insight! 258
        16.11.1 Does Epithelialization of the Tract or Anal
                 Glands Have Any Role in Persistent Fistula!...... 258
16.12   How to Select a Hybrid Procedure.................... 258
        16.12.1 What to Do and When to Do It? 258
16.13   Core Tips While Performing Fistula Surgery............. 268
16.14   Your Queries! My Answers! 269
16.15   Case Presentations 271
16.16   Conclusion...................................... 277
References... 277

17 Role of Lasers in Pilonidal Sinus........................ 279
    17.1   Introduction 279
    17.2   Epidemiology..................................... 279
    17.3   Location 279
    17.4   Risk Factors of Pilonidal Sinus 280
    17.5   Etiology 280
            17.5.1   Bascom Theory 280
            17.5.2   Karydakis Theory.......................... 280
            17.5.3   Stelzner Theory 281
    17.6   Pathophysiology.................................. 281
    17.7   Histopathology................................... 281
    17.8   The Direction of the Sinus Tract 281
    17.9   Clinical Presentation of the Disease 281
            17.9.1   History 281
            17.9.2   Physical Examination....................... 282
    17.10   Navicular Area................................... 283
    17.11   Classification of Pilonidal Sinus 284
    17.12   Imaging 286
    17.13   Differential Diagnosis 286
    17.14   Management of Pilonidal Sinus Disease 287
            17.14.1 Minimally Invasive Techniques for Pilonidal
                     Sinus: Newer Surgical Modalities 287

17.15 Video-Assisted Laser Ablation of the Pilonidal Sinus
        (VALAPS) 287
        17.15.1 Principle.. 287
        17.15.2 Device for Video-Assisted Endoscopy........... 288
        17.15.3 Device for Pit Excision 288
        17.15.4 Energy! Dosage! Fiber! 288
        17.15.5 Technique............................... 288
        17.15.6 Postoperative Care......................... 290
        17.15.7 Results of VALAPS 290
        17.15.8 Results of Minimally Invasive Procedures........ 292
17.16 Discussion 292
17.17 Case Presentation....................................... 293
        17.17.1 Opinion 294
17.18 Your Queries, My Answers 294
References.. 295

18 **Role of Lasers in Anal Fissures** 299
    18.1   Introduction 299
    18.2   Historical Aspect 299
    18.3   Epidemiology...................................... 299
    18.4   Etiology of Anal Fissure 300
    18.5   Risk Factors 300
    18.6   Pathophysiology of Anal Fissure 300
    18.7   Types of Anal Fissures............................. 301
    18.8   Classification of Anal Fissures Based on Morphology 301
            18.8.1 Characteristics of Superficial Anal Fissure 302
            18.8.2 Characteristics of Deep Anal Fissure........... 302
    18.9   Grading of Anal Fissures 302
    18.10 Location of Anal Fissure 303
    18.11 Anatomical Considerations: Why Anal Fissures
           Are Painful?....................................... 304
    18.12 Why Does a Sentinel Pile Form in an Anal Fissure?....... 304
    18.13 Clinical Evaluation of Anal Fissure................. 305
            18.13.1 History 305
            18.13.2 Physical Examination..................... 305
            18.13.3 Inspection............................... 305
            18.13.4 Palpation 305
            18.13.5 Digital Rectal Examination (DRE) 305
            18.13.6 Proctoscopy 305
    18.14 Role of Anal Manometry in the Diagnosis of
           Anal Fissure....................................... 305
    18.15 Differential Diagnosis of Anal Fissure.............. 306
    18.16 Complications of Anal Fissure...................... 306
    18.17 Why Is an Anal Fissure Described as an Ischemic
           Ulcer?... 306
    18.18 Management of Anal Fissures 306
            18.18.1 Dietary Modification 306
            18.18.2 Sitz Bath................................ 307
            18.18.3 Medical Management...................... 307
            18.18.4 Surgical Management 308

18.19   Laser Lateral Internal Sphincterotomy 310
18.20   How Much Sphincter Should Be Divided? 311
18.21   Why Should Posterior Sphincterotomy Not Be Done? 312
18.22   Results of Closed Versus Open Lateral Internal
        Sphincterotomy 312
18.23   Anal Fissure in Crohn's Disease 313
        18.23.1 Management. 313
18.24   Management of Anal Fissure in HIV. 313
18.25   A Word About Relapsing and Refractory Fissures 313
18.26   Discussion 313
18.27   Case Presentation. 314
        18.27.1 Opinion 314
18.28   Your Query, My Answer 315
References. 316

19   **Postoperative Management of Anorectal Wounds** 319
19.1   Introduction 319
19.2   Aims and Objectives 319
19.3   Why Is Wound Care Necessary After Anorectal
        Surgeries?. 319
19.4   Healing Phases of Wound 319
19.5   Postoperative Wound Care After Anorectal Surgery 320
        19.5.1   Ice Packs 320
        19.5.2   Sitz Bath. 320
        19.5.3   Topical Ointments After Surgery. 321
        19.5.4   Use of Laxatives. 322
19.6   Wound Cleaning. 322
        19.6.1   The Best Cleansing Agent: Povidone-Iodine
                 or Water!. 322
        19.6.2   Cleaning of the Wound After Fistula
                 and Fissure Surgery 323
        19.6.3   Cleaning of Wounds After Pilonidal Sinus 323
19.7   Special Dressings for Anal Fistula and Pilonidal
        Sinus Wounds. 323
        19.7.1   Hemoglobin Spray. 323
        19.7.2   Dried Amnion Chorion Granules with PHMB. . . . 324
        19.7.3   Use of Silver Dressings for Pilonidal Sinus. 325
19.8   Discussion 325
References. 326

Hemorrhoids 329

Fistula in Ano 331

Pilonidal Sinus 333

Fissure in Ano 335

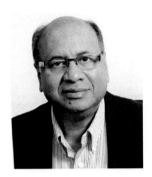

Kamal Gupta, MS FACS FAIS FACRSI graduated from Punjab University, Chandigarh, India. He was trained in Berlin, Germany, in lasers, but after that, he developed many procedures in lasers for minimally invasive proctology. He has done a traveling fellowship from St. Mark's Hospital, London, UK, awarded by the Association of Colon and Rectal Surgeons of India.He is the Consultant Surgeon and Laser Proctologist. He has trained more than 400 surgeons across India and abroad in laser proctology and has delivered numerous oral presentations. He has demonstrated live surgeries in laser proctology at national and international conferences. He is currently an executive committee member of the Association of Colon and Rectal Surgeons of India, vice president, Punjab Chapter of the Association of Surgeons of India, and president, Jalandhar City Chapter of The Association of Surgeons of India (ASI).

Lasers in Surgery: From Past to Present

"If you do not need the lasers, don't use them."

Leon Goldman

Key Concepts

- A laser is a source emitting high-intensity light, a parallel electromagnetic energy beam of a specific wavelength that can be concentrated on a focal spot.
- Commonest used lasers in surgery are CO_2, Nd: YAG, Argon, and Diode laser. A diode laser is used in proctology and endovenous ablation of varicose veins.
- The tissue interactions are photoablation, photodisruption, photochemical, photothermal, and plasma-induced ablation.
- The factors that impact tissue interaction are the laser wavelength, target tissue characteristics, and exposure time.
- Photothermal mechanisms work by converting the light into heat energy. The laser light is absorbed by chromophore in the tissue (protein, water, and hemoglobin), leading to tissue denaturation or destruction. Protein denaturation starts from 65 °C to 80 °C.
- Sharp conical glass tip fiber is used for hemorrhoids, radial fiber for fistula and pilonidal sinus and bare fiber for fissures.
- A wavelength of 1470 nm is 60 times more effective than 980 nm.

1.1 Introduction

LASERS celebrated its sixtieth anniversary in 2020 [1]. Laser is a vital development of the twentieth century. In 1917, Einstein was the first to describe that laser light was possible [2]. Over the years, the laser has become an integral part of medical and surgical applications, including Ophthalmology, Cardiology, Dermatology, Gastroenterology, and Proctology.

"Light Amplification through Stimulated Emission of Radiation" is the acronym of LASER. Lasers are high-intensity light sources that emit a parallel electromagnetic energy beam of a specific wavelength that can be focused on a focal spot captured by a lens [3]. A laser is an energy source that uses cutting laser beam power to make cuts in tissues to remove a lesion on the surface without much blood loss [4].

© The Author(s), under exclusive license to Springer Nature Singapore Pte Ltd. 2022
K. Gupta, *Lasers in Proctology*, https://doi.org/10.1007/978-981-19-5825-0_1

1.2   History of Lasers

Dr. Theodore was the first to demonstrate the "Ruby Laser" in 1960, 43 years after Einstein proposed his quantum theory of radiation [5]. In 1961, the University of Cincinnati built the first-ever laboratory for medical lasers and examined the safety of the then-new technology. The earliest experimental investigations on employing an "optical maser" were reported by Baxter in 1994 [6] and Zaret et al. in 1961 [7]. Campbell et al. reported treating patients with retinal detachment 2 years later, in 1963 [8]. In 1962, Goldman described the first medical application for tattoo removal [9].

Because of their unique qualities, lasers have been employed widely in surgery. McGuff used a Ruby-Laser to ablate atherosclerotic plaques for the first time in cardiovascular surgery in 1963 [10]. In 1964, Kumar Patel of Bell Labs devised a Carbon Dioxide laser (CO_2 laser) [11], and many surgeons used it to treat anorectal disorders. The invention of an argon laser and the Nd:YAG laser followed, and cutaneous laser research centered on them for the next two decades [12]. By proposing the theory of selective photothermolysis in 1980, Dr. Parrish revolutionized cutaneous laser surgery [12, 13].

1.3   Classification

The classification is based on various parameters, power levels, and hazards. The classification based on parameters is as follows (Table 1.1):

LASERs are categorized into four groups as per the hazard and the power level by the "American National Standards Institute" (ANSI)

Table 1.1 Classification based on various parameters

Medium	Solid	Gas	Semi-conductor
Laser technique	Non-contact	Contact	
Nature	Pulsed-wave	Continuous-wave	
Wave-length	Visible	Ultraviolet	Infrared
Power	Low power	Intermediate power	High power

Table 1.2 Classification according to power level and hazards

Class	Power level	Example	Dangerous and safety
Class I	Very low	Laser printer, CD players, supermarket reader	No effect on eye and skin
Class II	Low	Laser pointer	Safe to skin
Class III-a	Low	Laser pointer, low LLLT	Safe to the skin, not to the eyes
Class III-b	Medium	LLLT	
Class IV	Hot	Hot laser (surgical)	

[14]. An overview of the classification is listed below (Table 1.2):

1.4   Laser Light Characteristics

Laser has different properties as compared to ordinary light [15], as shown in (Table 1.3):

A brief synopsis of medical lasers in different medical applications is compiled in Table 1.4.

Carbon Dioxide Laser
The innovative technology of CO_2 laser transmits energy by mirrors and does not pass through a fluid [12]. A carbon dioxide laser is an effective tool for removing tumors and treating anorectal conditions like hemorrhoids and fistula [12]. A CO_2 laser generates an infrared beam with a wavelength ranging between 9.4 and 10.6 μm [16]. It has low coagulation properties. It is not recommended to treat active herpes, warts, and bacterial infections within the area [12]. The most common applications are ENT, maxillo-facial, and plastic surgery.

Argon Laser
Fruhmorgen and colleagues first proposed using an argon laser for endoscopic treatment of a bleeding lesion in 1976 [17]. These lasers coagulate the upper GI tract lesions, arteriovenous malformations, and benign and malignant lesions. Because the radiation from this source barely

Table 1.3 Characteristics of laser light

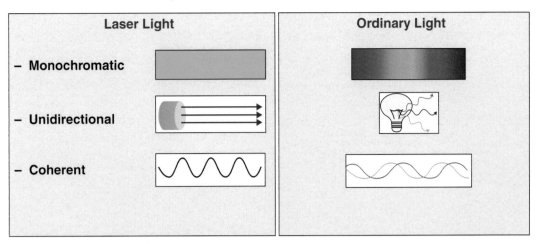

Table 1.4 Types of lasers used for medical applications

Medium	Type of laser	Medical application
Gas	Helium and neon	Biostimulation, physiotherapy, targeting beam.
	Argon	Ophthalmology, general surgery, dermatology, photodynamic therapy, otorhinolaryngology, tissue welding, gastroenterology, dentistry.
	CO_2	Dermatology, photodynamic therapy, ophthalmology.
	Metal vapor excimer	Dermatology, dentistry, ophthalmology.
Liquid	Tunable dye	Gynecology, ophthalmology, photodynamic therapy, dermatology.
Solid	Ruby	Dermatology
	Nd: YAG	Orthopedics, urology, gastroenterology, tissue welding, gynecology, neurosurgery, otorhinolaryngology, general surgery.
	Er: YAG	Gynecology, dermatology, ophthalmology, dentistry.
	Ho: YAG	Gynecology, orthopedics (tissue ablation), dentistry.
	KTP	Otorhinolaryngology, gastroenterology, gynecology.
Semi-conductor	Diode	Biostimulation, ophthalmology, tissue welding, proctology.

penetrates 1 mm of tissue, it is most effective in healing mucosal lesions [17]. It causes surface vessels to clot.

Neodymium-YAG Laser

In 1960, an Nd-YAG laser was first used in anorectal surgeries [18]. Because these lasers' light passes through optical fibers, it is used in the operating channel of most endoscopic equipment [18]. Although the cut is poor, the Neodymium/YAG laser coagulates well [12]. It is ideal for deeper and exophytic lesions since it pierces 3–4 mm into a tissue. The Nd-YAG laser has several advantages:

mild postoperative pain, no sphincter injury, no stenosis, and faster healing [19].

Diode Laser

Diode lasers, which have mW power, are widely employed in anorectal surgery and varicose vein treatment (Fig. 1.1). They are more widely employed in proctology than solid and gas lasers to deliver low energy. The diode laser emits an infrared beam.

The laser beam is delivered to the target tissue by optical fiber. A diode laser can be utilized in two different modes.

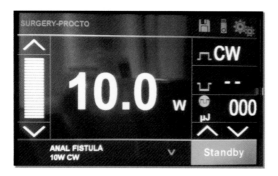

Fig. 1.1 Diode laser

Table 1.5 Laser delivery systems

Delivery method	Laser type
Fiber optic	Argon, Nd: YAG, Er: YAG, ho: YAG, diode, excimer, KTP, krypton, helium-neon, dye
Flexible waveguide	CO_2
Articulated arm	CO_2
Direct delivery	Helium-neon, diode, excimer

- **Continuous Mode:** The laser produces a constant light beam with no or slight power variation over time [20].
- **Pulsed Mode:** Energy from a laser is delivered in the form of a single pulse. The frequency, also called pulse repetition rate, is calculated in pulses per second [20].

1.5   Thermal Relaxation Time

The thermal relaxation time is the time taken for a target to dissipate nearly 63% of thermal energy [21, 22]. It varies depending on the target chromophore's size, ranging from a few nano-seconds (tattoo particles) to hundreds of milliseconds (leg venules) [21]. Because huge areas take a long time to cool, the larger the chromophore, the longer the thermal relaxation time [23].

When a laser is used in continuous mode, it heats the tissue exceeding its thermal relaxation time. Excess heat spreads to nearby tissues, causing collateral damage. Transfer of heat to neighboring tissues is restricted when light emits in short pulses, and so is the thermal relaxation time of the target [24].

1.6   Delivery Systems

The monochromatic beam of coherent light emitted from a laser should be of high intensity to achieve its aim. Many delivery techniques depend on target accessibility, desired spot size, operating power, and wavelength, as shown in Table 1.5 [25].

1.7   Laser and Tissue Interaction

Once laser energy is delivered, tissue interaction determines its application in clinical procedures [26]. Five tissue interactions are described:

1.7.1   Photothermal Interactions

In surgical applications, thermal interactions play a crucial role. The extent and scale of the thermal effect depend on the incident light energy, laser beam geometry, and thermal and optical properties of the tissue.

The thermal effects range from coagulation and protein denaturation to vaporization [27, 28]. The figure below demonstrates the schematic course of thermal interactions with tissue (Fig. 1.2).

The mechanism of photothermal energy is based on converting heat from light energy due to absorption by tissue chromophore (protein, water, and hemoglobin), leading to the destruction or denaturation of tissues. The relationship between tissue location and the thermal effects is shown in Fig. 1.3 [27]. According to the duration, degree, and absorption of heat, thermal action could result in vaporization, coagulation, or hyperthermia, as summarized in Table 1.6. Irreversible impacts like carbonization and denaturation result in thermal damage, which can cause edema, pain, and inflammation [27].

The short wavelengths (200–600 nm) have superficial penetration because of the absorption patterns. The longer wavelengths (650–1200 nm) have deeper tissue penetration [29, 30]. The pen-

Fig. 1.2 Schematic process of thermal interactions with tissue

```
┌──────────────────┐   ┌──────────────────┐   ┌──────────────────┐
│ Laser and optical│   │  Thermal tissue  │   │                  │
│ tissue parameters│   │    parameters    │   │  Type of tissue  │
└────────┬─────────┘   └────────┬─────────┘   └────────┬─────────┘
         │                      │                      │
         ▼                      ▼                      ▼
┌──────────────────┐   ┌──────────────────┐   ┌──────────────────┐
│  Heat generation │──▶│  Heat transport  │──▶│   Heat effects   │
└──────────────────┘   └──────────────────┘   └────────┬─────────┘
                                                        │
                                                        ▼
                                              ┌──────────────────┐
                                              │  Tissue Damage   │
                                              └──────────────────┘
```

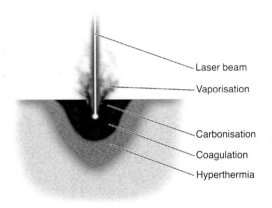

Laser beam
Vaporisation
Carbonisation
Coagulation
Hyperthermia

Fig. 1.3 Thermal effects

Table 1.6 Laser radiation and different thermal effects

Temperature	Biological changes
>300 °C	Melting
>150 °C	Carbonization
100 °C	Vaporization, thermal decomposition (ablation)
80 °C	Permeabilization of membranes
60–65 °C	Denaturation of proteins and collagen, coagulation
50 °C	Reduction in enzyme activity
45 °C	Hyperthermia
37 °C	Normal

etration depth decreases when the spot size decreases, which results in a high superficial treatment effect.

Effects of Photothermal Interactions

1. **Hyperthermia**—A moderate rise in temperature from 41 °C to 45 °C (or even 50 °C) is seen in just a few minutes. With an increase in temperature of more than 50 °C, a significant reduction is observed in the enzyme activity, which leads to reduced energy transfer and immobility of cells. A significant tissue percentage will undergo necrosis if the state of hyperthermia lasts for a few minutes.

2. **Coagulation**—Occurs due to denaturation of collagens and proteins, leading to cell necrosis. Once protein denaturation begins, it seals blood vessels, resulting in dearterialization. A temperature of 50 °C to 80 °C produces desiccation, and the tissue visibly becomes pale, and at 80 °C, the collagen denatures. The tissue matrix is removed, and the scarring process becomes evident. Coagulation is irreversible necrosis leading to tissue destruction [26, 31, 32].

3. **Vaporization**—Vaporization of cellular water occurs above a temperature of 100 °C, resulting in cells' destruction. Increasing temperature levels results in higher pressure as water in a cell expands in volume. The expansion results in localized microexplosions, also referred to as thermomechanical effects. Above 100 °C, volatilization transforms the tissue into smoke relatively quickly, in nearly 1/10th of a second, leaving a region of coagulative necrosis on its edges [33].

4. **Carbonization and Melting**—Tissues are cooled to avoid carbonization, usually with gas or water. If all water molecules vaporize and laser exposure continues, the temperature rises. Carbonization occurs at a temperature higher than 150 °C, which can be observed by

the escape of smoke and the blackening of adjacent tissues. Finally, melting could occur at a temperature above 300 °C, depending on the target tissues.

1.7.2 Photochemical Interactions

Interaction of laser with photosensitizing agents defines the concept of PDT (Photodynamic Therapy), and photochemical interactions have a vital role in this process. Presently, the primary use of photodynamic therapy is to treat malignant tissues. This process occurs when light energy induces or stimulates a chemical reaction in tissues. These reactions occur with low-density power and longer exposure time. Specific parameters for laser result in radiation distribution inside a tissue estimated by scattering. In most cases, visible range wavelengths are used as they have higher efficiency and higher penetration depth [26].

1.7.3 Photodisruption (Photoacoustic) Interactions

Significant usage for photoacoustic interaction was developed in urology and ophthalmology. Photodisruption is tissue disruption with high-power ionizing laser pulses. The Nd: YAG Q-switch laser operating on 1064 nm is applied in photodisruption of secondary cataracts in ophthalmology. A pulsed dye laser is used to fragment impacted ureter stones [34].

1.7.4 Photoablation Interactions

A laser light's energetic photons decompose the molecules by breaking the bonds, causing photoablation. It provides a very accurate tissue ablation that can be predicted [35]. Further, there is no heat injury to tissue during vaporization or coagulation. The inquest on whether photoablation is a photochemical or a photothermal process has been debated in research dated back to the 1980s. Niemz (2007), in a literature review,

stated that photoablation must be regarded as a distinct interaction mechanism that can be distinguished from photothermal and photochemical processes [35].

1.7.5 Plasma-Induced Ablation

When adequate laser parameters are used, plasma-induced ablation can result in highly well-defined and clean tissue removal with no thermal or mechanical damage. The type of interaction for plasma-induced ablation is used in refractive corneal surgery, caries therapy, and diagnostic purposes [35].

1.8 Interaction Parameters

The properties of the target tissue, the wavelength used in a laser, and equipment settings (exposure time and power density) all influence tissue interactions. Characteristics of the tissue are represented by its thermal and optical properties, as listed in Table 1.7.

When a laser beam falls on a tissue, the four primary interactions are reflection, scattering, absorption, and transmission [36], as shown in Fig. 1.4. The above parameters share a common datum: energy density characteristics, which are in the range of 1–1000 J/cm^2. Hence, laser exposure time is considered the most crucial parameter in controlling tissue interaction [35].

- **Absorption**: Some tissue molecules called chromophores absorb photons and convert into thermal energy from light energy. Protein,

Table 1.7 Factors affecting interaction mechanisms

Tissue parameters		Laser parameters
Optical	Thermal	
Transmission	Heat capacity	Mode of operation
Reflection	Heat conduction	Focal spot size
Absorption	(Extent of vascular flow)	Beam profile
Scattering		Power and energy density
		Exposure time
		Wavelength

Fig. 1.4 Interaction of laser light and tissue

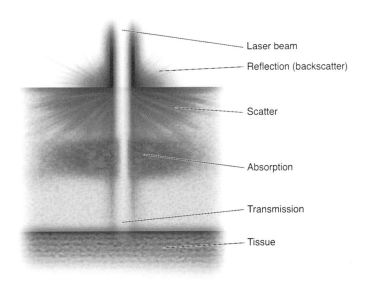

- Laser beam
- Reflection (backscatter)
- Scatter
- Absorption
- Transmission
- Tissue

water and hemoglobin are the three main chromophores.
- **Reflection**: The beam bounces off a surface without interaction or penetration [36].
- **Transmission**: Laser energy could pass from superficial tissues to interact with deep tissue. Tissue transmission is conducted using diode lasers [36].
- **Scattering**: When laser energy enters a target tissue, it scatters in different directions [36].

1.9   The Optical Fibers: Size, Structure, and Power Density

A beam is delivered to the target tissue through an optical fiber attached to a diode laser source. The core sizes used in proctology are 400–600 microns, and in some, it is up to 1000 microns [37]. Typical numerical apertures are in the range of 0.22 or above. The emission of light from the fiber depends on the fiber tip structure. The standard and simple fiber have a bare tip with front emission, like a flashlight.

Interaction of the tissues with a laser changes with power density. Laser energies are converted into heat energy inside a tissue, depending on power density. One can decrease or increase temperature through two methods

- By decreasing or increasing the power on the laser unit
- By decreasing or increasing the spot size

Reducing the power will reduce the rate of tissue impact, and reducing the distance increases the tissue impact. Hence, the higher the power density, the faster is the tissue impact.

1.10   Types of Fibers to Be Used in Proctology

Three types of fibers are used:

1. **Sharp conical glass tip fiber for hemorrhoids**
   The sharp tip enables easy insertion into the pile mass. The light can be diverged at a wide angle, causing the transmission of energy widely. The reduction in the power density allows controlled application with a slow rise in temperature inside the pile mass. The front emission controls the bleeding source by ensuring coagulation (Fig. 1.5).
2. **Radial fiber with round glass tip for fistula and pilonidal sinus**
   A fiber with radial emission is used for the fistula and pilonidal sinus. The radial pattern

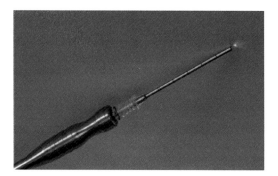

Fig. 1.5 Conical glass tip fiber

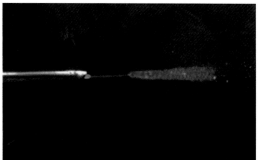

Fig. 1.7 Bare fiber

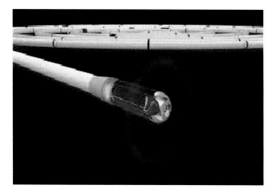

Fig. 1.6 Fistula and sinus probe

reduces the power density and ensures a more controllable and gradual rise in the surrounding temperature. The radial pattern ensures uniform illumination of 360-degree single or multiple rings in all directions. The radial fiber is encapsulated in the cap and made blunt to allow easy insertion into a fistula tract or sinus without damaging the surrounding tissue (Fig. 1.6).

3. **Bare tip fiber for fissure**

The bare fiber is used for cutting the tissue and maintaining hemostasis. By spraying the laser beam 1 mm away from the target tissue, hemostasis can be maintained due to the coagulation property of bare fiber. The bare fiber emits V-shaped energy. It causes slightly more pain postoperatively (Fig. 1.7).

1.11 A Comparative Study of the Various Wavelengths of Diode Laser

980 Versus 1470 nm

A wavelength of 1470 nm is more effective as it works under water as a medium [38]. The literature review reports severe anal pain in some patients treated with 980 nm [33, 38], attributed to higher laser energy. In a study on 35 patients that underwent the FiLaC procedure, Giamundo et al. reported a lower pain score with a wavelength of 1470 nm [38]. Laser energy of 1470 nm wavelength provides an optimal absorption curve in water, resulting in protein denaturation and local tissue shrinkage [39]. When there is no residual water content in the tissue and the temperature rises above 100 °C, vapors of white smoke are observed [39].

1.12 Tips Before Use of Lasers

A laser diode must be used by a professional with proper training. Below are the listed parameters that the operator must consider before using a laser:

- Energy per pulse
- Pulse duration
- Energy density
- Frequency
- Output power

Sometimes tiny fragments of carbon tissue stick on the fiber tip. These could absorb the laser beam and result in overheating. Therefore, removing the charred layer on the tip of fiber using wet gauze is necessary [33]. Laser light should be used with pinpoint accuracy.

1.13 Laser Safety

The safety of everyone involved in the procedure, from patient to surgeon to all the staff in the operating room, is of utmost importance because of the wide wavelength range, delivery methods, and maximum power levels available in present-day medical lasers. Laser-related hazards include direct exposure to beam, beam reflection, fire, and smoke due to vaporization (containing chemical toxins and pathogens). The standard safety steps are necessary for electronic and electrical equipment [40]. The probable hazards are given in Table 1.8:

The laser can cause biological damage [12].

- Burns or thermal damage occurs when tissue is heated to a point where protein denaturation takes place.

Table 1.8 Grouping the laser hazards

Laser radiation hazards	Skin	Burning sensation from acute reflected or direct beam exposure
		Carcinogenesis (With different wavelengths)
	Eye	Retinal or corneal burns (With different wavelengths)
		Retinal injury
		Cataracts
Secondary hazards	Excessive noise	
	Cryogenic coolant hazards	
	X-radiations from the higher voltage power supply	
	Fire hazards (flammable materials exposed to a beam)	
Chemical hazards	Smoke from laser-induced or vaporization reactions	
	Chemical lasers, dye, and excimer with toxic substances	
Electrical hazards	Shock risk from appliances operating on high power	

- Mainly photochemical damage happens with UV light shorter than 400 nm wavelength absorbed in the lens and the cornea, causing injuries at relatively low powers.

1.13.1 Safety Measures While Using Laser Fibers

The fibers used in proctology have a quartz cap connected to the fiber body. There are two ways of connecting the cap to the fiber body, gluing and fusing. If a manufacturing defect occurs or any significant deviation error occurs, the glue may heat up, and the cap may detach and remain in the tissue. This is a very devastating condition. Hence, before inserting the fiber, one must thoroughly check the fiber and cap [12].

1.13.2 Precautions

While using a laser, it is advisable to use special goggles to prevent light from entering the retina. Wavelengths between 400 and 1400 nm may result in the retina heating up and might cause burns. This is because the eye absorbs laser light through the lens and the cornea [40, 41].

1.14 Laser Versus Cautery

One frequently asked question is whether electrosurgical cautery can be used instead of a laser as both emit heat energy. Well, the answer is no. The explanation is as follows:

- The laser emits controlled energy at around 65–80 °C, which is not so in the cautery. The conduction paths cannot be controlled [42].
- A laser is a noncontact tool, whereas cautery works with tissue contact. Chances of injury to the sphincters are high with cautery compared to laser energy.
- Laser energy into the fistula tract causes no collateral damage, whereas cautery leads to lateral spread of current.

- The thermal trauma caused by the laser is comparatively low, and hyperthermic impacts are reversible and minimal [42]. The temperature at the cautery tip is 300 °C to 400 °C as compared to 80 °C to 100 °C at the laser tip.

1.15   Your Queries! My Answers!

1. **How to check the fiber for repeated use?**
   In general, the pattern of laser beam should be uninterrupted. The pattern can be checked by looking at the aiming beam pattern before inserting the fiber into the patient (Fig. 1.8a, b).
2. **How many times can a laser fiber be used?**
   It depends on the equipment being used. Ideally, the fibers are for single use only. If there is no locking mechanism, the fiber can be used multiple times. Do ensure to check the laser beam pattern before each use. If you feel the tip or cap is shaky, do not use it.
3. **What if the cap detaches in the pile mass?**
   The only solution is the excision of the pile mass, as it can be challenging to find the glass tip.
4. **How to clean the fiber?**
   Take a wet gauge piece. Hold the fiber straight and gently clean it upside down, starting from the tip. After cleaning, roll the fiber and keep it in the sterilized chamber. Also one can sterilize the fiber by ETO.

1.16   Discussion

Gone are the times when the surgical fraternity used to say, "Big Surgeons, Give Big Incisions." In the last three decades, minimally invasive surgical techniques have become very popular worldwide amongst surgeons and patients, as they offer enhanced recovery without creating large surgical wounds. The best examples are laparoscopic surgery and endovenous laser ablation of varicose veins (EVLA).

Lasers are extensively used for minimally invasive surgical procedures in proctology. In the last decade, techniques for treating anorectal disorders have changed drastically, with lasers replacing surgical knives. Of course, the criticism about using lasers continues as most surgeons still argue about the long-term efficacy. Thirty years ago, when I was doing my residency, surgeons used to pass similar comments about laparoscopy. The time has changed, but the mindset has not.

Laser surgery has become a popular and acceptable tool in the surgical armamentarium. However, owning lasers does not make one a Laser surgeon. One must master the technology and understand the mechanism of action of the lasers. The dependency of lasers on wavelength, size of the target tissue, power density, and dosage are some of the crucial factors that are mandatory for a thorough understanding of lasers.

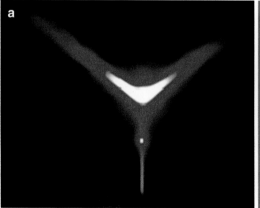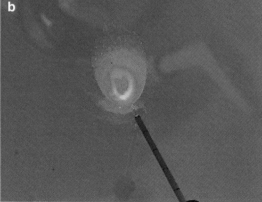

Fig. 1.8 (**a**) Laser beam as emitted by a new fiber. (**b**) Laser beam as emitted by fiber after multiple uses

Substantial literature is available worldwide on the use of lasers to treat benign anorectal diseases. Lasers in anorectal surgery have yielded excellent results with advantages of minimum discomfort, shorter operation duration, short hospital stay, negligible perianal wounds, early return to the work, and cost-effectiveness.

Laser hemorrhoidoplasty has proven effective in hemorrhoids and maintains the anatomical integrity of anal cushions. DLPL (Distal Laser and Proximal Ligation) and FiLaC (Fistula Laser Closure) are the novel techniques used for sphincter-saving in anal fistula treatment. Pilonidal sinus and fissure in ano are the other commonly treated conditions. We, as surgeons, should strive to implement this efficient modern technique in minimally invasive proctology surgery to alleviate the patients suffering from painful anorectal disorders.

1.17 Terminology

Blanching—Skin blanching happens when skin becomes pale or white due to applied pressure to a skin area [43].

Desiccation—To remove moisture from a tissue [44].

Volatilization—Volatilization is when a dissolved sample is vaporized [45].

Mono-chromatic—The light of the same wavelength [46].

Coherent—Light having the same frequency and wavelength [46].

Brightness—Extremely high-intensity

Highly focused—Concentrated with pinpoint accuracy [46].

Unidirectional—One direction [46].

References

1. History of laser 1960–2019 Melinda Rose and Hank Hogan. June 2019. Photonics Media. https://www.photonics.com/Articles/A_History_of_the_Laser_1960_-_2019/a42279
2. Einstein A. Zur quantentheorie der strahlung. 1916. http://www.ing-buero-ebel.de/strahlung/Original/Einstein.pdf.
3. Wright VC. Laser surgery: using the carbon dioxide laser. Can Med Assoc J. 1982;126(9):1035–9.
4. Stoppler MC. Medical definition of laser surgery. https://www.rxlist.com/laser/definition.htm.
5. Maiman T. Stimulated optical radiation in Ruby. Nature. 1960;187:493–4.
6. Baxter GD. Therapeutic lasers: theory and practice. New York: Churchill Livingstone; 1994.
7. Zaret MM, Breinin GM, Schmidt H, Ripps H, Siegel IM, Solon LR. Ocular lesions are produced by an optical maser (laser). Science. 1961;134(3489):1525–6.
8. Campbell CJ, Rittler MC, Koester CJ. The optical maser as a retinal coagulator: an evaluation. Trans Am Acad Ophthalmol Otolaryngol. 1963;67:58–67.
9. Gianfaldoni S, Tchernev G, Wollina U, Fioranelli M, Roccia MG, Gianfaldoni R, Lotti T. An overview of laser in dermatology: the past, the present and … the future (?). Open Access Maced J Med Sci. 2017;5(4):526–30. https://doi.org/10.3889/oamjms.2017.130.
10. Choy DS. History of lasers in medicine. Thorac Cardiovasc Surg. 1988;36(S2):114–7.
11. Kalpan I. The CO_2 laser is a versatile surgical modality. A review article. https://www.jstage.jst.go.jp/article/islsm/16/1/16_1_25/_pdf.
12. Khammam FA, Mossa AF, Issa NA. Hemorrhoids treatment using CO_2 laser (10600 nm). Int J Dev Res. 2019;9(7):28702–10.
13. Silvast WT. Laser fundamentals. Cambridge: Cambridge University Press; 1996.
14. Laser Hazard Classification. Haward campus services. Environmental health and safety. https://www.ehs.harvard.edu/sites/default/files/laser_hazard_classification_2018_0.pdf.
15. Takac S, Stojanović S. Osobine laserskog svetla [Characteristics of laser light]. Med Pregl. 1999;52(1–2):29–34.
16. https://www.lkouniv.ac.in/site/writereaddata/siteContent/202003251324429199nkpandey_CO2_Laser.pdf.
17. Frühmorgen P, Bodem F, Reidenbach HD, Kaduk B, Demling L. Endoscopic laser coagulation of bleeding gastrointestinal lesions with a report of the first therapeutic application in man. Gastrointest Endosc. 1976;23(2):73–5.
18. Plapler H. A new method for hemorrhoid surgery: an experimental model of diode laser application in monkeys. Photomed Laser Surg. 2008;26(2):143–6.
19. Zahir KS, Edward RE, Vecchia A. Use of the Nd-YAG laser improves the quality of life and economic factors in the treatment of hemorrhoids. May 2000. https://www.researchgate.net/publication/12504654_Use_of_the_Nd-YAG_laser_improves_quality_of_life_and_economic_factors_in_the_treatment_of_hemorrhoids.
20. Belikov AV, Skrypnik AV, Shatilova KV. Comparison of diode laser in soft tissue surgery using continuous-wave and pulsed modes in vitro. Front Optoelectron. 2015;8(2):212–9.
21. Yadav RK. Definitions in laser technology. J Cutan Aesthet Surg. 2009;2(1):45–6. https://doi.org/10.4103/0974-2077.53103.

22. Choi B, Welch AJ. Analysis of thermal relaxation during laser irradiation of tissue. Lasers Surg Med. 2001;29(4):351–9.
23. Patil UA, Dhami LD. Overview of lasers. Indian J Plast Surg. 2008;41(Suppl):S101–13.
24. Goldberg DJ. Current trends in intense pulsed light. J Clin Aesthet Dermatol. 2012;5(6):45–53.
25. Verdaasdonk RM, van Swol CF. Laser light delivery systems for medical applications. Phys Med Biol. 1997;42(5):869–94. https://doi.org/10.1088/0031-9155/42/5/010.
26. Van Gemert MJ, Welch AJ. Clinical use of laser-tissue interactions. IEEE Eng Med Biol Mag. 1989;8(4):10–3.
27. Ansari MA, Erfanzadeh M, Mohajerani E. Mechanisms of laser-tissue interaction: II. Tissue thermal properties. J Lasers Med Sci. 2013;4(3):99–106.
28. Roenigk RK. Laser: when is it helpful, unequivocal, or simply a marketing tool. Cutis. 1994;53(4):201–10.
29. Farkas JP, Richardson JA, Hoopman J, Brown SA, Kenkel JM. Micro-island damage with a nonablative 1540-nm Er: glass fractional laser device in human skin. J Cosmet Dermatol. 2009 Jun;8(2):119–26. https://doi.org/10.1111/j.1473-2165.2009.00441.x.
30. Farkas JP, Hoopman JE, Kenkel JM. Five parameters you must understand to master control of your laser/light-based devices. Aesthet Surg J. 2013;33(7):1059–64.
31. Clayman L, Kuo P, editors. Lasers in maxillofacial surgery and dentistry. New York: Thieme; 1997.
32. Svelto O. Ray and Wave propagation through optical media. In: Svelto O, editor. Principles of lasers. Boston: Springer; 1998. p. 129–60.
33. Fornaini C, Merigo E, Sozzi M, Rocca JP, Poli F, Selleri S, Cucinotta A. Four different diode lasers comparison on soft tissues surgery: a preliminary ex vivo study. Laser Ther. 2016;25(2):105–14.
34. Wright CH, Barrett SF, Welch AJ. Laser-tissue interaction. In: Vij DR, Mahesh K, editors. Medical applications of lasers. Boston: Springer; 2002. p. 21–58.
35. Niemz MH. Laser-tissue interactions, vol. 322. Berlin: Springer-Verlag; 2007.
36. Pohlaus SR. Lasers in dentistry: minimally invasive instruments for the modern practice. Provider. 2012;501:211886. https://www.dentalcare.com/en-us/professional-education/ce-courses/ce394/tissue-interactions-and-biological-effects
37. Multidiode™ Surgical Series 980/1064/1470. Multidiode™ Surgical Series 4G: the gold standard of a multidisciplinary surgical laser. https://www.inter-medic.net/en/producto/surgical-series/.
38. Giamundo P, Geraci M, Tibaldi L, Valente M. Closure of fistula-in-ano with laser-FiLaC™: an effective novel sphincter-saving procedure for complex disease. Color Dis. 2014;16(2):110–5.
39. Matsuura Y, Takehira M, Joti Y, Ogasahara K, Tanaka T, Ono N, Kunishima N, Yutani K. Thermodynamics of protein denaturation at temperatures over 100 °C: CutA1 mutant proteins substituted with hydrophobic and charged residues. Sci Rep. 2015;5:15545.
40. Sliney DH. Laser safety. Lasers Surg Med. 1995;16(3):215–25.
41. Laser safety glasses: the ugly truth about laser radiation exposure by Katie. https://blog.universal-medicalinc.com/laser-safety-glasses-the-ugly-truth-about-laser-radiation-exposure/.
42. Marsano LS. Principles of electrocautery. 2013. https://louisville.edu/medicine/departments/medicine/divisions/gimedicine/physician-resources/lectures/procedures/electrocautery.
43. Christiansen S. What is blanching of the skin? https://www.verywellhealth.com/blanching-skin-5114565.
44. Davis CP. Medical definition of desiccate. https://www.rxlist.com/desiccate/definition.htm.
45. Scheunert I. Ecotoxicological testing. In: Corn M, editor. Handbook of hazardous materials. San Diego, CA: Academic Press; 1993. p. 223–32. https://www.sciencedirect.com/science/article/pii/B9780121894108500249.
46. Definition and properties of laser light. https://ehs.oregonstate.edu/laser/training/definition-and-properties-laser-light.

"Those who have dissected or inspected many bodies have at least learned to doubt, while others who are ignorant of anatomy and do not take the trouble to attend it are in no doubt at all."

Giovanni Morgagni

Key Concepts

- The anal canal plays a crucial role in maintaining continence.
- In the anal canal, there are three zones: lower, upper, and middle.
- The proctodeum and hindgut junction form a transverse line that gives it a saw tooth appearance known as a dentate/pectinate line.
- Above and below this line, there is a dissimilarity in arterial and venous supply, lymphatic drainage, and nerve supply.
- The anal canal mucosa has three layers—endothelium, lamina propria, and muscular mucosae.
- An intersphincteric groove is formed when the internal anal sphincter (IAS) ends higher than the external anal sphincter (EAS).
- The muscles of the pelvic floor include the external anal sphincter. This striated muscle surrounding the inferior portion of the anal canal is under voluntary control.
- Normally the anorectal angle is 90°, but at the time of defecation, it becomes 120°.

2.1 Introduction

The anal canal is the digestive system's endpoint, and it plays a crucial part in continence. It is susceptible to a variety of diseases because of its unique anatomy. It begins at the anorectal ring, distal to the rectal ampulla, and ends at the anus, where the stratified squamous epithelium joins the perianal skin. It is entirely extraperitoneal [1].

The anal canal is generally defined as a surgical or anatomical anal canal. Milligan Morgan [2] introduced this concept.

The anatomical anal canal extends between the anal verge and the dentate line. In contrast, the surgical anal canal extends between the anal margin and anorectal ring (Fig. 2.1). It is estimated that the anal canal is 1.5–2.5 cm in length anteriorly, 2–3 cm laterally, and 3–4 cm posteriorly [3]. It expands in accordance with the shape and size of the feces, and its diameter fluctuates between 1.2 and 3.5 cm during defecation [3]. The EAS ("External anal sphincter"), IAS ("Internal anal sphincter"), and puborectalis comprise the anal canal. The anal cushions and inner and outer

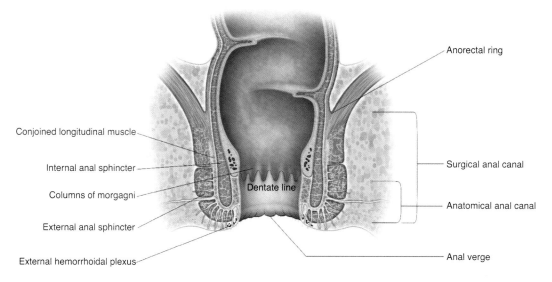

Fig. 2.1　Anal canal anatomy

involuntary anal sphincters keep the anterior-posterior slit in the anal canal closed. The anal canal is slightly longer in males, approximately 4.4 cm, and shorter in females, around 4 cm. The anorectal junction is defined by the forward convexity of the rectum's perineal flexure, which is located 2–3 cm in front of and somewhat below the coccyx's tip. In men, this corresponds to the apex of the prostate [4].

2.2　Anatomical Relations of Anal Canal

The anatomical relations are explained in Tables 2.1 and 2.2 and Figs. 2.2 and 2.3.

Table 2.1　Anatomical relation of the anal canal in males (Fig. 2.2)

Anteriorly	Posteriorly	Laterally
Urogenital diaphragm	Anococcygeal ligament	Ischium and ischiorectal fossa on either side with ischiorectal fat
Urethra	Coccyx and sacrum	
Bulb of penis		

Table 2.2　Anatomical relation of the anal canal in females (Fig. 2.3)

Anteriorly	Posteriorly	Laterally
Perineal body	Anococcygeal ligament	Ischium and ischiorectal fossa on either side with ischiorectal fat
Urogenital diaphragm	Coccyx and sacrum	
Posterior wall of the vagina		

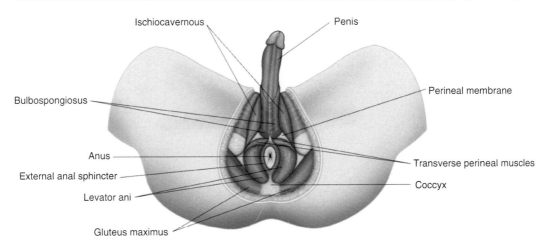

Fig. 2.2 Male perineum

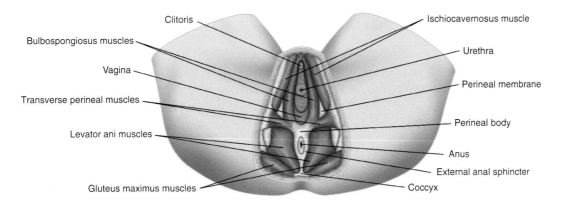

Fig. 2.3 Female perineum

2.3   Urogenital Triangle

Gorsch asserts that the urogenital triangle (Fig. 2.4) has three superimposed musculoskeletal planes [3]:

1. The superficial group contains
   (a) Bulbospongiosus
   (b) Superficial transverse perineal muscle
   (c) Ischiocavernosis muscle
2. The middle group contains
   (a) Sphincter urethrae membranous muscle
   (b) Deep, transverse perineal muscle
3. The deep group contains
   (a) Pubococcygeus and puborectalis muscles in the pelvic portion

Fig. 2.4 Urogenital
triangle

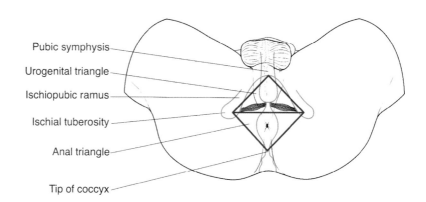

Pubic symphysis

Urogenital triangle

Ischiopubic ramus

Ischial tuberosity

Anal triangle

Tip of coccyx

2.4   Interior of Anal Canal

It is divided into three zones (Fig. 2.5):

1. Between the anorectal ring and the dentate
   line is the upper columnar zone, which
   comprises
   (a) Anal columns of Morgagni
   (b) Anal valves
   (c) Anal sinus/crypts

   (d) Pectinate/Dentate line
   (e) Anal papillae
   (f) Anal cushions
2. Between the dentate line and intersphincteric
   groove (White line of Hilton), there is a middle or intermediate zone lined by anoderm
   and is about 15 mm long.
3. The lower cutaneous zone is between the
   White line of Hilton and the anal verge. The
   thickness of anal verge is 8 mm.

Fig. 2.5 Anal canal interior

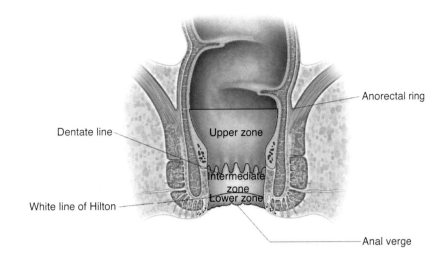

2.5   Upper Columnar Zone: Contents

2.5.1   Morgagni Columns

These are 12–16 vertical folds produced by the infoldings of the mucous membrane. These folds are known as columns of Morgagni (Fig. 2.6) [5]. They are formed as this part of the anal canal is stretchable. A mucosal membrane lines this section of the anal canal, endodermal in origin, and comprised of cuboidal cells. Because of the overlapping anal cushions, which contain internal hemorrhoidal plexus, they have a rich purple color. The epithelium develops into columnar cells above towards rectal mucosa and is pink in color. These columns accommodate the anal canal and sphincteric part, which contract and dilate [3].

2.5.2   Anal Valves

Small transverse folds of the mucous membrane known as anal valves connect the lower ends of Morgagni columns (Fig. 2.7) [6]. The anal crypt or sinus is a small pocket located above each valve. The underlying anal gland ducts open into the anal crypts and are sources of perianal abscesses and fistulas [7].

2.5.3   Anal Crypts and Anal Glands

Each anal crypt is connected to the anal glands. The anal glands are approximately 6–8 in number, and primarily they are located posteriorly [8]. The anal crypts, according to Gorsch, are small recesses that protrude between adjacent anal columns and behind the anal valves and differ in number, form, and depth [3]. The larger and more persistent crypts are commonly seen lateral to the posterior commissure and are often supposed to cause anal fissure and fistulas [3].

2.5.4   Dentate Line

The anal valves form a transverse line that gives it a saw tooth appearance. This line is known as the pectinate or dentate line [9, 10]. This line is crucial for appreciating the anal canal epithelium [7]. Above the dentate line, the lining is of endoderm comprising cuboidal cells. The anoderm is a nonkeratinized squamous epithelium that extends between the dentate line and the anal verge. It lacks features like glands and hair follicles [7]. When palpated, it is also delicate and pain-sensitive. On the dentate line are present anal papillae. Table 2.3 summarizes the differences in artery supply, lymphatic drainage, venous drainage, and nerve supply above and below the dentate line [11] (Fig. 2.8).

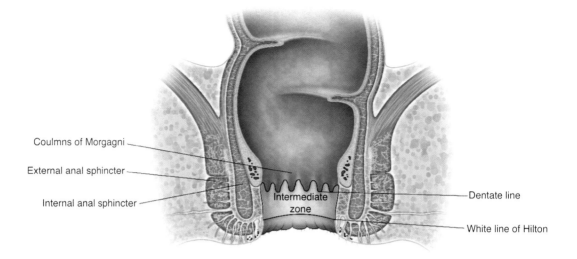

Coulmns of Morgagni

External anal sphincter

Internal anal sphincter

Intermediate zone

Dentate line

White line of Hilton

Fig. 2.6 Morgagni columns

Fig. 2.7 Diagram showing anal valves

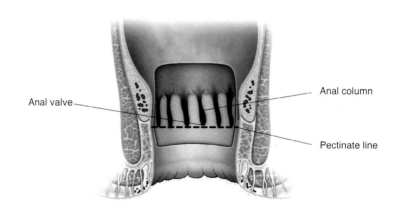

Anal valve

Anal column

Pectinate line

Table 2.3 Dentate line summarized

	Below the dentate line	Above the dentate line
Arterial blood supply	Inferior rectal artery	Superior and middle rectal artery
Venous drainage	Inferior rectal vein (systemic)	Superior rectal vein (portal)
Lymphatic drainage	Superficial inguinal nodes	Internal iliac nodes
Innervations	Somatic (Pudendal nerve)	Autonomic

2.5.5   Anal Papillae

These are remnants of the embryonic anal membrane and represent the junction of the proctodeum with the hindgut. These are present as small epithelial projections at the dentate line. In 60% of cases, 1–3 papillae are present, and in 40%, the number is from 4 to 6. The usual length of papillae is 1.0–5.0 mm. Due to their hyperplastic tendency, constant irritation, injury, or infection can cause enlargement, a condition known as "Hypertrophic Anal papillae" (Fig. 2.9) [12].

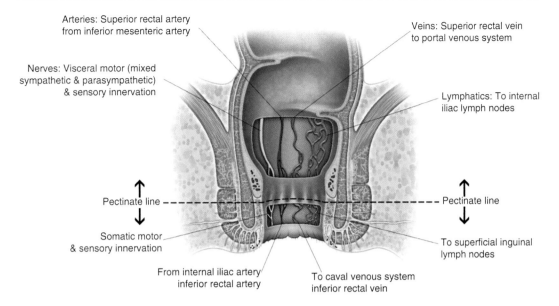

Arteries: Superior rectal artery from inferior mesenteric artery

Veins: Superior rectal vein to portal venous system

Nerves: Visceral motor (mixed sympathetic & parasympathetic) & sensory innervation

Lymphatics: To internal iliac lymph nodes

Pectinate line

Pectinate line

Somatic motor & sensory innervation

To superficial inguinal lymph nodes

From internal iliac artery inferior rectal artery

To caval venous system inferior rectal vein

Fig. 2.8 Dentate line

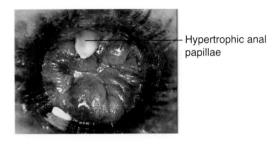

Hypertrophic anal papillae

Fig. 2.9 Hypertrophic anal papillae

2.5.6 Anal Cushions

The term "anal cushions" was described by Thomson in 1975 [13, 14]. According to Thomson, the submucosa inside the anal canal forms a discontinuous series of cushions instead of a continuous ring.

There are three columns of these cushions along the anal canal—right anterior, right posterior, and left lateral, popularly known as 3, 7, and 11 o'clock positions (Fig. 2.10) [13]. These cushions represent well-shaped, deep purple, hemi-spherical masses that protrude towards the anal canal lumen. Each cushion has a submucosa containing loose connective tissue, elastic muscle fiber, and anorectal vascular plexus consisting of arterioles and venules. The vascular plexus inside the cushions gives the surgical anal canal a purple color. The vertical mucosal folds of Morgagni superimpose the cushions.

The anal cushions are held in their normal position by the muscle fibers of ligament of Treitz. These fibers originate from conjoined longitudinal muscle (CLM), pierce the internal sphincter, and play a vital role in anchoring anal cushions (Fig. 2.11).

Histology of Mucosa Covering Anal Cushions
The anal canal mucosa has three layers—muscularis mucosae, lamina propria, and endothelium. The vessels cross muscularis mucosae to enter lamina propria. Due to momentary displacement during defecation, the mucosa may become lax

Fig. 2.10 Positions of
anal cushions

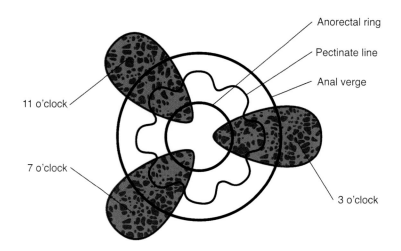

Fig. 2.11 Muscles of
Treitz

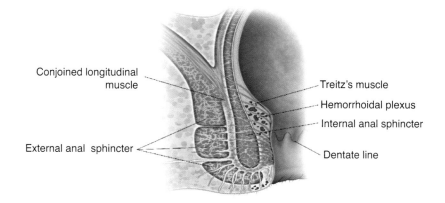

and friable. A portion of this laxed mucosal moiety might get pinched between the pectinate line and the passing stool. Trauma due to straining or passing hard stool may cause damage to the capillaries present in the lamina propria leading to bleeding [15] (Fig. 2.12).

2.5.7   Anal Transitional Zone (ATZ)

ATZ is a mucosal strip above the dentate line 0.5 to 1.0 cm long. The epithelium transforms to a single layer of columnar cells cephalad to this region and macroscopically develops the rectal mucosa's typical pink color [16] (Fig. 2.13).

Surgical Significance of Anal Transition Zone
Sensory nerves in the anal canal were described by Duthei and Gairns in 1960. This showed a high level of sensitivity to touch, temperature, and pain. Sensation and innervation are lacking in the mucosa [17, 18].

• The external anal sphincter contraction and internal anal sphincter relaxation are related to rectum's distention. Rectal contents may be sampled by the anal mucosa in ATZ which differentiates between gas, liquid, and solid stools.

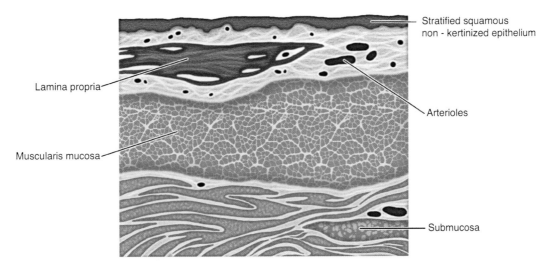

Fig. 2.12 Histology of anal cushions

Fig. 2.13 Anal
transition zone (ATZ)

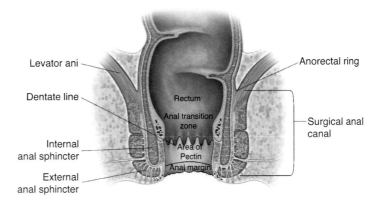

2.6   Intermediate Zone

Between the dentate line and the white line of Hilton is the intermediate zone. The intermediate zone is separated from the lower zone by a line known as the "White line of Hilton" [19]. It is approximately 1–1.5 cm long and lined with anal mucosa (anoderm). The mucosa over here is less mobile than in the upper zone. This area is known as the "area of pectin." This area of pectin is lined by stratified squamous nonkeratinized epithelium [20] (Fig. 2.14).

Surgical Significance of White Line of Hilton
- Because of its white color, the bottom limit of the pectin is known as the "White line of Hilton" [19].
- This is seen at the intersphincteric groove.
- The stratified squamous epithelium that lines it is pale, thin, glossy, lacks sweat glands, and indicates the lower limit of pectin.
- Internal anal sphincter in pectin region is spastic according to Goligher et al. [21]. Anal fissures usually extend between the anal verge and the dentate line for this reason.

Fig. 2.14 Intermediate
zone

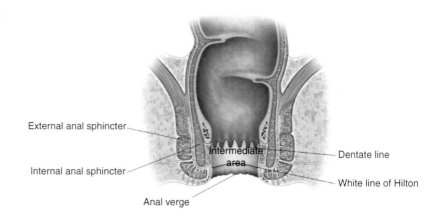

External anal sphincter

Internal anal sphincter

Intermediate area

Dentate line

White line of Hilton

Anal verge

2.7   Lower Cutaneous Zone

The lower zone is known as "Zona Certanea" [20]. It is about 8 mm long and extends between the anal verge and the Hilton's white line. It is lined by stratified squamous keratinized epithelium and looks like pigmented skin with sebaceous glands, hair follicles, and sweat glands (Fig. 2.15). Inferiorly, it blends with perianal skin.

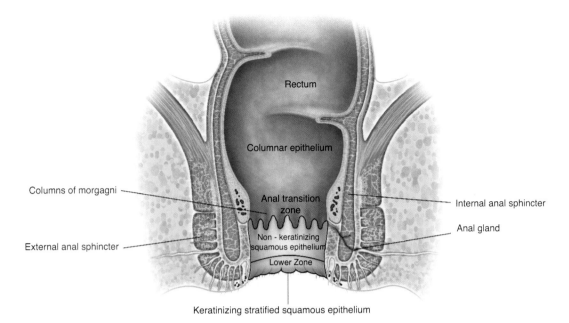

Fig. 2.15 Lower cutaneous zone

2.8   Internal Anal Sphincter (IAS)

IAS is the consolidation of rectum's circular muscle layer in distal 2.5–4 cm (Fig. 2.16) [22].

2.8.1 Origin and Insertion

The IAS may be felt 1.2 cm distal to the dentate line on physical examination. It is a smooth muscle that arises from the rectum's inner circular layer. The intersphincteric groove is between the external and internal anal sphincter [7].

2.8.2 Thickness

When measured endosonographically, it is 3 mm thick and represents a hypoechoic circular band [23].

2.8.3 Importance

About 50–80% of the resting anal tone is maintained by IAS [24].

2.8.4 Innervation

This muscle is innervated by para-sympathetic and sympathetic fibers from the splanchnic nerves and inferior pelvic plexus (S2–S4) [25]. The pudendal nerve does not innervate the IAS.

2.8.5 Blood Supply

The internal pudendal artery supplies the internal anal sphincter.

Fig. 2.16 IAS, CLM (conjoined longitudinal muscle), EAS, and anorectal ring

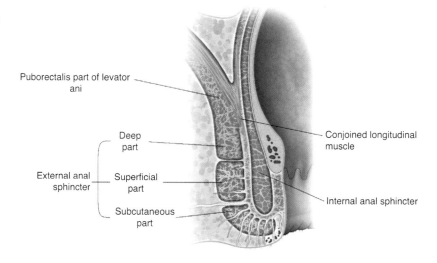

Table 2.4 Salient features of the internal anal sphincter

Salient features	
Control	Involuntary
Insertion	The rectum's inner circular layer
Termination	Approximately 6 mm above anal verge
Thickness	3 mm
Nerve supply	Pelvic splanchnic nerves (S4)
Functions	• Keeps anal canal and orifice closed • Helps in the mechanism of defecation

2.8.6 Functions

It helps maintain continence by controlling involuntary liquid stool and gas loss [25].

2.8.7 Features

Table 2.4 lists the most important characteristics of the IAS.

2.9 Conjoined Longitudinal Muscle (CLM)

CLM [7] is the blending of the puborectalis with the rectum's longitudinal muscle coat. This muscle connects the external and internal anal sphincters. It gets inserted in the perianal skin to form corrugator cutis ani (Fig. 2.16). When it descends,

it becomes fibroelastic, forming fan-shaped medial extensions that cross the IAS and contribute to the Treitz ligament, a group of smooth muscles in the submucosa [16].

2.9.1 Thickness

Approximately 2.5 mm [26].

2.9.2 Functions

The CLM acts as a skeleton for the external and internal anal sphincter complex, providing support and connecting them. CLM and extensions divide adjacent tissues into subspaces [27]. According to Shafik et al., the conjoined longitudinal muscle has a minimal role in maintaining continence [28]. Because of its fan-shaped insertion in the perianal skin, along with fibers of the subcutaneous segment of the EAS, it is responsible for septa formation where external hemorrhoidal plexus is present.

2.10 EAS (External Anal Sphincter)

The pelvic floor muscle includes EAS. It is a striated muscle covering an inferior section of the anal canal and is under voluntary control.

This muscle is relaxed at the time of defecation, allowing the passage of feces (Fig. 2.16).

2.10.1 Origin and Insertion

It extends from the skin and fascia surrounding the anus and the entire anal canal. The attachment of the superficial part of the EAS into the coccyx forms the anococcygeal ligament posteriorly. Anteriorly it is inserted into the perineal body [29].

There are three anatomic components to this sphincter: subcutaneous, superficial, and deep [29].

2.10.1.1 Subcutaneous Part

Corrugator cutis ani is formed by inserting the subcutaneous portion into the perianal skin along with the CLM fibers. It surrounds the anal verge. The typical creases seen externally around the anus are the results of the fibers of the EAS. The inferior fibers extend past the IAS. The anal canal mucosa covers it on the inner side and the lower aspect is covered by the anal skin.

2.10.1.2 Superficial Part

It is an elliptical ring of muscle fibers surrounding the internal sphincter's lower region. Its two divergent parts encircle the anal canal's middle half. It is inserted anteriorly into the perineal body and posteriorly into the coccyx through the anococcygeal ligament.

2.10.1.3 Deep Part

The deep part becomes continuous with puborectalis to form an anorectal sling. According to some authors, the EAS is a single type 1 skeletal muscle that contracts on twitching [28]. Instead of three parts, superficial, subcutaneous, and deep, there are two parts of an EAS: lower and upper. The upper portion extends up to the lower part of the IAS, and the lower part extends beyond the IAS [6].

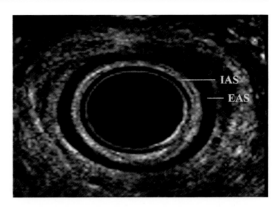

Fig. 2.17 Endoscopic appearance of IAS and EAS

2.10.2 Thickness

Endosonographically, the EAS is hyperechoic with a mean thickness of 6 mm (Fig. 2.17) [23].

2.10.3 Relations of External Anal Sphincter with Muscles of Perineum

Partially blends with
1. Puborectalis muscle
2. Superficial transverse perineal muscle
3. The layer of pelvic diaphragm covering the inferior aspect of the levator ani
4. Conjoined longitudinal muscle [29]

A space between the external anal sphincter and the internal anal sphincter is called intersphincteric space. Anal glands are present in this space. Their blockage can lead to fistula or abscess formation. Surgically this space may be assessed on bi-digital examination.

2.10.4 Innervation

The external anal sphincter receives somatic innervations from the inferior anal nerve, a branch of the pudendal nerve (S2–S4).

2.10.5 Blood Supply

The external anal sphincter is supplied by inferior rectal arteries, which are terminal branches of the internal pudendal artery originating from the internal iliac artery.

2.10.6 Functions

The EAS maintains approximately 25–30% of the resting tone [30]. It is under voluntary control, and at the time of defecation, it acts as a piston for easy evacuation.

> **Surgical Significance of the EAS**
>
> Shafik in 1975 postulated the "**Triple Loop System**" of the EAS in which each loop is a separate sphincter [28]. Three main U-shaped loops comprise external anal sphincter, as described by Shafik. The upper loop is comprised by the deep external sphincter and the puborectalis, which inserts on the pubis. The superficial part forms the middle loop, which is inserted in coccyx. Subcutaneous part forms the lower loop, which is connected to the perianal skin (Fig. 2.18).

> Any one of the three loops may serve as a sphincter for solid stools, but not for flatus or liquid.

2.10.7 Features

See Table 2.5.

Table 2.5 Salient features of EAS

Salient features	
Insertion	Posteriorly into the anococcygeal ligament Anteriorly into the perineal body
Divisions	Subcutaneous Superficial Deep
Thickness	6 mm
Innervation	Inferior anal nerve Pudendal nerve - a branch of (S2–S4) [29]
Blood supply	Inferior rectal arteries
Functions	Voluntary control for defecation Helps to support the pelvis along with the perineal muscles

Fig. 2.18 Triple loop system

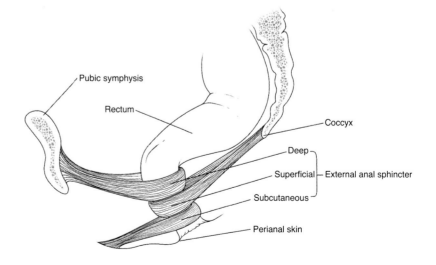

Pubic symphysis

Rectum

Coccyx

Deep

Superficial ⎤ External anal sphincter

Subcutaneous ⎦

Perianal skin

2.11   Blood Supply to Anal Canal

2.11.1   Arterial Supply

Three arteries supply the anal canal—the superior, the middle, and the inferior hemorrhoidal artery (Fig. 2.19) [31]. An extension of the inferior mesenteric artery, the SHA "Superior hemorrhoidal artery" divides into two branches at the third sacral vertebral level (S3) [32]. These branches follow the extramural, transmural, and submucosal course within the rectal wall to form corpus cavernosum recti. Of variable origin, the paired middle hemorrhoidal arteries supply to the distal and middle rectum. They may arise from the internal iliac artery's anterior division, or the inferior vesical artery, or both. According to some authors, it is present only in 40–60% of cases [33, 34]. The inferior hemorrhoidal artery originates from the internal pudendal artery, a branch of the internal iliac artery's anterior division.

2.11.2   Venous Supply

The veins follow the arterial supply. The superior hemorrhoidal vein continues as the inferior mesenteric vein to join the splenic vein [16]. The internal iliac veins receive drainage from inferior and middle hemorrhoidal veins. A portocaval anastomosis is formed through communication between the hemorrhoidal plexuses. However, hemorrhoidal engorgement is an uncommon occurrence. Instead, true rectal varices may develop in portal hypertension (Fig. 2.20).

Surgical Significance

Venous flow between anal canal and the rectum is facilitated by systemic and portal circulation. Always differentiate between rectal varices and hemorrhoids in cases of bleeding per rectum (Fig. 2.21). The terms hemorrhoidal/rectal arteries and veins refers to the same vessels.

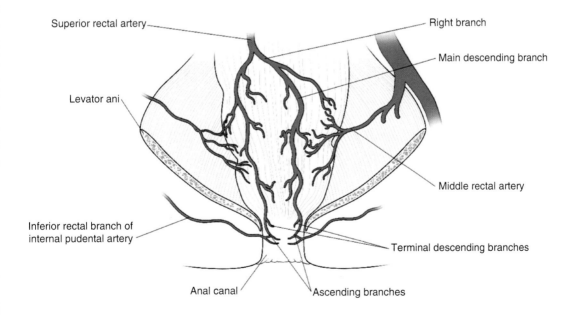

Fig. 2.19 Arterial blood supply of anal canal

Fig. 2.20 Venous
supply of anal canal

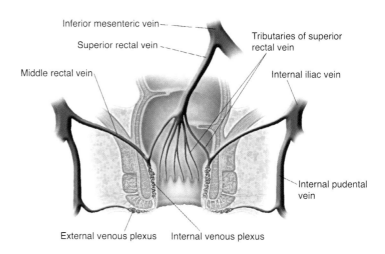

Inferior mesenteric vein
Superior rectal vein
Middle rectal vein
Tributaries of superior rectal vein
Internal iliac vein
Internal pudental vein
External venous plexus   Internal venous plexus

Fig. 2.21 Portal—
systemic circulation in
the distal part of the
rectum

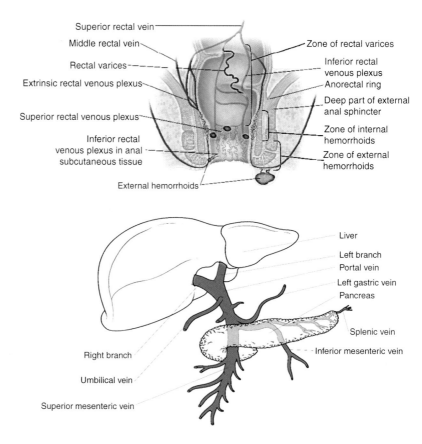

Superior rectal vein
Middle rectal vein
Rectal varices
Extrinsic rectal venous plexus
Superior rectal venous plexus
Inferior rectal venous plexus in anal subcutaneous tissue
External hemorrhoids
Zone of rectal varices
Inferior rectal venous plexus
Anorectal ring
Deep part of external anal sphincter
Zone of internal hemorrhoids
Zone of external hemorrhoids

Liver
Left branch
Portal vein
Left gastric vein
Pancreas
Splenic vein
Inferior mesenteric vein
Right branch
Umbilical vein
Superior mesenteric vein

2.12   Escape Valve Mechanism: A Significant Finding

A study by Goligher in 1980 and Shafiq in 1984 [21, 28] established that free communication is present between the portal and systemic flow via superior, inferior, and middle hemorrhoidal veins supplying the internal iliac veins which return blood to the heart via the inferior vena cava. During defecation, the rectum contracts, allowing portal venous circulation to flow into systemic. This system acts as a natural escape valve mechanism whenever there is an abnormal elevation in the portal vein pressure [21]. On the other hand, systemic blood cannot return to portal blood. The above theory explains why hemorrhoids are not common in portal hypertension patients.

2.13   Anal Canal Lymphatic Drainage

Above the dentate line the lymphatics drain into the internal iliac lymph nodes and distal to dentate line into superficial inguinal lymph nodes (Fig. 2.22) [16].

Fig. 2.22 The anal canal lymphatic drainage

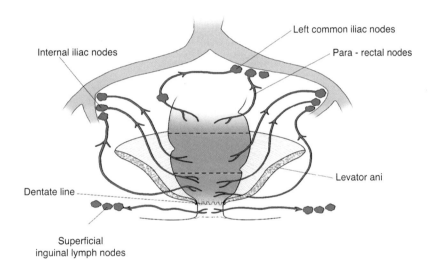

2.14 Anal Canal Innervation

Painless hemorrhoids are due to the absence of somatic innervation in the distal rectum, unless they are suddenly incarcerated, prolapsed, strangulated, or thrombosed. Bilateral somatic fibers of the inferior rectal nerves transfer the pain from thrombosed external hemorrhoids or anal fissures to the anal canal under the dentate line. Visceral afferent fibers do provide sensory innervation to the distal rectum. These fibers connect to the inferior hypogastric plexus (Fig. 2.23) [16].

2.14.1 Above Dentate Line

- Para-sympathetic (S-2, S-3, S-4)
- Sympathetic (L-5)

2.14.2 Below Dentate Line

- The pudendal nerve's inferior rectal branch (S-2 and S-3)
- Perineal branch (S-4)

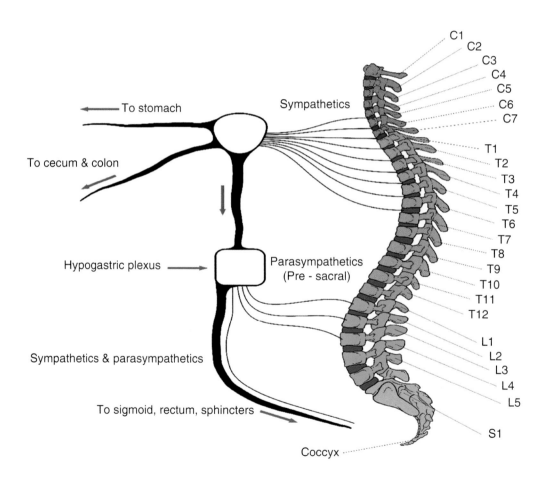

Fig. 2.23 Anal canal innervation

2.15 Anal Canal Histology

It consists of the following zones [20].

- Simple columnar epithelium in the rectum
- Cuboidal cells in the area of columns of Morgagni
- Stratified columnar epithelium in the anal glands
- Stratified squamous nonkeratinized epithelium in anoderm
- Stratified squamous keratinized epithelium in the lower zone

2.16 Pelvic Floor Muscles

2.16.1 Levator Ani

Levator ani forms the pelvic floor and has three components: iliococcygeus, puborectalis, and pubococcygeus (Fig. 2.24) [35].

(a) Pubococcygeus

It enters the coccyx from the pubic bones' posterior surfaces, lateral to the puborectalis. It participates in the formation of an anococcygeal ligament.

(b) Iliococcygeus

It arises from the coccyx and the ischial spine, the lateral aspect of S3–S4, and the anococcygeal raphe.

(c) Puborectalis

A strong striated muscular loop in the shape of a U originates from pubic bones' posterior to the rectum fibers. It joins the deep part of EAS to form an anorectal ring.

In the midline, the pelvic floor is "defective." The "Levator Hiatus" [36] is a defect that consists of an elliptical gap between the two pubococcygeus muscles that is subdivided into the anal hiatus (dorsal) and urogenital hiatus (ventral) by prerectal fibers. The rectum passes via anal hiatus. In men, the urogenital hiatus is

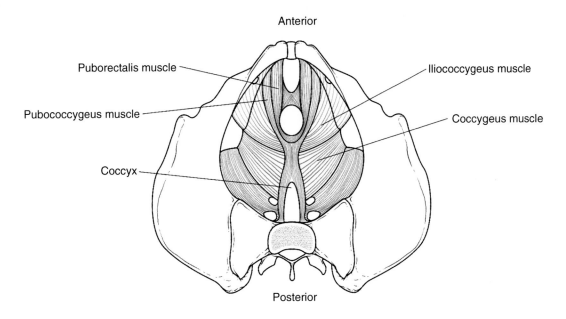

Fig. 2.24 Pelvic floor muscles

the passage of the urethra, whereas, in females, it is the passage of the vaginal canal.

2.16.2 Blood Supply

Inferior gluteal, pudendal arteries, and inferior vesical.

2.16.3 Innervation

The sacral roots (S-2, S-3, and S-4) on the pelvic surface and the pudendal nerve (perineal branch) [13].

2.16.4 Functions

It extends stability and support to abdominopelvic visceral organs [37].

2.16.5 Features

Table 2.6 represents the salient features of the levator ani muscle.

Surgical Significance
- Women who have a levator ani injury account for 55% of cases of pelvic organ prolapse.
- Sixteen percent of women without pelvic floor injuries may have a prolapse of the rectum.

Table 2.6 Salient features of levator ani muscles

Salient features	
Formed by	Puborectalis Pubococcygeus Iliococcygeus
Origin/insertion	**Puborectalis** **Origin**—Pubic bones **Insertion**—Coccyx, forming a puborectalis ring, posterior to the rectum **Pubococcygeus** **Origin**—Posterior surface of bodies of the pubic bone **Insertion**—Coccyx forming anococcygeal **Iliococcygeus** **Origin**—Ischial spine **Insertion**—Coccyx, lateral aspect of S3–S4 and anococcygeal raphe
Blood supply	Inferior gluteal, pudendal arteries, and inferior vesical
Innervation	Nerves from sacral plexus, pudendal nerve branch, coccygeus plexus fibers
Venous drainage	Correspondingly the accompanied arteries
Function	Maintains intra-abdominal pressure and helps in respiration Supporting abdominopelvic visceral organs

Fig. 2.25 Anorectal
ring

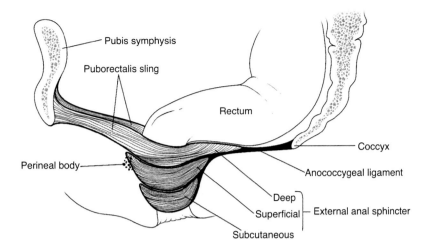

2.17   Anorectal Ring

Puborectalis muscle is related to two anatomic structures—the anorectal angle and ring. The puborectalis, the uppermost fibers of an external and the internal anal sphincter, fuse to form it. Milligan Morgan invented the term anorectal ring, a muscular ring located at the anorectal junction [38]. The anorectal ring can easily be palpated after inserting a finger into the anal canal and rotating laterally like a hook at the anorectal junction (Fig. 2.25) [39].

Surgical Significance
- Anorectal ring maintains gross fecal continence.
- The surgical division of this ring while treating fistula or abscess, results in fecal incontinence.

2.18   Anorectal Triangle

Musculature in the anal triangles includes:

- The external and internal anal sphincters
- The pyriformis and pelvic diaphragm muscles are formed from the levator ani and ischiococcygeus muscles [3]

Surgical Significance

The deep muscle strata and the sphincters are intricately interconnected. The levators coordinate the functioning of the sphincters by supporting and fixing the pelvic diaphragm [3].

Sitting   Squatting

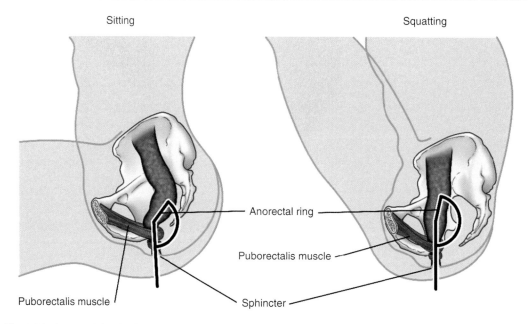

Fig. 2.26 Anorectal ring in sitting and squatting positions

2.19   Anorectal Angle

The anorectal junction is U-shaped, formed by a puborectalis muscle sling. Normally the anorectal angle is 90°, but at the time of defecation, it becomes 120°. The anorectal angle and the puborectalis are responsible for ensuring fecal continence (Fig. 2.26) [40, 41].

2.20   Physiology of Anal Canal and Defecation

Anal cushions and external and internal anal sphincters comprise the anal sphincter complex for continence mechanisms. Anal cushions maintain about 15–20% of resting anal pressure, the internal anal sphincter maintains about 50–55%, whereas external anal sphincter maintains the rest [42, 43].

Both physiological and anatomical factors control the defecation process. The desire to defecate and the act of defecation are two different physiological processes. The sensory stimuli that produces a desire to defecate are in rectal wall musculature. The distal anal canal contains the intrinsic sensory nerves that help to differentiate liquid from solid parts. Extrinsic receptors may sense rectal distention in the rectal wall, stimulating the defecation process. Rectal distension leads to the rectoanal inhibitory reflex causing the external sphincter contraction and IAS relaxation.

The physiology of defecation is shown in the flow chart below (Table 2.7).

Take-Home Message
- A surgeon dealing with anorectal diseases must understand the anal canal anatomy. In-depth knowledge can help surgeons perform challenging surgeries effectively and help decrease complications during surgery.
- While treating hemorrhoids, dentate line is a crucial landmark. Above the dentate line, innervation is by the sympathetic nervous system and below by the pudendal nerve. The groove between external and internal anal sphincters is easily palpable and is a marker for lateral internal sphincterotomy in anal fissure. The anoderm is as an area between an anal verge and the dentate line. When palpated, it is also delicate and pain-sensitive. Preservation of ano-

Table 2.7 Physiology of defecation

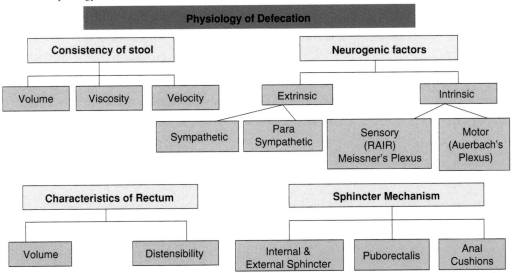

derm is of utmost importance during hemorrhoidectomy as its excision can lead to anal stenosis or stricture formation. Anal sphincter relaxation and contraction are the primary causes of the rectoanal inhibitory reflex during defecation. Opening of the anal ducts into the crypts is an important landmark in fistula surgery as the fistula is formed by obstruction of the anal glands. Preservation of the sphincters during fistula surgery is possible only when the exact anatomy of the anal canal is known.

References

1. Lindberg MR, Lamps LW. Anus and anal canal. https://doi.org/10.1016/B978-0-323-54803-8.50059-0.
2. Milligan ET, Morgan CN. Surgical anatomy of the anal canal: with special reference to anorectal fistulae. Lancet. 1934;2:1150–6.
3. Noll CM, Stanton FD. Anatomy - anus, and rectum. https://www.topratedoctor.com/anal-rectal-anatomy.html. Anal Rectal Anatomy INDEX-Doctors and clinics.
4. Dev M. Anatomy & physiology of rectum. Obstetrics & Gynaecology Dr. SMCSI Medical College. https://www.slideshare.net/MinnuDev/anatomyphysiology-of-rectum.
5. Haubrich WS. Morgagni of the foramen and columns of Morgagni. Gastroenterology. 2002;123(2):424.
6. Standring S. Gray's anatomy - the anatomic basis of clinical practice, Section 8. 40th ed. UK: Elsevier Health Sciences; 2008. p. 1156. ISBN 9780702047534
7. Lee JM, Kim NK. Essential anatomy of the anorectum for colorectal surgeons focused on the gross anatomy and histologic findings. Ann Coloproctol. 2018;34(2):59–71.
8. Seow-Choen F, Ho JMS. Histoanatomy of anal glands. Dis Colon Rectum. 1994;37:1215–8.
9. Gordon PH. Anorectal anatomy and physiology. Gastroenterol Clin N Am. 2001;30(1):1–13.
10. The anal canal - structure - arterial supply. Teach Me Anatomy. https://teachmeanatomy.info/abdomen/gi-tract/ana.
11. Kapoor VK, Gest TR. Anal canal anatomy. 2016. https://emedicine.medscape.com/article/1990236-overview.
12. Schutte G, Tolentino M. A study of anal papillae. Dis Colon Rectum. 1962;5:217–23.
13. Thomson H. Piles: their nature and management. Lancet. 1975;2(7933):494–5.
14. Lohsiriwat V. Anatomy, physiology, and pathophysiology of hemorrhoids. In: Hemorrhoids; 2018. p. 9–17.
15. Margetis N. Pathophysiology of internal hemorrhoids. Ann Gastroenterol. 2019;32(3):264–72.
16. Marcio J, Jorge N, Habr-Gama A. Anatomy and embryology of the colon, rectum, and anus. 4.
17. Duthie HL, Gairns FW. Sensory nerve-endings and sensation in the anal region of man. Br J Surg. 1960;47:585–95.
18. Duthie HL, Bennett RC. The relation of sensation in the anal canal to the functional anal sphincter, a possible factor in anal continence. Gut. 1963;4:179–82.

19. Ewing MR. White line of Hilton. Proc R Soc Med. 1954;47(7):525–30. PMCID: PMC1918929. PMID: 13185975
20. Karunaharamoorthy A, Mytilinaios D. Anal canal. 2021. https://www.kenhub.com/en/library/anatomy/the-anal-canal.
21. Goligher JC, Leacock AG, Brossy JJ. The surgical anatomy of the anal canal. Br J Surg. 1995;43:51–61.
22. Sands LR, Sands DR. Ambulatory colorectal surgery. 2008. p. 13. https://books.google.co.in/books.
23. Min Ju Kim. Transrectal ultrasonography of anorectal diseases: advantages and disadvantages. Ultrasonography. 2015;34(1):19–31. https://doi.org/10.14366/usg.14051. Published online 2014 November 19. PMCID: PMC4282231. PMID: 25492891
24. Bernstein WC. What are hemorrhoids, and what is their relationship to the portal venous system? Dis Colon Rectum. 1983;26:829–34.
25. Lestar B, Penninckx F, Kerremans R. The composition of anal basal pressure. An in vivo and in vitro study in man. Int J Color Dis. 1989;4(2):118–22.
26. Hass PA, Fox TA Jr. The importance of the perianal connective tissue in the surgical anatomy and function of the anus. Dis Colon Rectum. 1977;20:303–13.
27. Moore KL, Dalley AF, Agur AMR. Clinically oriented anatomy. 7th ed. Philadelphia, PA: Lippincott Williams & Wilkins; 2014.
28. Shafik A. A new concept of the anatomy of the anal sphincter mechanism and the physiology of defecation. III. The longitudinal anal muscles: anatomy and role in sphincter mechanism. Investig Urol. 1976;13(4):271–7.
29. Pirie E, Rad A. External anal sphincter. https://www.kenhub.com/en/library/anatomy/external-anal-sphincter.
30. Quigley EM. Disorders of the pelvic floor and anal sphincters; a gastroenterologist's perspective. Revista Médica Clínica Las Condes. 2013;24(2):293–8.
31. Guntz M, Parnaud E, Bernard A, Chome J, Regnier J, Toulemonde JL. Vascularisation sanguine du canal anal [Vascularization of the anal canal]. Bull Assoc Anat (Nancy). 1976;60(170):527–38. French. PMID: 1028448.
32. Aigner F, Bodner G, Gruber H, Conrad F, Fritsch H, Margreiter R, et al. The corposum caverosum recti. Dis Colon Rectum. 1964;7:398–9.
33. Aigner F, Bodner G, Conrad F, Mbaka G, Kreczy A, Fritsch H, et al. The superior rectal artery and its branching pattern with regard to its clinical influence on ligation techniques for internal hemorrhoids. Am J Surg. 2004;187(1):102–8.
34. Ayoub SF. Arterial supply of the human rectum. Acta Anat. 1978;100:317–27.
35. Didio LJA, Diaz-Franco C, Schemainda R, Bezerra AJC. Morphology of the middle rectal arteries: a study of 30 cadaveric dissections. Surg Radiol Anat. 1986;8:229–36.
36. Gowda SN, Bordoni B. Anatomy, abdomen and pelvis, levator ani muscle. In StatPearls [Internet]. StatPearls Publishing. 2021.
37. Bremer RE, Barber MD, Coates KW, Dolber PC, Thor KB. Innervation of the levator ani and coccygeus muscles of the female rat. Anat Rec Part A. 2003;275(1):1031–41. https://doi.org/10.1002/ar.a.10116.
38. Andromanakos N, Filippou D, Karandreas N, Kostakis A. Puborectalis muscle and external anal sphincter: a functional unit? Turk J Gastroenterol. 2020;31(4):342–3. https://doi.org/10.5152/tjg2020.19208. Published online 2020 April 01. PMCID: PMC7236642
39. Naunton Morgan C, Thompson HR. Surgical anatomy of the anal canal with special reference to the surgical importance of the internal sphincter and conjoint longitudinal muscle. Ann R Coll Surg Engl. 1956;19(2):88–114.
40. Brown CG, Mohsen N S. Evaluation of pelvic floor dysfunction with dynamic MRI. J Am Osteopath Coll Radiol. 2017;6(3):13–11.
41. Altomare DF, Rinaldi M, Vegila A, Gugliemli A, Sallustio PL, Tripoli G. Contribution of posture to the maintenance of anal continence. Int J Colorectal Dis. 2001;16(1):51–4. https://doi.org/10.1007/s003840000274. PMID: 11317698
42. Madrid DM, Hani A, Costa VA, Leguizamo AM, Puentes G, Ardila A. How to perform and interpret high resolution anorectal manometry. Rev Col Gastroenterol. 2019; https://doi.org/10.22516/25007440.411.
43. Tsang CBS, Seow-Choen F. Anal incontinence. In: Holzheimer RG, Mannick JA, editors. Surgical treatment: evidence-based and problem-oriented. Munich: Zuckschwerdt; 2001.

Anal Cushions and Pathophysiology of Hemorrhoids

3

"The anal canal is lined by cushions of specialized submucosal tissue which assist the continence mechanism."

Hamish Thomson

Key Concepts

- Hemorrhoids are inflamed or swollen anal cushions that line the anal canal. The three primary cushions are found at the right posterior, right anterior, and left lateral positions. They correspond with the superior hemorrhoidal artery branches.
- The anatomy of anal cushions can be described in terms of two components: nonvascular and vascular.
- The vascular component consists of the internal hemorrhoidal plexus formed by the superior hemorrhoidal artery (SHA). It comprises arterioles and venules, forming an arteriovenous network without interposed capillaries, commonly referred to as CCR (corpus cavernosum recti).
- The superior hemorrhoidal artery branches pass the rectal wall's muscular layer above the levator ani, reach the submucosa, and form CCR.
- The superior hemorrhoidal artery and its branching pattern determine the ligation techniques for internal hemorrhoids.
- Anal cushions can bleed, prolapse, or become thrombosed.
- For the surgical management of hemorrhoids, there is a paradigm shift from conventional surgeries to minimally invasive procedures.
- A hybrid procedure combining hemorrhoidal artery ligation and laser hemorrhoidoplasty is the futuristic approach for hemorrhoids.

3.1 Introduction

Hemorrhoids are swollen or inflamed anal cushions lining the anal canal. Chronic constipation is the most prevalent cause in middle and old age. The estimated global prevalence of hemorrhoids is between 2.9% and 27.9%, of which over 4% are symptomatic [1, 2]. Though hemorrhoids are prevalent in the general population, many patients may find it uncomfortable and embarrassing to consult a surgeon [3].

K. Gupta, *Lasers in Proctology*, https://doi.org/10.1007/978-981-19-5825-0_3

3.2   Anatomy of Anal Cushions and Hemorrhoids

Thomson was allocated a thesis for his master's degree in surgery on "Origin and Explanation of Hemorrhoids." In 1975, based on anatomical studies, he described the complex structure of hemorrhoids and named it "Anal Cushions" [4]. It proved to be the turning point in hemorrhoidal disease history. Crapp and Alexander Williams coined "Vascular Cushions" to assess the therapeutic options of hemorrhoidal disease in 1975 [5].

Inside the anal canal, the three primary cushions may be found at the right posterior, left lateral, and right anterior positions. These cushions are deep purple, hemispherical masses extending toward the lumen of the upper surgical canal. They correspond to the superior hemorrhoidal artery branches [4]. Sometimes, an additional cushion is present posteriorly and is referred to as an accessory cushion (Fig. 3.1) [4].

The anatomy of anal cushions can be described in terms of two components; nonvascular and vascular. Both these components are essential in the etiopathogenesis of hemorrhoids.

3.2.1   Nonvascular Component of Anal Cushions

It consists of four anatomical features that maintain the anal cushions in their normal position, which are as follows [6–8]:

First—The connective tissue, which is present between the sinusoids.

Second—The fibers of the ligament of Treitz pierce the internal anal sphincter (IAS) and significantly contribute to anchoring the anal cushions. The weakening and disintegration of these fibers lead to prolapse. The Treitz muscle has two parts: first is the anal submucosal muscle, which fixes the "cushions to the internal anal sphincter, and the second is the mucosal suspensory ligament," fixing sinusoids to the conjoined longitudinal muscle (CLM) [9].

Third—A sphincter-like structure is present in the terminal arterioles. This sphincter-like structure reduces the arterial inflow, therefore allowing adequate venous drainage. These sphincters are absent or nearly flat in patients with hemorrhoids, leading to the arteriovenous plexus hyperperfusion.

Fourth—The small caliber of the terminal branches of the supplying arteries. Hypervascularization may cause venous stasis in people with hemorrhoids.

3.2.2   Vascular Component of Hemorrhoids

It consists of the internal hemorrhoidal plexus formed by the superior hemorrhoidal artery branches. It comprises arterioles and venules, forming an arteriovenous network without interposed capillaries. Lacking muscular walls and lined by endothelium, these are present in the hollow spaces of the anal cushions and are called sinusoids [10, 11]. These sinusoids lead to the formation of fenestrations (Fig. 3.2). They have been termed

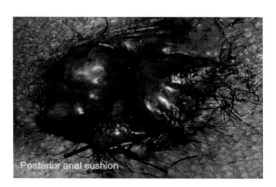

Fig. 3.1 Accessory anal cushion

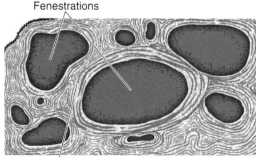

Fig. 3.2 Histology of sinusoids and formation of fenestrations

corpus cavernosum recti because they make a spongy network similar to the erectile tissue of the penis. The sinusoids act as a three-way crossroads, taking "blood from the superior hemorrhoidal artery and middle hemorrhoidal arteries, oxygenating the nonvascular portion of the cushion, and releasing venous blood" to the superior and middle hemorrhoidal vein [8]. The sinusoids strengthen the activity of the anal cushions and result in anal continence by aiding the closure of the anal canal.

The corpus cavernosum recti hyperplasia has been suggested to cause hemorrhoids [11]. The superior and the middle hemorrhoidal arteries constitute the primary vascular supply of anal cushions. Although the middle hemorrhoidal artery supplies the anal cushions, it does not participate in forming corpus cavernosum recti.

3.3   Functions of Anal Cushions

The anal cushions accomplish the following functions:

- Facilitates anal closure to maintain continence
- Maintains 15–20% of resting anal pressure
- Protects sphincter mechanism during defecation

3.4   Superior Hemorrhoidal Artery (SHA) and Formation of Corpus Cavernosum Recti (CCR)

The superior hemorrhoidal artery contributes significantly in the formation of the corpus cavernosum recti [12] (Fig. 3.3a). At the S3 vertebra level, the SHA divides into two branches: left and right. The left does not branch out further, whereas the right gives three to five branches [13, 14]. The superior hemorrhoidal artery branches cross the rectal wall's muscular layer above the levator ani, reaches the submucosa, and form the corpus cavernosum recti. A few branches of the SHA follow the extramural, transmural, and intramural course and participate in forming the CCR [15–17]. It is pertinent to remember that the

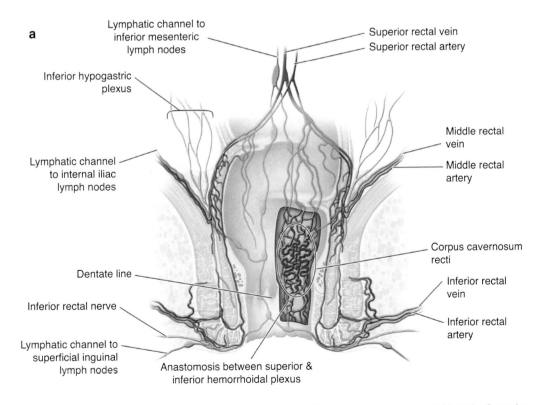

Fig. 3.3 (a) Diagrammatic representation of corpus cavernosum recti formation and posterolateral branch of superior hemorrhoidal artery. (b) Superior hemorrhoidal artery and posterolateral branches

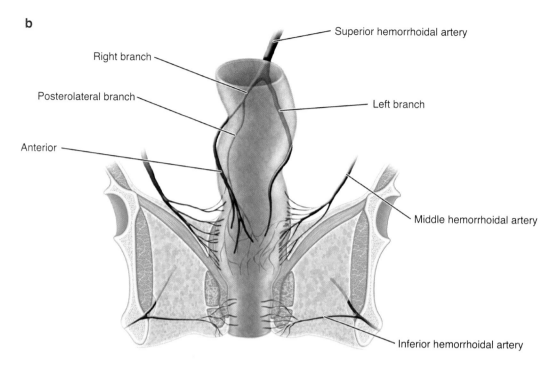

b

Superior hemorrhoidal artery

Right branch

Posterolateral branch

Left branch

Anterior

Middle hemorrhoidal artery

Inferior hemorrhoidal artery

Fig. 3.3 (continued)

posterolateral branches are too high at the ano-rectal ring level. Thus, it is impossible to ligate them while performing hemorrhoidal artery ligation (Fig. 3.3b).

Aigner et al. [15] studied the superior hemorrhoidal artery branching pattern and its clinical impact on internal hemorrhoid ligation procedures. They demonstrated that the superior hemorrhoidal artery was the sole contributor to the corpus cavernosum recti formation. The superior hemorrhoidal artery branches did not course precisely at 3, 7, and 11 o'clock positions. Further, the superior hemorrhoidal artery bifurcated in 82% of the cases, starting at about 12 cm above the dentate line, and trifurcated in 12% [15, 18–20] (Fig. 3.4).

The superior, inferior, and middle hemorrhoidal arterial branches form anastomoses in the submucosa, making rectal ischemia uncommon (Fig. 3.5a, b). The hemorrhoidal venous plexus drains parallel to the arterial supply [21].

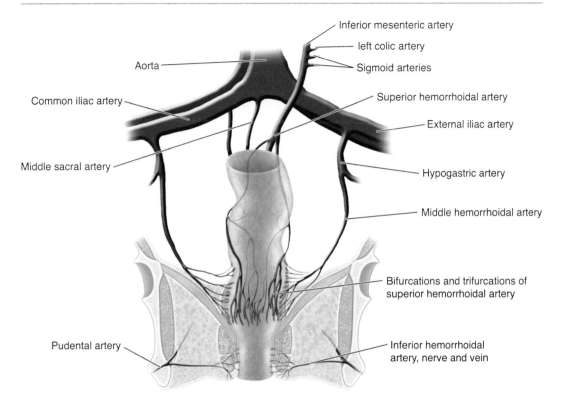

Fig. 3.4 Bifurcation and trifurcation of the superior hemorrhoidal artery branches

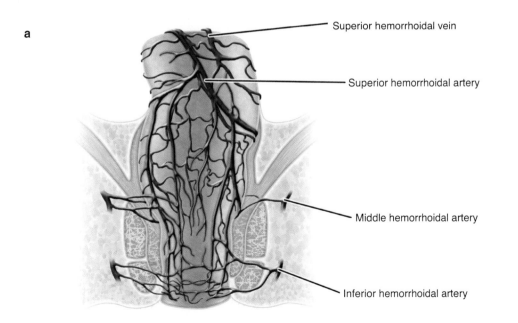

Fig. 3.5 (**a**) Anastomosis between superior hemorrhoidal artery and inferior hemorrhoidal artery as seen after removal of mucosa. (**b**) Anastomosis between superior and inferior hemorrhoidal plexus

b

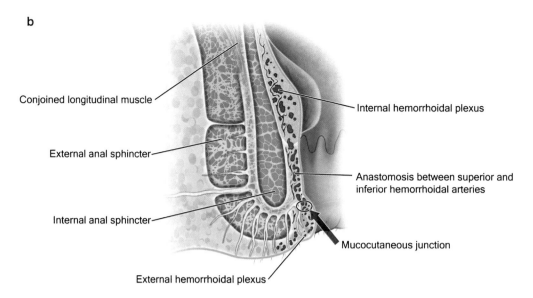

Conjoined longitudinal muscle

Internal hemorrhoidal plexus

External anal sphincter

Anastomosis between superior and inferior hemorrhoidal arteries

Internal anal sphincter

Mucocutaneous junction

External hemorrhoidal plexus

Fig. 3.5 (continued)

3.5　Physiological Significance of Anal Cushions and Their Relation to Defecation

The anal cushions and internal anal sphincter aid each other during defecation. When the sphincter is relaxed, the pressure is reduced. This allows blood to flow from the anal cushions to the superior and middle hemorrhoidal veins, thus reducing their size. As the fecal matter descends, it causes dilatation of the anal canal. Consequently, Treitz's muscle contracts, the anal cushions slide down, and the internal anal sphincter is protected from injury caused by fecal matter [18]. After defecation, anal cushions return to their normal position. They are refilled with blood and regain their normal size to maintain anal continence [6] (Fig. 3.6).

Any anatomical and physiological change causes a cascade of events, resulting in hemorrhoids. A brief description of the prevailing theories is discussed below to understand this better.

Low pressure

High pressure

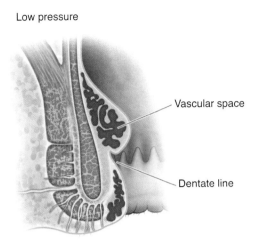

Vascular space

Dentate line

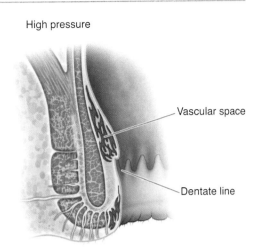

Vascular space

Dentate line

Fig. 3.6 Surgical significance of anal canal physiology

3.6 Pathophysiology of Hemorrhoids

Understanding the pathophysiology of hemorrhoids has spurred advancements in the surgical management of hemorrhoids. Different theories have been prevalent since ancient times, but the widely accepted theories are as follows:

- Sliding anal lining theory
- Hypervascularization theory
- Theory of straining and constipation

3.6.1 Sliding Anal Cushion Theory

A widely accepted theory is Thomson's "theory of sliding anal cushions," originally known as the "sliding anal lining theory." Perianal connective tissue and conjoined longitudinal muscle are essential fibroelastic elements that keep the anal cushions anchored. Haas and colleagues [22] postulated that as a person ages, the muscular element decreases, and the connective tissue element increases. Around the age of 30, the connective tissue fibers around the blood vessels start to disintegrate and loosen, and the veins become

distended [23]. Anal cushions are enlarged due to the hemorrhoidal tissue getting detached from the internal sphincter to move down. Goligher [24, 25] further endorsed the sliding anal cushion theory in 1986. Based on this theory, Goligher proposed the classification of internal hemorrhoids.

3.6.2 Hypervascularization Theory

In morphological and hemodynamic research published in 2006, Aigner et al. claimed that the arterial blood supply of the internal hemorrhoidal plexus is linked to hemorrhoid pathogenesis [15]. The terminal branches of the SHA supplying the anal cushions exhibited a threefold larger caliber, higher peak velocity, more blood flow, and greater acceleration in hemorrhoids patients compared to healthy persons, resulting in hypervascularization [15].

In addition, individuals with grade 3 and 4 hemorrhoids were shown to have larger vessels with a greater flow than those with grade 1 and 2 hemorrhoids. These abnormalities persisted after surgical excision of hemorrhoids, indicating link between hypervascularization and subsequent recurrence [15].

3.6.3 Theory of Straining and Constipation

The relevance of a low-fiber diet in the etiology of hemorrhoid illness was recognized by Burkitt et al. [26]. Constipation is exacerbated by repeated and prolonged straining while passing hard stools, contributing to hemorrhoid protrusion.

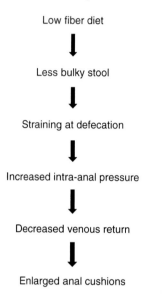

Low fiber diet

⬇

Less bulky stool

⬇

Straining at defecation

⬇

Increased intra-anal pressure

⬇

Decreased venous return

⬇

Enlarged anal cushions

In summary, four core pathophysiological events can be universally recognized regardless of the origin of hemorrhoids [17]:

- First is the sliding process of anal cushions.
- The second is the deterioration of the connective tissue of the anal cushions.
- Thirdly, there is a decrease in venous return from the sinusoids to the superior and middle rectal veins.
- Fourth is the stagnation of blood inside the dilated plexus.

3.7 Correlation Between Anal Tone and Formation of Hemorrhoids

Whenever a patient suffers from a hemorrhoidal disease, there is always an abnormality in anorectal physiology. According to Gass et al. [27],

the higher the anal tone of the sphincter, the greater the protrusion and herniation of hemorrhoids. "Sun et al. [20] found that the resting anal pressure in individuals with prolapsing or nonprolapsing hemorrhoids was significantly greater than healthy individuals." Sun et al. [20], Elgendi et al. [28], as well as Ho et al. [29] concluded that the pressure becomes normal after hemorrhoidectomy.

The hemorrhoidal disease causes increased anal tone in individuals with hemorrhoids. The presence of an increased anal tone is not an etiological factor in the formation of hemorrhoids [23, 28].

Many surgeons are often in dilemma whether lateral internal sphincterotomy should be performed during hemorrhoids surgery or not. Lateral internal sphincterotomy has no advantage in hemorrhoidal surgery. It should only be performed when there is an associated anal fissure.

3.8 The Fate of Anal Cushions

The anal cushions may:

- Bleed
- Prolapse
- Thrombose

3.9 Classification of Hemorrhoids

Hemorrhoids are classified as follows:

- Internal hemorrhoids
- External hemorrhoids
- Mixed (Interno-External) hemorrhoids

3.9.1 Internal Hemorrhoids

They develop from the superior hemorrhoidal plexus above the dentate line. They are painless because they are covered with insensate mucosa. They can get thrombosed and prolapse to varying

Grade 1

Grade 2

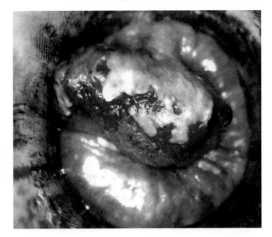

Grade 3

Grade 4

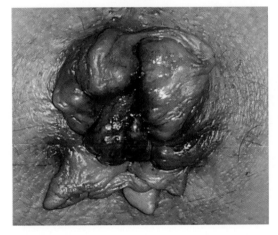
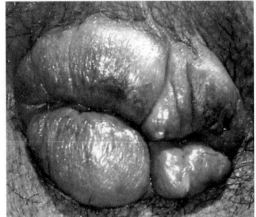

Fig. 3.7 Classification of internal hemorrhoids (Goligher's classification). Grade (1) Prominent blood vessels. Grade (2) Hemorrhoids present up to the anal verge. Grade (3) Pro- lapsed hemorrhoids which are manually reducible. Grade (4) Prolapsed hemorrhoids which are not reducible

degrees, which is the basis for their classification into different grades (Fig. 3.7).

Grade I—Piles that do not prolapse and remain inside (presence of prominent blood vessels/prolapse of mucosal moiety) [4]

Grade II—Pile masses come out while passing motion but reduce on their own

Grade III—Pile masses prolapse during defecation, but the patient has to reduce it manually

Grade IV—Pile masses remain outside and are irreducible

ACRSI (Association of Colon and Rectal Surgeons of India 2016 Guidelines) [10]
(Table 3.1)

When a single pile mass is present, the most common position is 11 o'clock. In my opinion, it forms due to the peculiar anatomy of the anal sphincters. The external sphincter is elliptical, while the internal sphincter is round. Loose areolar tissue is present in between, weakening the Treitz muscle (Fig. 3.8).

Table 3.1 Classification of hemorrhoids as per ACRSI guidelines

Grade	Characteristics
I	Remains within the anal canal
II	Protrudes while defecation and decreases rapidly
III	Protrudes during defecation but needs manual repositioning
IV	Remains prolapsed outside; external hemorrhoids
Each primary grade (I to IV) of hemorrhoids is further categorized based on the "number of hemorrhoids and the presence of circumferential hemorrhoids or thrombosis by using the suffixes (A to D), as mentioned below.	
A	Single hemorrhoidal tissue
B	Two pile masses but with a circumference of <50%
C	Circumferential piles that occupy >50% of the anal canal's circumference
D	Gangrenous or thrombosed piles (complicated)

Fig. 3.8 Shape of external and internal anal sphincters

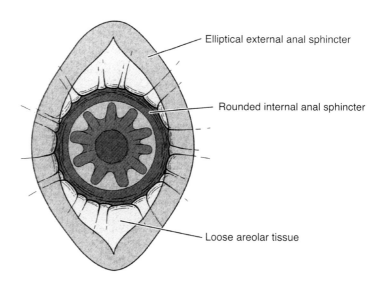

Elliptical external anal sphincter

Rounded internal anal sphincter

Loose areolar tissue

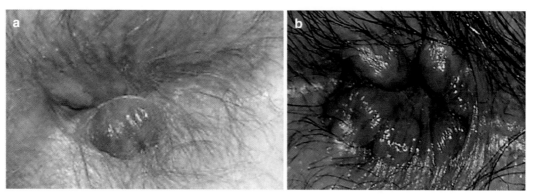

Fig. 3.9 (**a**) Formation of thrombosis from external hemorrhoidal plexus. (**b**) Formation of bulges from external hemorrhoidal plexus

3.9.2 External Hemorrhoids

These appear below the dentate line and are caused by the inferior hemorrhoidal plexus.

They may become thrombosed and ulcerated (Fig. 3.9a, b). Sometimes bulges may be seen around the anal orifice, portraying external hemorrhoids due to dilatation of inferior hemor-

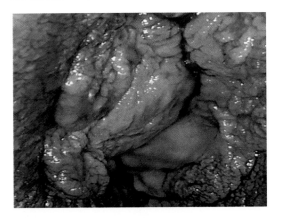

Fig. 3.10 Interno-external hemorrhoids

rhoidal plexus. Varicose veins and hemorrhoids co-exist in around 30% of the patients [30].

3.9.3 Mixed Hemorrhoids

They are interno-external hemorrhoids resulting from an anastomosis between the inferior and superior hemorrhoidal plexus (Fig. 3.10). They may prolapse, thrombose, or ulcerate.

3.10 Rectal Varices and Hemorrhoids

Rectal varices are dilated portosystemic communications that pass from the middle rectum to the anorectal junction. Clinically the rectal varices are present above the anorectal ring as bluish-colored longitudinal columns, whereas hemorrhoids are seen as bulges at 3, 7, and 11 o'clock below the anorectal ring. The superior, inferior, and middle rectal veins form two plexus: an external and internal venous plexus. Approximately 10 cm cephalad to the dentate line, the superior rectal vein bifurcates into two branches to enter the rectum via the lateral rectum wall. The inferior and middle hemorrhoidal veins enter the inferior vena cava [21].

The superior and inferior veins flow in opposing directions from the intrinsic rectal venous plexus. The inferior group forms the inferior rectal veins. External hemorrhoids are formed as a result of the dilatation of these veins. The superior rectal veins drain the upper portion of the anal canal. Their dilatation in the anal columns forms internal hemorrhoids, and dilatation of these veins in the rectum forms rectal varices [21].

Take-Home Message

- Various authors have described hemorrhoids as primary and secondary depending on their position [31], primary at 3, 7, and 11 o'clock, and secondary at other positions. In my opinion, secondary is a misnomer. Instead, they should be called accessory hemorrhoids, formed where superior hemorrhoidal artery branches are present. Secondary hemorrhoids nomenclature should be used if hemorrhoids are present secondary to some disease, e.g., carcinoma rectum.

- Several theories have been postulated about the prolapse of hemorrhoids, but the most accepted theories are the sliding anal cushion theory by Thomson and the hypervascularization theory by Aigner.

- Depending on the clinical presentation of the disease, the treatment option varies. The treatment of hemorrhoids aims to fix the vascular and the nonvascular components of the anal cushions. Failure of conservative management or office procedures is an indication of surgical intervention.

- Today, there is a paradigm shift from conventional surgeries to minimally invasive procedures. The end of the twentieth century is marked by the development of many new procedures like Diathermy hemorrhoidectomy by Alexander Williams in 1991 [32], DGHAL (Doppler-guided Hemorrhoidal Arterial ligation) by Morinaga in 1995 [33], and Stapled hemorrhoidopexy by Longo in 1998 [34]. Recent developments include laser hemorrhoidoplasty. Both DGHAL and laser hemorrhoidoplasty are minimally invasive surgical approaches for treating hemorrhoids with fewer postoperative complications [1].

- A hybrid procedure that combines finger-guided hemorrhoidal artery ligation and laser hemorrhoidoplasty to treat hemorrhoids is always preferred.

References

1. Johanson JF, Sonnenberg A. The prevalence of hemorrhoids and chronic constipation. An epidemiologic study. Gastroenterology. 1990;98(2):380–6.
2. Rogozina VA. Gemorroĭ [Hemorrhoids]. Eksp Klin Gastroenterol. 2002;4:93–134.
3. Lawrence A, McLaren ER. External hemorrhoid. In: StatPearls. Treasure Island, FL: StatPearls Publishing; 2021.
4. Thomson WH. The nature of hemorrhoids. Br J Surg. 1975;62(7):542–52.
5. Alexander-Williams J, Crapp AR. Conservative management of hemorrhoids. Part I: injection, freezing, and ligation. Clin Gastroenterol. 1975;4(3):595–618.
6. Lohsiriwat V. Treatment of hemorrhoids: a coloproctologist's view. World J Gastroenterol. 2015;21(31):9245–52.
7. Lohsiriwat V. Hemorrhoids: from basic pathophysiology to clinical management. World J Gastroenterol. 2012;18(17):2009–17.
8. Yang HK. The pathophysiology of hemorrhoids. In: Hemorrhoids. Berlin: Springer; 2014. p. 15–24.
9. Zoulamoglou M, Kaklamanos I, Zarokosta M, et al. The ligament of Parks as a key anatomical structure for safer hemorrhoidectomy: anatomic study and a simple surgical note. Ann Med Surg (Lond). 2017;24:31–3.
10. Agarwal N, Singh K, Sheikh P, Mittal K, Mathai V, Kumar A. Executive summary—the Association of Colon & Rectal Surgeons of India (ACRSI) practice guidelines for the management of hemorrhoids-2016. Indian J Surg. 2017;79(1):58–61.
11. Blarucha AE, Wald A. Anorectal diseases. In: Yamada T, editor. Textbook of gastroenterology. 5th ed. West Sussex: Wiley-Blackwell; 2009. p. 1717.
12. Agbo SP. Surgical management of hemorrhoids. J Surg Tech Case Rep. 2011;3(2):68–75.
13. Smith M. Hemorrhoidectomy: past and present. Dis Colon Rectum. 1961;4:442–4.
14. Pilcher JE. Guy de Chauliac and Henri de Mondeville. A surgical retrospect. Ann Surg. 1895;21(1):84–102.
15. Aigner F, Gruber H, Conrad F, et al. Revised morphology and hemodynamics of the anorectal vascular plexus: impact on the course of hemorrhoidal disease. Int J Color Dis. 2009;24(1):105–13.
16. Soop M, Wolff BG. "Total" hemorrhoidectomy: the whitehead hemorrhoidectomy and modifications. In: Khubchandani I, Paonessa N, Azimuddin K, editors. Surgical treatment of hemorrhoids. London: Springer; 2009. p. 95–100.
17. Margetis N. Pathophysiology of internal hemorrhoids. Ann Gastroenterol. 2019;32(3):264–27.
18. Milligan ET, Morgan CN, Jones L, Officer R. Surgical anatomy of the anal canal, and the operative treatment of hemorrhoids. Lancet. 1937;230(5959):1119–24.
19. Aigner F, Bodner G, Gruber H, et al. The vascular nature of hemorrhoids. J Gastrointest Surg. 2006;10(7):1044–50.
20. Sun Z, Migaly J. Review of hemorrhoid disease: presentation and management. Clin Colon Rectal Surg. 2016;29(1):22–9.
21. Sharma M, Rai P, Bansal R. EUS-assisted evaluation of rectal varices before banding. Gastroenterol Res Pract. 2013;2013:619187.
22. Haas PA, Fox TA, Haas GP. The pathogenesis of hemorrhoids. Dis Colon Rectum. 1984;24:442–50.
23. Sandler RS, Peery AF. Rethinking what we know about hemorrhoids. Clin Gastroenterol Hepatol. 2019;17(1):8–15.
24. Gao XH, Wang HT, Chen JG, Yang XD, Qian Q, Fu CG. Rectal perforation after the procedure for prolapse and hemorrhoids: possible causes. Dis Colon Rectum. 2010;53(10):1439–45.
25. Goligher J. Surgery of the anus, rectum, and colon. 5th ed. London: Bailliere Tindall; 1984.
26. Burkitt DP. Varicose veins, deep vein thrombosis, and hemorrhoids: epidemiology and suggested etiology. Br Med J. 1972;2(5813):556–61.
27. Gass OC, Adams J. Hemorrhoids; etiology and pathology. Am J Surg. 1950;79(1):40–3.
28. El-Gendi MA, Abdel-Baky N. Anorectal pressure in patients with symptomatic hemorrhoids. Dis Colon Rectum. 1986;29(6):388–91.
29. Ho YH, Seow-Choen F, Goh HS. Haemorrhoidectomy and disordered rectal and anal physiology in patients with prolapsed hemorrhoids. Br J Surg. 1995;82(5):596–8.
30. Ekici U, Kartal A, Ferhatoglu MF. Association between hemorrhoids and lower extremity chronic venous insufficiency. Cureus. 2019;11(4):e4502.
31. Riss S, Weiser FA, Schwameis K, et al. The prevalence of hemorrhoids in adults. Int J Color Dis. 2012;27(2):215–20.
32. Sharif HI, Lee L, Alexander-Williams J. Diathermy haemorrhoidectomy. Int J Color Dis. 1991;6(4):217–9.
33. Morinaga K, Hasuda K, Ikeda T. A novel therapy for internal hemorrhoids: ligation of the hemorrhoidal artery with a newly devised instrument (Moricorn) in conjunction with a Doppler flowmeter. Am J Gastroenterol. 1995;90(4):610–3.
34. Longo A. Treatment of hemorrhoidal disease by reducing mucosa and hemorrhoidal prolapse with a circular stapling device: A new procedure. In: Proceeding of the 6th World Congress of Endoscopic Surgery. 1998. p. 777–784.

"Diagnosis is not the end, but the beginning of practice."

Martin Fischer

Key Concepts

- Hemorrhoids may present with bleeding, prolapse, mucosal discharge as chief clinical complaints.
- Hemorrhoidal bleeding is usually bright red and painless.
- The best diagnostic tool for a patient with hemorrhoids is a thorough history and differential diagnosis to rule out other causes.
- Proper positioning of the patient is essential in the physical examination; the left lateral is the preferred position.
- Painful rectal bleeding may indicate a fissure in ano.
- It is imperative to note the color of the blood that can vary from black to bright red.
- Sigmoidoscopy should be advised in every patient above 50 presenting with bleeding per rectum.
- If there is a family history of colorectal cancer, every patient above the age of 40 should be subjected to a complete colonoscopy.

4.1 Introduction

Generally speaking, for patients, all anorectal problems are hemorrhoids. A clinician must listen to the patient's complaints calmly, thoroughly examine the perianal region, and diagnose. A thorough and systemic approach helps attain an appropriate diagnosis.

4.2 Clinical Features

4.2.1 Bleeding

The most common symptom is rectal bleeding, even before hemorrhoids prolapse [1]. It may be in the form of dripping in the toilet, spurt, or wiping with tissue paper after defecation [1, 2]. Hemorrhoidal bleeding is usually bright red and painless (Fig. 4.1a, b).

4.2.2 Prolapse

Another common symptom of hemorrhoids is prolapse (Fig. 4.2a, b). Internal hemorrhoids are classified depending on the degree of prolapse [3].

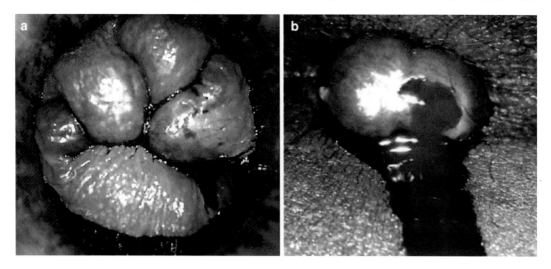

Fig. 4.1 (**a**) Active bleeding as seen in second-degree internal hemorrhoids. (**b**) Active bleeding as seen in external hemorrhoids

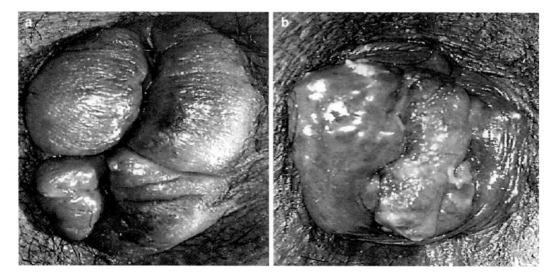

Fig. 4.2 (**a**) Prolapse of hemorrhoids. (**b**) Prolapse of hemorrhoids with edema

4.2.3 Thrombosis

A part or whole of the anal cushion may become thrombosed [4] (Fig. 4.3a, b).

4.2.4 Mucus Discharge

The columnar mucosa is sometimes exposed to the outer environment when the prolapse is substantial enough to extend beyond the anal canal. It leads to irritation and secretes mucus [5].

4.2.5 Pain

Pain with bleeding per rectum during bowel movements is usually attributed to a fissure in ano [6]. Bleeding, extreme pain, and occasional symptoms of systemic disease indicate strangulation of hemorrhoidal masses [7].

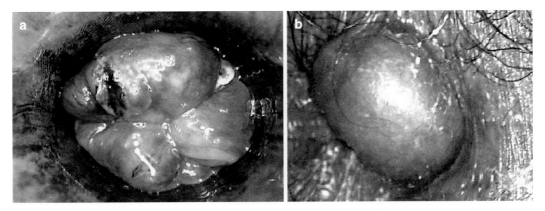

Fig. 4.3 (**a**) Thrombosed internal hemorrhoids. (**b**) Thrombosed external hemorrhoids

4.2.6   Pruritus Ani

The inflamed mucosa produces mucus that causes perineal irritation, itching, and soiling [8].

4.2.7   Feeling of Lump

Prolapsed internal hemorrhoids are manifested by rectal fullness or feeling of incomplete evacuation [1].

4.3   History for Evaluation of Hemorrhoids

The most important diagnostic tool is taking a proper history of the patient. While taking history, evaluate the patient, focusing on the following aspects:

- Gender/Age—Common in both the sexes. The patients are between 25 and 75 years of age.
- Dietary habits—Lack of fiber diet is one of the predisposing factors in the development of hemorrhoids.
- Severity, extent, and duration of symptoms
  - Prolapse
  - Bleeding
  - Presence or absence of pain
- History of bowel habits
  - Frequency
  - Consistency
  - Ease of evacuation
  - Constipation
- Family history of colorectal cancer
- Social-economic history
- Any history of weight loss/trauma
- As previous surgery in the anorectal region may alter the physiological and anatomical function of the anorectum, a detailed history should be taken.

4.4   Physical Examination

Proper positioning of the patient is essential in the physical examination. The preferred position is left lateral. The buttocks must project over the table's edge. The knees and hips are flexed to bring the knees closer to the patient's chest.

4.4.1   Inspection

Pull the buttocks apart gently. Inspect the anus, perianal area, perineum, and gluteal folds. Look for conditions like external hemorrhoids or prolapsing internal hemorrhoids, skin tags, anal fissures, fistulas, abscess, anal cancer, warts, and condyloma. Infection, especially fungal or dermatitis, or scratch marks due to itching, may be seen. Look for any scar from previous surgery. The patient may say, "something comes out of the anal orifice at the time of defecation." Ask the patient to strain. This will assist in differentiating prolapsed hemorrhoids from rectal prolapse. The presence of sulci indicates hemorrhoids, whereas the presence of concentric folds indicates prolapse rectum (Fig. 4.4a, b).

4.4.2   Palpation

The perianal region must be palpated for any swelling before a digital rectal examination (DRE). While assessing the swelling, observe the patient's facial expression. Any indurated painful swelling on one side of the anus with brawny edema might indicate an abscess.

4.4.3   Digital Rectal Examination (DRE)

A gentle digital examination is done wearing disposable gloves. The patient should be instructed to open his mouth and breathe slowly and deeply. Then, the gloved finger, lubricated with jelly, is inserted in the anus with a gentle push and rotated all over to look for abnormalities. Remember that it is the digit and not the tip of the finger that goes inside. Patients with fissures may have spasm of the sphincters and complain of pain during the digital examination. In such cases, Xylocaine 5% is inserted in the anus with the help of Foley's catheter and left for 15 min. After that, the patient

is again taken for DRE. While performing DRE, look for anal tone, hypertrophic anal papillae, rectal polyp, benign and malignant growth, and prostate in males. At the end of the rectal examination, it is advisable to look at the examining finger for the presence of feces, blood, pus, or mucus (Tables 4.1 and 4.2).

Table 4.1   Normal structure palpable on DRE

Structure in female	• Perineal body
	• Cervix (felt through vaginal wall)
	• Ovaries
Structure in male	• Prostate (anterior)
	• Seminal vesicles (anterior)
Structure palpable in both sexes	• Coccyx and sacrum
	• Ischial spine
	• Anorectal ring
	• Intersphincteric groove
	• Ischiorectal fossa

Table 4.2   Points to remember before DRE

• Always explain to the patient before doing DRE
• Female patients may feel shy to undergo DRE. Always examine such patients in the presence of a nurse
• Be gentle while inserting a finger
• In the left lateral posture, examine the patient
• Cover the rest of the parts completely
• Use gloves to examine the patients
• The lighting in the room should be good

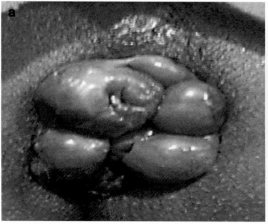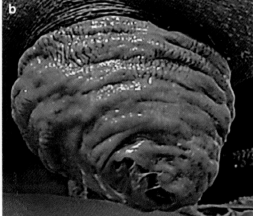

Fig. 4.4   (**a**) Prolapsed hemorrhoids showing presence of sulci. (**b**) Concentric folds as seen in rectal prolapse

Contraindications of DRE
- Patients with severe neutropenia
- Anal stricture
- Acute anal fissure
- Thrombosed external piles

4.4.4 Proctoscopy

DRE alone is insufficient to detect or exclude internal hemorrhoids. For confirmation of the diagnosis, a proctoscopy is always necessary. Always be gentle before inserting the proctoscope. Ask the patient to relax, take a deep breath, and insert a well-lubricated proctoscope. Take out the obturator to view the interior of the anal canal for a clear vision. The red-purple mucosa with piles will bulge into the proctoscope [9] (Fig. 4.5). Sometimes, hypertrophic anal papillae are seen. Look for hyperemic rectal mucosa to rule out inflammatory bowel disease.

4.4.5 Symptoms, Signs, Examination Findings and Differential Diagnosis at a Glance

Refer to Tables 4.3, 4.4 and 4.5.

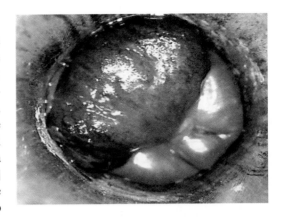

Fig. 4.5 Hemorrhoids as seen through proctoscopy

Table 4.3 Symptoms, signs, examination of hemorrhoids (local and proctoscopy)

Symptoms and Signs			
First-degree	Second-degree	Third-degree	Fourth-degree
Painless Bleeding per rectum bright red. Burning in the anal region may or may not be present	Painless bleeding per rectum bright red	Painless Bleeding per rectum bright red	Painless /Painful bleeding per rectum, bright red and in a spurt, drops, or seen on the toilet paper
Bleeding can be in spurts, drops, or sometimes on the toilet paper	Protruding of the hemorrhoidal mass during defecation/ straining which reduces on its own	Protruding of the hemorrhoidal mass during defecation/straining, which the patient has to reduce manually	Prolapsed and irreducible hemorrhoids lying outside the anal canal
Only prolapse of mucosal moiety as seen on proctoscopy	Anemia may or may not be present	Mucus discharge	Mucus discharge may be present
		Anemia may or may not be present	A feeling of incomplete evacuation

Table 4.4 Examination: Local (L/E) and Proctoscopy examination (P/E)

Examination: Local (L/E) and Proctoscopy examination (P/E)			
L/E Does not show anything outside	**L/E** Does not show anything outside locally	**L/E** May show hemorrhoidal masses locally that reduces manually	**L/E** Shows prolapsed hemorrhoidal masses locally, which is not reducible
P/E Small bulges in the lumen of the anal canal due to the laxed mucosal moiety	**P/E** Small bulges in the lumen of the anal canal can be seen	**P/E** Bulges in the lumen of the anal canal seen	**P/E** Bulges are seen protruding outside the anal canal that are irreducible

Table 4.5 Differential diagnoses of hemorrhoids [10, 11]

Diagnosis	Clinical features	Findings
Anal cancer	Pain in the anal area and, in severe instances, loss of weight	Ulcerating lesion of the anus
Anal condylomas	Anal intercourse history anal mass without bleeding	Cauliflower like lesions
Colorectal cancer	Blood in stool, weight loss, changing bowel habits, abdominal pain, family history	Abdominal mass or tenderness
Anal fissure	Tearing pain and bleeding with bowel movement	Examining the anal canal in a fissure is painful
Perianal abscess	Pain onset gradually	In contrast to the rectal mucosa, this mass is covered with sensitive skin
Inflammatory bowel disease	Constitutional signs, abdominal pain	Abdominal mass or tenderness
Rectal polyp	Changing stool color, rectal bleeding, excess mucus, pain, iron deficiency anemia, changing bowel habits (i.e., frequency), abdominal pain	Mushroom-like growth in the anal canal
Skin tags	No bleeding	Around the anus, tags are visualized
Rectal prolapse	Pain, blood and mucus, constipation, incomplete evacuation, difficulty in passing motion, protrusion of the rectum through the anus	Concentrically arranged mucosal folds should easily distinguish complete rectal prolapse

4.5 Evaluation and Clinical Correlation of Anorectal Symptoms

4.5.1 Rectal Bleeding

Bleeding per rectum is one of the most familiar complaints of anorectal patients requiring medical or surgical intervention. Most patients with painless rectal bleeding are patients with hemorrhoids [12]. Painful rectal bleeding may indicate a fissure in ano. When bleeding is associated with diarrhea, inflammatory bowel disease should always be considered (Table 4.6). Rectal cancer can exhibit symptoms of painful bleeding and tenesmus. It is imperative to note the color of the blood that can vary from black to bright red [12].

- Dark, mahogany, or maroon color may indicate carcinoma rectum or bleeding from the upper GI tract.
- No frank blood in the stool but positive occult blood indicates the necessity of a gastrointestinal evaluation.

4.5.2 Pain

Continuous pain which is not associated with defecation is indicative of anorectal abscess or thrombosed hemorrhoids. Pain associated with defecation is suggestive of anal fissure. Deep-seated throbbing pain with difficulty in sitting indicates a perianal abscess. An intermittent deep-seated pain unrelated to defecation indicates proctalgia fugax. Pain in the coccyx area associated with discharge from an opening in the coccyx region indicates pilonidal sinus. Continuous pain may indicate pudendal nerve entrapment syndrome. The carcinoma rectum may be associated with tenesmus. In Levator ani syndrome, the patient reports dull pain in the rec-

Table 4.6 Causes of rectal bleeding [12]

Anal causes	Rectal causes	Colonic causes	General causes
Hemorrhoids	Angiodysplasia	Diverticular disease	Clotting deficiencies
Anal fissure	Ischemia	Infective	Anticoagulants
Anal fistula	Infective	Inflammatory • Ulcerative colitis • Crohn's disease	Uremia
Perianal hematoma	Inflammatory	Intussusception	
Condylomas	Solitary rectal ulcer syndrome	Neoplasia	
Trauma	Neoplasia	Angiodysplasia	
Malignancy			

Table 4.7 Summary of correlation between pain and bleeding PR [14]

Findings	Possibility
Painless bleeding PR	Hemorrhoids
Painful bleeding PR	Anal fissure
Bleeding PR with pain and tenesmus	Carcinoma anus or rectum

Table 4.8 Common causes of rectal discharge [16]

Discharge of mucus	Discharge of pus
Rectal prolapse	Perianal Crohn's disease
Hemorrhoids	Anal fistula
Solitary rectal ulcer syndrome	Anal tuberculosis
Villous adenoma	Syphilis and gonorrhea
Carcinoma of the rectum	Anal neoplasm
Proctitis	Condyloma

tum that worsens as he sits [13]. It usually persists for 20 min after defecation (Table 4.7).

4.5.3 Perianal/Rectal Mass

They may include perianal abscesses, external hemorrhoids, condylomas, skin tags, and anal carcinoma. The possibility of neoplasm should always be kept in mind irrespective of age. Approximately 80% of rectal neoplasms are within the range of digital examination [11, 12]. It is always necessary to assess mobility and persistence of growth. Local tenderness may indicate the presence of fissure, abscess, or hematoma.

4.5.4 Mucus Discharge

Mucus discharge from the anal area is one of the complaints of anorectal diseases. A purulent discharge may indicate perianal and anal sepsis. A blood-stained mucus discharge associated with diarrhea indicates Ulcerative colitis or Crohn's disease [15]. A copious secretion is always indicative of neoplasia. These types of secretions lead to skin irritation and pruritus (Table 4.8).

4.6 Diagnostic Evaluations

4.6.1 Sigmoidoscopy

The distal colon is inspected up to 40 cm from the anal verge using a sigmoidoscope introduced into the anal canal. A solitary rectal ulcer should always be ruled out, typically present anteriorly about 8 cm from the anal verge. If required, a therapeutic procedure is carried out [17].

4.6.2 Colonoscopy

According to the ASCRS (American Society of Colon and Rectal Surgeons) clinical practice recommendations, patients experiencing hemorrhoidal symptoms like prolapse and rectal bleeding should have a comprehensive endoscopic examination of the colon and rectum [18]. It is an essential investigation in evaluating rectal bleeding that may not be from hemorrhoids and may help exclude other risk factors like malignancy of the colon or rectal bleeding with no prominent clinical findings on anorectal examination [14].

ASCRS Clinical Practice Guidelines for Sigmoidoscopy and Colonoscopy

Sigmoidoscopy should be advised in every patient above age of 50 presenting with bleeding per rectum. In case there is a family history of colorectal cancer, all patients above the age of 40 years should be subjected to complete colonoscopy [18].

Although hemorrhoids are not cause of anemia, yet all the young patients with bleeding per rectum should be subjected to colonoscopy irrespective of age.

When no source of bleeding is seen on anorectal examination, the bleeding is unusual for hemorrhoids, anemia or occult blood present in the stool, or possibility of colonic neoplasia exist, a total colon examination through colonoscopy is recommended.

Table 4.10 Indication and contraindications of sigmoidoscopy [17]

Indications of sigmoidoscopy
• Evaluation of distal colon/sigmoid
Contraindications
• Acute diverticulitis
• Bowel perforation
• Fulminant colitis
• Active peritonitis
• Anal Fissure
• Cardiopulmonary instability

Take-Home Message

• A thorough examination of the anal region helps in making a definitive diagnosis. An essential clinical finding for determining the source of bleeding is observing the color of the blood. Colonoscopy or sigmoidoscopy should be considered mandatory while evaluating a patient with a rectal bleed.

4.7 Indications and Contraindications of Colonoscopy and Sigmoidoscopy (Tables 4.9 and 4.10)

Table 4.9 Indication and contraindications of colonoscopy [19]

Indications of colonoscopy
• Bleeding per rectum
• Evaluation of inflammatory bowel disease
• Screening of cancer
• Endoscopic removal of polyps
• Colonic stent placement
• Endoscopic submucosal dissection
Contraindications
• Uncooperative patients
• Suspected or known colonic perforation
• Inadequate sedation
• Clinically unstable patients
• Severe fulminant colitis and toxic megacolon
• Peritonism
• Inadequate bowel preparation
• Recent myocardial infarction

References

1. Lohsiriwat V. Hemorrhoids: from basic pathophysiology to clinical management. World J Gastroenterol. 2012;18(17):2009–17. https://doi.org/10.3748/wjg.v18.i17.2009.
2. Margetis N. Pathophysiology of internal hemorrhoids. Ann Gastroenterol. 2019;32(3):264–72. https://doi.org/10.20524/aog.2019.0355.
3. Sun Z, Migaly J. Review of hemorrhoid disease: presentation and management. Clin Colon Rectal Surg. 2016;29(1):22–9. https://doi.org/10.1055/s-0035-1568144.
4. Castillo AH. Thrombosed hemorrhoid: what is it, causes, diagnosis, treatment, and more. https://www.osmosis.org/answers/thrombosed-hemorrhoid.
5. Sandler RS, Peery AF. Rethinking what we know about hemorrhoids. Clin Gastroenterol Hepatol. 2019;17(1):8–15. https://doi.org/10.1016/j.cgh.2018.03.020.
6. Villalba H, Villalba S, Abbas MA. Anal fissure: a common cause of anal pain. Perm J. 2007;11(4):62–5. https://doi.org/10.7812/tpp/07-072.
7. Mir SA, Intikhab M, Tak SA, Wani M. Profile and management of complicated (strangulated) prolapsed internal hemorrhoids at a tertiary care hospital—a prospective study. Int J Contemp Med Res. 2019;6(5):E1–3.

8. Ansari P. Pruritus Ani. Clin Colon Rectal Surg. 2016;29(1):38–42.

9. Rigid proctosigmoidoscopy. https://www.jpma.org.pk/PdfDownload/5534.

10. Herold A. Differential diagnoses of hemorrhoidal disease. Hautarzt. 2020;71:269–74.

11. Gibson MC. Hemorrhoids differential diagnosis. https://www.wikidoc.org/index.php/Hemorrhoids_differential_diagnosis.

12. Sabry AO, Sood T. Rectal bleeding. In: StatPearls. Treasure Island, FL: StatPearls Publishing; 2022.

13. Waldman SD. Levator ani pain syndrome. In: Atlas of uncommon pain syndromes. 3rd ed. Philadelphia, PA: Elsevier Saunders; 2014.

14. Ferguson MA. Office evaluation of rectal bleeding. Clin Colon Rectal Surg. 2005;18(4):249–54. https://doi.org/10.1055/s-2005-922847.

15. Ungaro R, Mehandru S, Allen PB, Peyrin-Biroulet L, Colombel J-F. Ulcerative colitis. Lancet. 2017;389(10080):1756–70. https://doi.org/10.1016/S0140-6736(16)32126-2.

16. Pizzorno JE, Joiner-Bey H. The clinician's handbook of natural medicine. 3rd ed. St. Louis, MI: Elsevier; 2016.

17. Cappell MS, Friedel D. The role of sigmoidoscopy and colonoscopy in the diagnosis and management of lower gastrointestinal disorders: technique, indications, and contraindications. Med Clin North Am. 2002;86(6):1217–52. https://doi.org/10.1016/s0025-7125(02)00076-7.

18. Davis BR, Lee-Kong SA, Migaly J, Feingold DL, Steele SR. The American Society of Colon and Rectal Surgeons Clinical Practice guidelines for the management of hemorrhoids. Dis Colon Rectum. 2018;61(3):284–92.

19. Bhagatwala J, Singhal A, Aldrugh S, Muhammed Sherid M, Sifuentes H, Sridhar S. Colonoscopy—indications and contraindications. In: Ettarh R, editor. Screening for colorectal cancer with colonoscopy. London: IntechOpen; 2015.

"A lifestyle change begins with a vision and a single step."

Jeff Calloway

Key Concepts

- Hemorrhoids can affect people of all age groups.
- Patients with hemorrhoids may experience variations in their bowel habits, tenesmus, and fullness in the anal area.
- Most people are treated by dietary or conservative management.
- Lifestyle modifications, relieving constipation, avoiding straining, and fluid intake may help treat and prevent hemorrhoids.
- As the first-line treatment for symptomatic relief of grades 1 and 2, the recommended treatment is Micronized Purified Flavonoid Fraction (MPFF).
- Rubber band ligation of the hemorrhoidal tissue causes ischemia and necrosis of prolapsing mucosa, followed by scar fixation.
- Infrared coagulation is a nonoperative procedure that uses infrared energy for dearterialization, and submucosal fibrosis, which results in scar fixation.
- Sclerotherapy using sclerosants results in contraction and fibrosis of anal cushions, which relieves the engorgement of the venous plexus.

5.1 Introduction

Hemorrhoids have been described from ancient times. The ancient text narrates numerous treatment options ranging from ointments to surgical excision and ligation of this common disease. Insights into ancient text describe that the recommended treatment of hemorrhoids included, following a sensible lifestyle, appeasing Gods of hemorrhoids, and amulets of dried toads.

5.2 History

The first recorded mention of hemorrhoids dates back to 1700 BC when an ointment made from powdered, triturated, and roasted acacia leaves was used to cure hemorrhoids in an Egyptian papyrus [1]. In 1200 BC, the Egyptian "Chester Beatty Medical Papyrus" [2] wrote primarily about this ailment. Hemorrhoids are treated in four ways according to the ancient Sanskrit scripture Sushruta Samhita (fourth century BC to fifth century BC). They include conservative measures, application of Kshar chemical, heat cautery, and surgical excision of hemorrhoids (Shastrakarma) [3]. Hippocrates (460–377 BC), as evidenced by his dissertations "On Fistula" and "On Hemorrhoids" [4], talked about anorectal disorders. Hippocrates used two methods to cure hemorrhoids: hot iron cauterization and chemical cauterization with alum and copper [3].

In his writings, Celsus (25 BCE–14 BCE) discussed ligature and ligature with excision procedures [5, 6]. Galen (130–200 AD) wrote extensively on hemorrhoids and proposed intermittent ligation of hemorrhoids for 2 h [6, 7].

In the realm of hemorrhoidal surgery, the Europeans saw a significant advancement. Some of the master surgeons of the European era in the thirteenth century include Lanfrank of Milan, John of Arderne, Guy de Chauliac, and Henri de Mondeville. During that time, however, little has been documented [6, 7]. Following that, barbers, also known as "Barber-Surgeons," took over the profession of surgery. The barber surgeon's period lasted approximately 350 years [7].

Sir Astley Cooper, in 1836, advocated only ligation after three of his patients died when hemorrhoids were removed [6, 7]. According to Copeland, increased anal tone, which was thought to cause hemorrhoids, was treated with rectal beguinage. In 1871, Mitchell (of Illinois) was the first to inject carbolic acid into hemorrhoids [7]. After that, the Whitehead procedure in 1882 stated removing the area bearing the piles and restoring the mucosal continuity with the anal skin [8], contributing a little to hemorrhoidectomy. Salmon created the groundwork for today's gold standard hemorrhoidectomy in 1835. Many new surgical procedures, which have since been modified, have been implemented to treat hemorrhoids better.

As patients are always fearful of surgery, conservative care remains the primary choice for treating hemorrhoids. A patient visits a surgeon only after the disease has progressed to an advanced stage.

5.3 Nonsurgical Management of Hemorrhoids

Nonsurgical hemorrhoid treatment comprises conservative management and office procedures. The mainstay of initial therapy includes lifestyle and dietary modifications. If none of these are effective, the next step is to follow an office-based treatment like infrared coagulation, sclerotherapy and rubber band ligation.

Nonsurgical hemorrhoids management includes

- Lifestyle and dietary modifications
- Medical management
- Office procedures

Indications
- Grade 1 and 2 hemorrhoids
- Nonthrombosed external hemorrhoids

5.3.1 Lifestyle and Dietary Modification

Changes in lifestyle and diet are first-line treatments for individuals suffering from grade I and grade 2 internal and nonthrombosed external hemorrhoids [9]. Increased dietary fiber intake, preventing straining during defecation, and spending less time on the commode are advised [9]. According to a recent meta-analysis [10], fiber supplements can moderately reduce overall bleeding symptoms and should be suggested early.

According to straining and constipation theory, fiber restores normal bowel movement frequency by increasing fecal mass, volume, and softness. Patients with constipation should consume fiber-rich foods such as oats, lentils, flex seeds, chia seeds, prunes, raisins, broccoli, spinach, figs, pears, grapes, orange, and papaya [11] (Table 5.1). The recommended dose of fiber intake is about 38 g in men and 28 g in women. Fiber supplements help reduce the bleeding and persisting symptoms risk by nearly 50%.

Table 5.1 Fiber diet chart

Fruits	Vegetables
Raspberries	Broccoli
Pear with skin	Tomato, peas
Apple with skin	Carrot, spinach
Banana, black grapes	Potato, beans
Orange, mausami, papaya	Bhindi, green lasun
Strawberries	Green salad
Dried figs, raisins, pulses	Plenty of water

However, they do not improve the itching, pain, and prolapse [12]. Fibers must be gradually titrated (for instance, increasing by 5 g each week) to minimize the gastrointestinal after-effects (like bloating and flatulence) up to 20–30 g every day [13].

Lifestyle modifications like improving fluid intake, relieving constipation, and avoiding straining may prevent hemorrhoids [13]. Fluid intake should be 1 L of water for every 20 kg of body weight. Adding bulk to the diet might help improve bowel habits. Both diarrhea and constipation are clinically potent causes and triggering factors for symptoms in hemorrhoidal disease, and their management is as valuable as the treatment of hemorrhoids [13].

Letter from America

Modifications in diet are comprised of acceptable amount of fiber and fluid consumption and proper instructions of defecation habits which in general are comprised of first-line primary treatment for patients with hemorrhoids symptomatic disease.

Recommendation Grade: Strong as per the moderate-quality indications, 1B [14].

5.3.2 Medical Management

Medical management aims to achieve the following:

- To decrease the inflammation
- To re-establish optimal hemodynamic and microcirculation

5.3.2.1 Role of Flavonoids

As the primary treatment, Micronized Purified Flavonoid Fraction (MPFF) is suggested for symptomatic relief of grade 1 and 2 and selected grade 3 hemorrhoids [15]. Flavonoids have a unique mode of dual-action. MPFF comprises 10% hesperidin and 90% diosmin [15]. They are used as oral medication for treating hemorrhoids [15].

Mechanism of Action
MPFF acts by

- Reducing the inflammation
- Decreasing hyperpermeability
- Increasing venous tone
- Facilitating lymphatic drainage [16]

The small size of flavonoids increases their solubility and absorption and shortens the onset of action. MPFF breaks the vicious cycle of chronic inflammation and protects the hemorrhoidal plexus [16, 17].

Hemorrhoidal Crisis
The hemorrhoidal crisis is a condition when hemorrhoids present with active bleeding, increased hemorrhoidal mass, and inflammation. In an acute hemorrhoidal attack, three tablets of 1000 mg MPFF can be prescribed daily for 4 days, followed by two tablets for 3 days. Afterward, one tablet of 1000 mg is recommended daily for 60 days as a maintenance dose. MPFF is also an effective adjuvant after surgical procedures, reducing lymphostasis [16, 17]. In acute hemorrhoidal disease, a mixture of flavonoids (diosmin, troxerutin, and hesperidin) were shown to control symptoms efficiently and manage both congestion and thrombosis of anal cushions [17]. Other venoactive medicines like Ginkgo biloba, Euphorbia prostrata, and Calcium dobesilate have not shown optimal results in managing hemorrhoids [18]. Calcium dobesilate was found to induce agranulocytosis [18].

Letter from America
Use of MPFF

Cochrane review—beneficial effect of MPFF on bleeding, pruritus, and recurrence [18].

Grade of recommendation: weak according to the evidence, 2B.

5.3.2.2 Topical Treatment of Hemorrhoids

There are various over-the-counter (OTC) hemorrhoidal remedies like astringents, topical anesthetics, corticosteroids, and zinc oxide (protectants). There is a lack of evidence supporting these OTC products' effectiveness. Topical ointment of nitroglycerin (0.4%) reduces rectal pain. However, it is used commonly in anal fissures [19]. Long-term usage of topical products, specifically preparations that contain steroids, must be avoided as they can cause allergy [20] (Grade of recommendation 2B).

5.3.2.3 Sitz Bath

Sitz baths often reduce itching, burning, and pain after a bowel movement for a temporary period. This relatively simple procedure involves filling up the bathtub with warm water (Fig. 5.1). The water used should be tap water and lukewarm (not exceeding 40–42 °C) [21]. The patient is asked to sit in the tub for around 15–20 min [21]. Shafik theorized that a warm Sitz bath via a neural pathway eased the pain by relaxing the internal anal sphincter [22]. This procedure minimizes the pain by reducing the anal pressure, increasing vasodilatation, and reducing edema [22].

5.3.3   Ambulatory Treatment (Office Procedures)

The commonly used office treatment procedures are:

- Infrared coagulation (IRC)
- Sclerotherapy
- Rubber band ligation (RBL)

The office procedures aim to relieve the symptoms by reducing the vascularity or size of hemorrhoidal tissue and increasing the hemorrhoidal tissue fixation in the rectal wall by scar fibrosis [23].

5.3.3.1 Infra-Red Coagulation

Infra-red coagulation was introduced as the mainstay procedure for treating hemorrhoids. Popularly known as IRC, this procedure was first described by Nieger [24] (Fig. 5.2). It is a painless, noninvasive, safe, and easy procedure that gives optimal results compared to other ambulatory treatment procedures.

Principle

Infrared energy is used to induce protein denaturation, leading to dearterialization. The shrinkage of the hemorrhoidal tissue occurs following submucosal fibrosis and scar fixation [25].

Indications

Grade 1 and 2 hemorrhoids.

Contraindications

Prolapsing hemorrhoids.

Technique

The tip of the infrared coagulator is pressed against the mucosa at the apex of the hemorrhoids, and the energy is released through the window of the proctoscope. The radiation is released in pulses. The duration of each pulse is 1.5s, given three times to each hemorrhoid. The penetration depth of infrared energy is approxi-

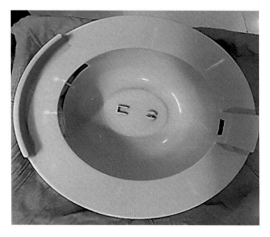

Fig. 5.1 Sitz bathtub

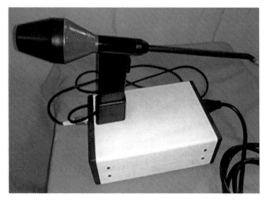

Fig. 5.2 Infrared equipment

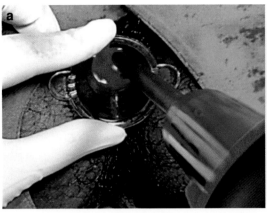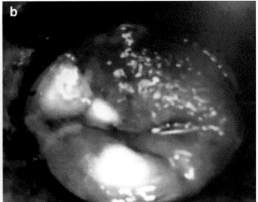

Fig. 5.3 (**a**) Activation of IRC beam at the apex of the hemorrhoids. (**b**) White eschar formation at the apex

mately 3 mm. A white round spot, equivalent to the diameter of the infrared probe, appearing at the application site indicates eschar formation due to tissue coagulation (Fig. 5.3a, b). Minor discomfort is felt after the completion of the procedure. All three hemorrhoidal masses can be simultaneously treated. If necessary, the procedure can be repeated after 2–3 weeks [25, 26].

Success Rate
The success rate following IRC is shown in Table 5.2. In a study conducted by Mohammad Reza Nikshoar, the postoperative pain score after infrared coagulation was less than the conventional surgery (2 vs. 6, respectively) [26]. In a comparative study between the two procedures, rubber band ligation versus infra-red coagulation for hemorrhoids, the visual analog score for rubber band ligation was more than the infrared coagulation [27].

Complications
If the thermal energy from the infrared beam is released at the dentate line, the patient would feel severe pain, and bleeding may occur due to sloughing.

Opinion
I prefer to do infrared coagulation in patients with symptomatic grade 1 hemorrhoids. The principle of IRC is protein denaturation leading to dearterialization. As the position of the superior hemorrhoidal artery branches is not con-

Table 5.2 Success rate of infrared coagulation

Journal	Success rate (%)	Bleeding
Brastisl Lek Listy P. J. Gupta [27]	80	15% (7 out of 46 had bleeding after IRC)
J Laser Med Sci Mohammad Reza Nikshoar [26]	80	IRC-5% Closed hemorrhoidectomy 30% [26]

stant, it is better to palpate the vessels before releasing energy. This approach will achieve better efficacy. To palpate the vessels, one needs to insert a half-cut proctoscope under general anesthesia (Propofol). The procedure is similar to finger-guided hemorrhoidal artery ligation, which will be discussed under laser hemorrhoidoplasty.

5.3.3.2 Sclerotherapy
John Morgan first attempted this procedure in 1896 using persulfate of iron [28]. In 1928, Blanchard recommended injecting 3–5 mL of almond oil with phenol (5%) above the pile mass and not into it [29]. Turell (1959) and Later Bacon (1949) came up with a method of directly injecting urea hydrochloride and quinine solution into the piles [30, 31].

Principle
Chemical agents create a scar fixation of the mucosa by fibrosis [32]. The principle is known as "Chemical Ablation." An inflammatory focus is created by

injecting the sclerosant solution into the submucosal tissue of internal hemorrhoids. It decreases vascularity, intravascular thrombosis, contraction, and fibrosis of the hemorrhoidal mass with cushion fixation in its normal anatomical position [23].

Indications
First- and second-degree internal hemorrhoids.

Contraindications
- External hemorrhoids
- Thrombosed internal hemorrhoids
- Gangrenous hemorrhoids

Common Reagents Used
- Sodium tetradecyl sulfate (Setrol)
- Polidocanol 3%
- Phenol with almond oil
- Aluminum potassium sulfate/Tannic acid (Latest in Japan) [33]

Technique
A sclerosant solution of about 0.5 mL is injected into the submucosal tissue of each internal hemorrhoidal mass, creating an inflammation focus. The patient is placed in the left lateral position. While injecting, make sure there is a wheal formation and not a bleb. If it is a bleb, it means the injection is very superficial. If there is no wheal formation, the needle has entered the sphincter complex while injecting the solution.

Foam sclerotherapy, popularly known as Tessari's method [34], is a procedure where 1 mL of solution is mixed with 4 mL of air [35, 36] (Fig. 5.4). The foam is then injected into the hemorrhoids. With foam, there is better diffusion using less quantity of the sclerosant. These days, phenol with almond oil is not used due to the large volume injected into each pile mass, and the results with this sclerosant are not satisfactory [35].

Complications
- Thrombosis and necrosis
- Burning
- Local abscess
- Bacteremia and sepsis
- Portal pyemia

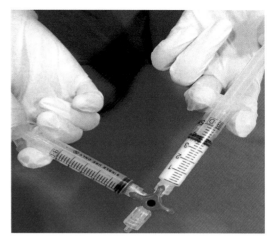

Fig. 5.4 Tessari's method

- Mild pain
- Pressure
- Bleeding

Injections into the deeper plane may lead to infection and abscess formation. Sloughing can be there:

- If the injection is too superficial
- Too much solution is injected into single hemorrhoid, or
- A second injection is given into hemorrhoids too soon after the first

Ideally, the injection should be repeated after 3 weeks. Failure to respond after three injections is an indication of surgical intervention.

Precautions
- During the procedure, one should always stay above the dentate line. While injecting the solution, always withdraw the syringe's piston to ensure that the solution is not inserted into the blood vessel.

  It is worth mentioning that sclerotherapy for varicose veins is done by injecting a sclerosant directly into the vein that converts the vein into a string of connective tissue in a process known as sclerosis [37]. The sclerosant destroys the endothelium of the vein, and the vein gets absorbed into the surrounding tissue and disappears over time [37]. In contrast, the sclerosant in hemorrhoids is directly injected into the pile mass, which leads to scarring and fibrosis.

- If injections are given too deep, they can lead to infection, prostatitis, urethral irritation, perirectal fibrosis, or severe sepsis [38].
- The injection should be given directly into the pile mass. Some authors recommend that the injection be given into the submucosa at the base of the hemorrhoidal tissue and should never be given in the hemorrhoids, as it may cause pain in the upper abdomen [32].

Success Rate
The success rate of sclerotherapy has been mentioned in Table 5.3.

5.3.3.3 Rubber Band Ligation
Barron, in 1964, modified the technique as an improvement of the outpatient ligature method, which was designed and practiced originally by Blasdell [40, 41] (Fig. 5.5a, b).

Table 5.3 Success rate of injection sclerotherapy

Journal	Success rate
Int J Surg Investig Kanellos [39]	57.6%
Journal of Investigative Surgery Pierluigi Lobasico [38]	78.8% (after a single session) 86% (after two sessions)

Principle
Hemorrhoidal tissue banding leads to ischemia of prolapsing mucosa followed by rectal wall scar fixation [41].

Indications
Internal hemorrhoids—Grades 1, 2, and a few grade 3 cases.

Contraindications
- External hemorrhoids
- Patients with hypertrophied anal papillae
- Strangulated hemorrhoids
- Internal thrombosed hemorrhoids
- Patient with large grade 4 hemorrhoids
- Patients on anticoagulants

Technique
The patient is placed in either the left lateral or jackknife posture as per the surgeon's preference. The procedure can be carried out with an endoscope with a retroflection or forward-view or done without the endoscope using a forceps ligator or a suction elastic band ligator. When a ligator is placed accurately, a rubber band is employed at the internal hemorrhoid base. It is vital to position the band 1–2 cm above the dentate line. The zone of anal transition includes a considerable amount of innervation, and placing the band in this area can cause a considerable amount of pain. In severe pain, it is advisable to remove the bands immediately. The number of bands placed may be from 1

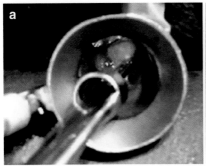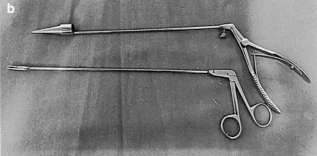

Fig. 5.5 (a) Rubber band ligation. (b) Barron band ligator

to 3 at any given time. Using multiple bands may lead to vasovagal reactions, urinary retention, and pain.

By applying a rubber band at the hemorrhoidal tissue base, the hemorrhoids are fixed high in the anal canal, rectifying the prolapse. By interrupting the blood flow, the size of the hemorrhoids decreases.

In the case of small hemorrhoids, the normal saline solution is injected into the banded pile mass to increase its volume. This tightens the noose around the neck and prevents the band from slipping [42]. Bulk agents or stool softeners are added. The patient should be informed that a few drops of blood may be seen for 5–7 days after the banding. After 2–4 weeks, an appointment should be made to evaluate the success of banding [42]. Patients can resume their regular diet after the procedure.

Complications of Rubber Band Ligation
- **Pain**—This is attributed to the placement of the rubber band near the dentate line and pressure exerted by the bands on the somatic nerves. Pain is ill-defined, throbbing, and might increase 4–6 h after the banding [43]. Sometimes the pain may be due to multiple bandings. Pain may worsen after a few days; in that case, a re-evaluation of the patient is required. Pain may be eased by mild analgesics, a warm Sitz bath, and avoiding hard stool by consuming bulk-forming or mild laxatives. Trichow et al. [44] recommended injecting a solution of local anesthesia into a hemorrhoidal bundle after rubber band ligation.
  Severe pain indicates that the band has been placed over the dentate line. Go for immediate band removal [45].
- **Slippage of Bands**—To prevent slippage, one may inject 1 mL of normal saline into the pile mass once the band is released [42].
- **Thrombosis**.
- **Massive Bleeding**—Incidence was reported in 7.5% of patients on anticoagulants [46].
- **Vasovagal Symptoms**.
- **Delayed Hemorrhage**—Approximate 1% of the patients may experience late bleeding [42].

Table 5.4 Results of rubber band ligation

Journal	Success rate
World journal of Gastrointest Surg Albuquerque A. [42]	69%
Dis Colon Rectum Indru Khubchandani [45]	80.1% (multiple ligation) 71.9% (single ligation)
Dis Colon Rectum V.S. Iyer [46]	80.2%

All three hemorrhoids can be banded in one session. However, the patient may require repeated sessions in grade 2 and a few cases of grade 3 hemorrhoids. The most prominent hemorrhoid is tackled first.

Precautions
Skin tags and hypertrophied anal papillae should not be treated by rubber band ligation.

Postprocedure Care
The patient should not strain while defecating. A fiber-rich diet should be advised to the patient.

Success Rate
The success rate of rubber band ligation is shown in Table 5.4.

5.4   A Word About Cryotherapy

Principle
"Ablation of the hemorrhoidal tissue with a freezing cryoprobe" at a temperature of minus 160 °C, using liquid nitrogen [47].

Advantages
It causes less pain as the sensory nerve endings are destroyed at very low temperatures. It was found that cryotherapy was linked to prolonged foul-smelling discharge [47]. This procedure has almost been abandoned now.

A comparative study between IRC, sclerotherapy, and rubber band ligation is shown in Table 5.5.

Table 5.5 Comparative results of IRC, sclerotherapy, and rubber band ligation

Procedure	Success rate
IRC [49]	46%
Sclerotherapy [38]	21.2% (single ST session) 14% (after the second session)
Rubber band ligation [49]	73%

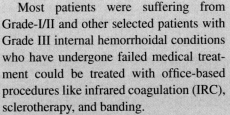

Letter from America
Office Procedures
    Most patients were suffering from Grade-I/II and other selected patients with Grade III internal hemorrhoidal conditions who have undergone failed medical treatment could be treated with office-based procedures like infrared coagulation (IRC), sclerotherapy, and banding.
    Grade of recommendation: Strong as per the high-quality evidence, 1A [48].

5.5 Discussion

Nonsurgical hemorrhoid treatment, which includes lifestyle and dietary modifications, is still the primary line of management of hemorrhoids. Hemorrhoids are most commonly caused by constipation and straining. Drinking enough liquids and eating a high-fiber diet help patients improve their condition. Changing bowel habits, sitting in the toilet for long periods, and converting toilets into libraries should be avoided.

Nugroho in 2011 [50] and Sitti in 2017 concluded that 66.6% of patients with hemorrhoids consumed low-fiber foods [51]. High-fiber foods can bind water in the colon to soften the stool's consistency, make the volume of the stool big, and stimulate the rectum nerves, resulting in a desire for defecation. The stool becomes easier to pass, and constipation and straining are reduced [14].

MPFF is a highly tolerated therapeutic option for internal hemorrhoids, and it is advised in patients with first-degree hemorrhoids and postoperatively [17].

All office procedures are performed above the dentate line [52], and the underlying principle is scar fibrosis. In infrared coagulation, dearterialization results in the reduction of hemorrhoids. Sclerotherapy leads to chemical ablation followed by scar fixation of the mucosa by fibrosis [53]. In the rubber band, ligation of the hemorrhoidal tissue results in necrosis or ischemia of prolapsing mucosa, followed by scar fixation in the rectal wall [52].

Studies have shown that rubber band ligation has advantages over other office procedures for treating grade 1 and 2 hemorrhoids. In comparison to rubber band ligation, infrared coagulation causes only small tissue coagulation resulting in minimal tissue injury of 2–3 mm depth [54]. This decrease in depth presumably causes less tissue fixation and scarring, increasing the possibility of recurrence and chances of offending tissue being incompletely destroyed [54]. Infrared coagulation has been linked to fewer complications [54, 55]. A comparative study by Johanson et al. reported that rubber band ligation had lasting efficiency but higher pain incidence after the procedure [54]. Marques et al. conducted a random crossover trial to compare the two procedures, RBL and IRC [55]. The complications, patient satisfaction, effectiveness, pain, and preference to treat the internal hemorrhoids were studied. They reported higher bleeding incidence immediately or 6/24 h after the rubber band ligation procedure than the infrared coagulation. The number of patients using analgesics were considerably higher in the rubber band ligation group than in the infrared coagulation group 24 h after treatment [56].

5.6 Which Is the Best Office Procedure Out of Sclerotherapy, Infrared Coagulation, and Rubber Band Ligation?

Research by Johansson et al. and MacRae [57] showed that rubber band ligation led to the least recurrent hemorrhoid symptoms and the lowest rate of repeat treatment [57]. As a result, rubber band ligation is advised as a primary nonoperative option for treating grade 1 and 2 hemorrhoids [57].

Rubber band ligation is the most common surgical process performed in the British assessment of over 900 colorectal and general surgeons, followed by sclerotherapy and hemorrhoidectomy [56].

Take-Home Message
- The flavonoids are quite effective for patients with one to two episodes of mild bleeding in grade 1 hemorrhoids. Although mentioned in the literature, I have never treated any patient with profuse active bleeding on flavonoids alone. Always an office procedure has been carried out along with prescribing flavonoids.
- As far as office procedures are concerned, the overall results mentioned in the literature favor rubber band ligation over infrared coagulation and sclerotherapy. However, I prefer sclerotherapy or infrared coagulation for grade 1 and 2 hemorrhoids, and the results are promising.
- Failed medical management of grade 2 and 3 hemorrhoids is an absolute indication for surgical intervention.

References

1. Vieni S, Latteri F, Grassi N. [Historical aspects of a frequent anal disease: hemorrhoids]. Chir Ital. 2004;56(5):745–8. Italian. PMID: 15553451.
2. Fenger C. Everything you ever wanted to know about the history of hemorrhoids. Denmark: Odense University Hospital; 2018.
3. Agbo SP. Surgical management of hemorrhoids. J Surg Tech Case Rep. 2011;3(2):68–75. https://doi.org/10.4103/2006-8808.92797. PMID: 22413048; PMCID: PMC3296437
4. Mosavat SH, Ghahramani L, Haghighi ER, Chaijan MR, Hashempur MH, Heydari M. Anorectal diseases in Avicenna's "canon of medicine". Acta Med Hist Adriat. 2015;13(Suppl 2):103–14. PMID: 26959635
5. Celsus. On medicine, Volume III: Books 7–8. In: Spencer WG, editor. Loeb Classical Library 336. Cambridge, MA: Harvard University Press; 1938.
6. Pata F, Gallo G, Pellino G, Vigorita V, Podda M, Di Saverio S, D'Ambrosio G, Sammarco G. Evolution of surgical management of hemorrhoidal disease: an historical overview. Front Surg. 2021;8:727059. https://doi.org/10.3389/fsurg.2021.727059.
7. Ellesmore S, Windsor ACJ. Surgical history of hemorrhoids. In: Mann CV, editor. Surgical treatment of hemorrhoids. London: Springer; 2002. https://doi.org/10.1007/978-1-4471-3727-6_1.
8. Wolff BG, Culp CE. The Whitehead hemorrhoidectomy. An unjustly maligned procedure. Dis Colon Rectum. 1988;31(8):587–90. https://doi.org/10.1007/BF02556790. PMID: 3042301
9. Elnaim ALK, Wong MPK, Sagap I. The perils of hemorrhoids treatment. IIUM Med J Malaysia. 2019;18(3).
10. Acheson AG, Scholefield JH. Management of hemorrhoids. BMJ (Clinical research ed). 2008;336(7640):380–3. https://doi.org/10.1136/bmj.39465.674745.80.
11. de Vries J, Miller PE, Verbeke K. Effects of cereal fiber on bowel function: a systematic review of intervention trials. World J Gastroenterol. 2015;21(29):8952–63. https://doi.org/10.3748/wjg.v21.i29.8952.
12. Kaidar-Person O, Person B, Wexner SD. Hemorrhoidal disease: a comprehensive review. J Am Coll Surg. 2007;204(1):102–17.
13. Schuster BG, Kosar L, Kamrul R. Constipation in older adults: a stepwise approach to keep things moving. Can Fam Physician. 2015;61(2):152–8.
14. Davis BR, Lee-Kong SA, Migaly J, Feingold DL, Steele SR. The American Society of Colon and Rectal Surgeons clinical practice guidelines for the management of hemorrhoids. Dis Colon Rectum. 2018;61(3):284–92.
15. Godeberge P, Sheikh P, Lohsiriwat V, Jalife A, Shelygin Y. Micronized purified flavonoid fraction in treating hemorrhoidal disease. J Comp Eff Res. 2021;10(10):801–13. https://doi.org/10.2217/cer-2021-0038. Epub 2021 Apr 30. PMID: 33928786
16. Mansilha A, Sousa J. Pathophysiological mechanisms of chronic venous disease and implications for venoactive drug therapy. Int J Mol Sci. 2018;19(6):1669.
17. Lyseng-Williamson KA, Perry CM. Micronised purified flavonoid fraction: a review of its use in chronic venous insufficiency, venous ulcers, and hemorrhoids. Drugs. 2003;63(1):71–100. https://doi.org/10.2165/00003495-200363010-00005. PMID: 12487623
18. Agarwal N, Singh K, Sheikh P, Mittal K, Mathai V, Kumar A. Executive summary - The Association of Colon & Rectal Surgeons of India (ACRSI) practice guidelines for managing Hemorrhoids-2016. Indian J Surg. 2017;79(1):58–61. https://doi.org/10.1007/s12262-016-1578-7.
19. Mott T, Latimer K, Edwards C. Hemorrhoids: diagnosis and treatment options. Am Fam Physician. 2018;97(3):172–9. PMID: 29431977
20. Topical steroid allergy and dependence. Prescrire Int. 2005;14(75):21–2. PMID: 15751172.
21. Tejirian T, Abbas MA. Sitz bath: where is the evidence? The scientific basis of a common practice. Dis Colon Rectum. 2005;48(12):2336–40. https://doi.org/10.1007/s10350-005-0085-x. PMID: 15981059
22. Shafik A. Role of warm-water bath in anorectal conditions. The "thermosphincteric reflex". J

Clin Gastroenterol. 1993;16(4):304–8. https://doi.org/10.1097/00004836-199306000-00007. PMID: 8331263

23. Sanchez C, Chinn BT. Hemorrhoids. Clin Colon Rectal Surg. 2011;24(1):5–13. https://doi.org/10.1055/s-0031-1272818.

24. Leicester RJ, Nicholls RJ, Mann CV. Infrared coagulation: a new treatment for hemorrhoids. Dis Colon Rectum. 1981;24(8):602–5. https://doi.org/10.1007/BF02605755. PMID: 7318625

25. Singal R, Gupta S, Dalal AK, Dalal U, Attri AK. Our experience in Government Medical College and Hospital is an optimal painless treatment for early hemorrhoids. J Med Life. 2013;6(3):302–6.

26. Nikshoar MR, Maleki Z, Nemati Honar B. The clinical efficacy of infrared photocoagulation versus closed hemorrhoidectomy in treatment of hemorrhoid. J Lasers Med Sci. 2018;9(1):23–6. https://doi.org/10.15171/jlms.2018.06.

27. Gupta PJ. Infrared coagulation: a preferred option in treating early hemorrhoids. Acta Cir Bras. 2004;19(1):74–8.

28. Čuk V, Šćepanović M, Krdžić I, Kenić M, Kovačević B, Čuk V. Where are we now in the treatment of hemorrhoids? Acta Medica Medianae. 2015;54(1):97–106.

29. Blanchard CE. Textbook of ambulant proctology. Youngstown: Ohio Medical Success Press; 1928. p. 134.

30. Bacon HE. The anus, rectum and sigmoid colon. 3rd ed. Philadelphia: Lippincott; 1949.

31. Turrell R. Diseases of the colon and anorectum. Philadelphia: Saunders; 1959. p. 888.

32. Lohsiriwat V. Hemorrhoids: from basic pathophysiology to clinical management. World J Gastroenterol. 2012;18(17):2009–17. https://doi.org/10.3748/wjg.v18.i17.2009.

33. Tomiki Y, Ono S, Aoki J, Takahashi R, Ishiyama S, Sugimoto K, et al. Treatment of internal hemorrhoids by endoscopic sclerotherapy with aluminum potassium sulfate and tannic acid. Diagn Ther Endosc. 2015;2015:517690.

34. Xu J, Wang YF, Chen AW, Wang T, Liu SH. A modified Tessari method for producing more foam. Springerplus. 2016;5:129. https://doi.org/10.1186/s40064-016-1769-5.

35. Weledji EP. Minor anorectal conditions in proctology. Austin J Surg. 2018;5(5):1142.

36. Yano T, Yano K. Comparison of injection sclerotherapy between 5% phenol in almond oil and aluminum potassium sulfate and tannic acid for grade 3 hemorrhoids. Ann Coloproctol. 2015;31(3):103–5. https://doi.org/10.3393/ac.2015.31.3.103.

37. Rabe E, Breu FX, Flessenkämper I, et al. Sclerotherapy in the treatment of varicose veins. Hautarzt. 2021;72:23–36. https://doi.org/10.1007/s00105-020-04705-0.

38. Lobascio P, Laforgia R, Novelli E, Perrone F, Di Salvo M, Pezzolla A, Trompetto M, Gallo G. Short-term results of sclerotherapy with 3% polidocanol foam for symptomatic second- and third-degree hem-

orrhoidal disease. J Investig Surg. 2021;34(10):1059–65. https://doi.org/10.1080/08941939.2020.1745964. Epub 2020 Apr 15. PMID: 32290709

39. Kanellos I, Goulimaris I, Vakalis I, Dadoukis I. Long-term evaluation of sclerotherapy for hemorrhoids. A prospective study. Int J Surg Investig. 2000;2(4):295–8. PMID: 12678531

40. Blaisdell PC. Office ligation of internal hemorrhoids. Am J Surg. 1958;96:401–4. https://doi.org/10.1016/0002-9610(58)90933-4. PMID: 13571517

41. Barron J. Office ligation of internal hemorrhoids. Am J Surg. 1963;105:563–70. https://doi.org/10.1016/0002-9610(63)90332-5. PMID: 13969563

42. Albuquerque A. Rubber band ligation of hemorrhoids: a guide for complications. World J Gastrointest Surg. 2016;8(9):614–20. https://doi.org/10.4240/wjgs.v8.i9.614. PMID: 27721924; PMCID: PMC5037334

43. Sajid MS, Bhatti MI, Caswell J, Sains P, Baig MK. Local anesthetic infiltration for the rubber band ligation of early symptomatic hemorrhoids: a systematic review and meta-analysis. Updates Surg. 2015;67(1):3–9.

44. Tchirkow G, Haas PA, Fox TA Jr. Injection of a local anesthetic solution into hemorrhoidal bundles following rubber band ligation. Dis Colon Rectum. 1982;25(1):62–3. https://doi.org/10.1007/BF02553555. PMID: 7056145

45. Khubchandani IT. A randomized comparison of single and multiple rubber band ligations. Dis Colon Rectum. 1983;26(11):705–8.

46. Iyer VS, Shrier I, Gordon PH. Long-term outcome of rubber band ligation for symptomatic primary and recurrent internal hemorrhoids. Dis Colon Rectum. 2004;47(8):1364–70.

47. Southam JA. Hemorrhoids treated by cryotherapy: a critical analysis. Ann R Coll Surg Engl. 1983;65(4):237–239.34.

48. Rivadeneira DE, Steele SR, Ternent C, Chalasani S, Buie WD, Rafferty JL, Standards Practice Task Force of The American Society of Colon and Rectal Surgeons. Practice parameters for the management of hemorrhoids (revised 2010). Dis Colon Rectum. 2011;54(9):1059–64.

49. Walker AJ, Leicester RJ, Nicholls RJ, Mann CV. A prospective study of infrared coagulation, injection, and rubber band ligation in treating hemorrhoids. Int J Color Dis. 1990;5(2):113–6. https://doi.org/10.1007/BF00298482. PMID: 2358736

50. Nugroho SP. Hubungan Antara Konsumsi Serat Makanan dengan Kejadian Hemoroid. Malang: Fakultas Kedokteran Universitas Muhammadiyah Malang; 2011.

51. Sitti HF. Hubungan diet dan kebiasaan duduk dengan hemoroid eksterna pada mahasiswa semester 7 Fakultas Kedokteran Universitas Hasanuddin. Makassar: Fakultas Kedokteran Universitas Hasanuddin; 2017.

52. Singer M. Hemorrhoids. The ASCRS textbook of colon and rectal surgery. New York: Springer; 2011. p. 175–202.

53. Ambrose NS, Morris D, Alexander-Williams J, Keighley MRB. A randomized trial of photocoagulation or injection sclerotherapy for the treatment of first- and second-degree hemorrhoids. Dis Colon Rectum. 1985;28:238–40.

54. Johanson JF, Rimm A. Optimal non-surgical treatment of hemorrhoids: a comparative analysis of infrared coagulation, rubber band ligation, and injection sclerotherapy. Am J Gastroenterol. 1992;87(11):1600–6.

55. Marques CF, Nahas SC, Nahas CS, Sobrado CW Jr, Habr-Gama A, Kiss DR. Early results of the treatment of internal hemorrhoid disease by infrared coagulation and elastic banding: a prospective randomized crossover trial. Tech Coloproctol. 2006;10(4):312–7. https://doi.org/10.1007/s10151-006-0299-5. Epub 2006 Nov 27. Erratum in: Tech Coloproctol. 2009 Mar;13(1):103. PMID: 17115317

56. Beattie GC, Wilson RG, Loudon MA. The contemporary management of hemorrhoids. Colorectal Dis. 2002;4(6):450–4.

57. MacRae HM, McLeod RS. Comparison of hemorrhoidal treatment modalities. A meta-analysis. Dis Colon Rectum. 1995;38:687–94.

Hemorrhoidectomy: The Gold Standard

"The Lord will smite thee with the botch of Egypt, and with the emerods, and with the scab, and with the itch."
Moses

Key Concepts

- The principle behind hemorrhoidectomy is ligation and excision.
- Hemorrhoidectomy is deemed the gold standard in the surgical management of hemorrhoids.
- Grades 3 and 4, thrombosed, strangulated, and interno-external hemorrhoids are the indications for hemorrhoidectomy.
- Salmon proposed an excision with a high ligation procedure in which the pile mass was separated at the mucocutaneous junction and extended beyond the anorectal ring.
- Milligan Morgan is a modification of Miles' technique. The upper end of excision is limited to the anorectal ring, and the lower end includes a part of the perianal skin.

6.1 Introduction

The word "ectomy" means surgical removal [1]. Hemorrhoidectomy means the surgical removal of hemorrhoids. The conventional Milligan-Morgan hemorrhoidectomy is globally considered a "Gold standard" for large, strangulated, or circumferential hemorrhoids [2, 3]. Different hemorrhoidectomy techniques have been developed over time. A brief description of the surgical procedures for hemorrhoids is discussed to understand the principle behind each technique.

6.2 Historical Background

Hemorrhoids are amongst the oldest diseases mentioned in the literature. The ancient era substantiates excision and ligation as one of the procedures for hemorrhoids. The modern era symbolizes a few outstanding surgeons; Salmon was the first to introduce anal stretching to treat hemorrhoids [4, 5]. He next conducted a hemorrhoid tissue excision procedure, which provided the basis for open hemorrhoidectomy [4, 5]. His technique was described by Allingham in 1888 [6]. However, the major innovation transpired in 1937 with the Milligan-Morgan hemorrhoidectomy [7]. It is a widely accepted procedure for treating hemorrhoids. Over the years, colorectal surgeons have gradually modified the technique to perfection.

K. Gupta, *Lasers in Proctology*, https://doi.org/10.1007/978-981-19-5825-0_6

6.3 Indications of Hemorrhoidectomy

- Grade 2 hemorrhoids (failure of medical management/office procedures)
- Grade 3 and 4 hemorrhoids
- Thrombosed internal hemorrhoids
- Strangulated hemorrhoids
- Interno-external hemorrhoids

6.4 Principle of Hemorrhoidectomy

The principle of hemorrhoidectomy is "ligation and excision." The pedicle ligation of hemorrhoids stops blood flow from the superior hemorrhoidal artery (SHA) branches to the anal cushions [8]. Ligation is followed by excision of the swollen and prolapsed anal cushions, known as "Hemorrhoids." Hemorrhoidectomy aims to preserve skin bridges (anoderm) between excised hemorrhoids to avoid anal stricture [9].

6.5 Modifications in Hemorrhoidectomy Over the Years

- Open hemorrhoidectomy (Milligan Morgan)
- Closed hemorrhoidectomy (Ferguson)
- Circumferential hemorrhoidectomy (Whitehead)
- Submucosal hemorrhoidectomy (Park)
- Anal dilatation (Lord)
- Thermal devices for hemorrhoidectomy
- Laser hemorrhoidectomy (CO_2 Laser)
- Radiofrequency ablation

6.6 Evolution of Hemorrhoidectomy

6.6.1 Excision and High Ligation

Salmon first introduced this technique in 1836 for hemorrhoids [10]. The technique was considered the safest and best operation for most cases of hemorrhoids [6]. Description of Salmon's

technique is well mentioned in Allingham's textbook "The diagnosis and the treatment of the rectum," published in 1888.

6.6.1.1 Technique

The pile mass was separated by starting the incision at the mucocutaneous junction and continued on either side of the hemorrhoid tissue. Ligation was done, and the hemorrhoid tissue was excised about 7.5 cm from the anal verge, proximal to the anorectal ring [6, 10].

6.6.1.2 Pitfalls of Salmon's Technique

The disadvantage of this technique was the creation of extensive raw areas leading to fibrosis and anal canal stenosis, the incidence being up to 20% [10].

Modification of Salmon's Open Hemorrhoidectomy

Many surgeons modified the technique because Salmon's hemorrhoidectomy was associated with a large granulation area in the anal canal. These modifications included:

- Miles technique
- Milligan-Morgan's technique

6.6.2 Miles' Hemorrhoidectomy (Excision with Low Ligation)

In 1919, Mile evolved a new technique of hemorrhoidectomy with low ligation up to the anorectal ring [10]. The principle was the removal of hemorrhoidal tissue and healing by secondary intention.

In this technique, the upper end of the excision was extended up to the anorectal ring and not proximal to the anorectal ring, as in Salmon's technique. However, the lower incision was at the mucocutaneous junction, similar to Salmon's technique.

6.6.2.1 Pitfalls of the Miles' Technique

In Miles' technique, the lower level of excision was also limited to the mucocutaneous junction, similar to Salmon's technique, which resulted in the formation of skin tags. The incidence reported was 34% [10].

6.6.3 Milligan-Morgan's Hemorrhoidectomy

In 1937, Milligan and Morgan modified Miles' technique, popularly known as Milligan Morgan's hemorrhoidectomy, which is considered the gold standard [7]. In this technique, the upper end of the excision was up to the anorectal ring, and the lower incision included the perianal skin to avoid postoperative skin tags.

6.6.3.1 Technique

The patient is placed in a lithotomy position under spinal anesthesia. Artery forceps is applied on the perianal skin at 3, 7 and 11 o'clock, and gentle traction is given to visualize the internal hemorrhoids. The incisions are so marked that sufficient bridges of intervening anoderm between the excised hemorrhoidal tissue are preserved. Dissection is started from the largest hemorrhoid, or if of similar size, then the one on the left lateral position.

A V-shaped incision starting at the distalmost external component is extended proximally in an elliptical manner. The hemorrhoidal tissue from the submucosal plane is raised and separated from the internal sphincter by blunt and sharp dissection, converging at the pedicle. The pedicle is securely ligated at the apex of the hemorrhoidal mass by an absorbable 2-0 polyglactin suture, and finally, the hemorrhoid tissue is excised [7].

Alternatively, an hourglass or dumbbell-shaped incision is taken around the hemorrhoidal mass to ensure that maximal anoderm is retained and dissection is completed as above. In this technique of excisional hemorrhoidectomy, after excision and ligation of the pedicle, the incision is kept open to heal by secondary intention, which may heal within 4–6 weeks. All the three hemorrhoids are excised similarly, ensuring adequate anoderm and mucosal tissue are retained between the excised hemorrhoids [7].

6.6.3.2 Pitfalls of Milligan-Morgan Hemorrhoidectomy

- Bleeding (Early and delayed)
- Pain
- Mucosal stenosis or anal canal stenosis
- Prolonged healing time [11]

In a study by J Watts et al. on healing after hemorrhoidectomy, the proportion of patients showing unhealed wounds 6 weeks after hemorrhoidectomy was 4% [10]. The incidence of stenosis and fibrosis after the procedure was 1% [10].

6.6.4 Ferguson's Closed Hemorrhoidectomy

Ferguson, in 1959, described this technique [12]. As with Milligan Morgan, the treatment involves complete excision of the pile mass, including the perianal skin. The excision is continued superiorly up to the anorectal ring. An interrupted fine catgut stitch was used to close the wound from the anorectal ring to the perianal skin [12], leaving a small margin for draining the collection (Fig. 6.1a–c). Nowadays, instead of catgut, polyglactin 3-0 suture is used.

6.6.4.1 Advantages of Ferguson's Over Milligan Morgan

Ferguson's technique outperforms Milligan Morgan in postoperative pain, bleeding, wound healing, and early mobilization. In Milligan Morgan's excisional hemorrhoidectomy, large wound areas are created, causing pain and delayed healing [13]. Scar retraction may result in anal stenosis.

Abdul Razaque Shaikh et al., on comparing the Milligan-Morgan and Ferguson methods for hemorrhoidectomy, found that it takes longer to recover after Milligan Morgan than Ferguson [14]. Arabman et al. suggested faster wound healing in Ferguson's [15].

One of the significant complications of hemorrhoidectomy is postoperative pain caused by internal sphincter spasms due to trauma, inflammation, and sensitive anoderm [16, 17]. A meta-a

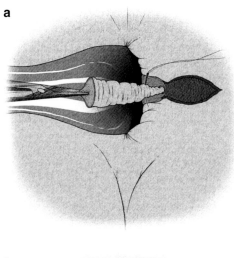

b

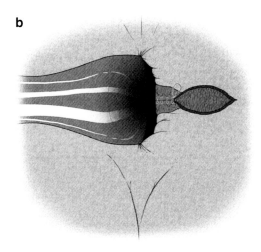

c

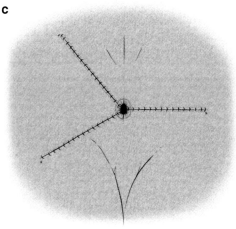

Fig. 6.1 (a–c) Ferguson's technique. (a) Pedicle ligation with excision of hemorrhoidal mass. (b) Continuous suturing of the raw area leaving about 5 mm of open wound at the end for drainage purposes. (c) Final wound as seen at the end of procedure

analysis of randomized controlled studies concluded that Ferguson's technique outperforms open hemorrhoidectomy in postoperative bleeding risk, pain, and wound recovery time [18]. A comparative study of both techniques is mentioned in Table 6.1.

6.6.5 Whitehead Hemorrhoidectomy

In 1882, Walter Whitehead recommended removing the entire pile-bearing mucous membrane ring with a circular incision. The whole section of dilated hemorrhoidal masses and the surrounding mucosa are excised, and the proximal end is sutured to the skin below [4].

6.6.5.1 Pitfalls of Whitehead Hemorrhoidectomy

Whitehead's study, published in 1887, found no incidences of ectropion or stenosis [21]. However, studies reported various complications after the procedure [22], as mentioned in Table 6.2. This procedure is almost abandoned now.

Table 6.1 Comparative study of Milligan Morgan and Ferguson

Journal	Postoperative pain	Anal stenosis	Retention of urine	Bleeding	Recurrence
Journal of Medical Science	Milligan Morgan-77%	Milligan Morgan-0%			
Borse [19]	Ferguson's-48%	Ferguson's-0%			
Pak J Med Sci	Milligan Morgan-lower	Milligan Morgan-	Milligan Morgan-11.81%	Milligan Morgan-3.63%	Milligan Morgan-3.63%
Shaikh A R [14]	Ferguson's-moderate	Ferguson's-2.91%	Ferguson's-3.88%	Ferguson's-	Ferguson's-0.97%
Nepal Med Coll J	Milligan Morgan-7.8				
Pokharel N [20]	Ferguson's-4.9				

Table 6.2 Complication after Whitehead hemorrhoidectomy

Stenosis	Up to 8.8%
Extreme pain	Up to 50%
Anal incontinence	2–12%
Fecal impaction	0.3%
Urinary retention	2–50%
Fistula or abscess formation	1.1%
Postoperative or intraoperative bleeding	0.03–6%
Ectropion or wet anus	The exact incidence not mentioned
Wound healing complications	1–2%
Infection [21, 22]	0.5–5.5%

6.6.6 Submucosal Hemorrhoidectomy (Park's Procedure)

Though hemorrhoidectomy was considered the gold standard for treating hemorrhoids, postoperative pain remained one of the significant consequences of the surgery. According to Park, severe anal canal scarring, the endoanal tube insertion, and the inclusion of the fiber of the internal anal sphincter in the pedicle stitch caused anal stenosis and postoperative pain [23]. To reduce such complications, Park developed submucosal hemorrhoidectomy in 1950 [24].

Because of its complexity and length, considerable blood loss, and danger of incontinence, the submucosal reconstructive hemorrhoidectomy procedure [25] has never been popular. The results are mentioned in Table 6.3.

6.6.7 Rise and Fall of Lord's Procedure

Lord et al. in 1968 suggested anal dilatation [26] based on the assumption that internal hemorrhoids result from circular constricting bands in the anal canal or lower rectal wall. These interfere with normal defecation, and subsequently, the intrarectal pressure rises during the act of defecation, leading to venous congestion and hemorrhoid formation.

6.6.7.1 Principle
The procedure is based on the etiopathogenesis theory that hemorrhoids occur due to increased anal tone.

6.6.7.2 Indications
- Second-degree hemorrhoids
- Anal fissure

6.6.7.3 Technique
Under general anesthesia, the constricting bands are broken down by vigorously stretching the anal canal and lower rectum by inserting four fingers of both hands into the lumen and dilating in all directions [26]. The dilatation achieved during surgery is preserved using bulk-forming laxatives and an anal dilator of 4 cm diameter.

However, this procedure fell to disgrace due to a high incontinence rate (52%) [27].

Table 6.3 Results of submucosal hemorrhoidectomy

Journal	Recurrence	Anal skin tag	Anal stenosis	Gas incontinence
Epub Rosa G [25]	1.6%	1.6%	1%	0.8%
Surgical treatment of hemorrhoids Milito et al. [23]	7%	6.5%	1.6%	3.2%

Table 6.4 Comparative study of bipolar diathermy with ultrasonic scalpel

Bipolar diathermy				
Type of device	VAS score on postoperative first day	Urinary retention	Wound edema	Reactive hemorrhage
Bipolar diathermy	2 [28]	6.7%	16.7%	No
Ultrasonic scalpel	3 [28]	16.7%	20.0%	One patient

6.7 Thermal Devices in Hemorrhoidectomy

The most common complication of hemorrhoidectomy is postoperative pain. Surgeons have been looking for a procedure associated with minimal pain and less morbidity for a while. Replacement of scissors and the introduction of thermal coagulating devices for hemorrhoidectomy are advancements in this field. Various thermal coagulating devices like bipolar diathermy, ligasure, and harmonic scalpel are used.

6.7.1 Bipolar Diathermy in Hemorrhoidectomy

The diathermy forceps get energy from a bipolar electrothermal device [28]. There is localized coagulation with minor heat spread, causing less postoperative pain [28].

6.7.1.1 Indication
- Second- to fourth-degree hemorrhoids

6.7.1.2 Technique
With bipolar diathermy, the anal cushions are excised without ligature of the vascular pedicles [28]. A V-shaped incision is made in the skin along the hemorrhoid base up to the pedicle, followed by excision.

6.7.1.3 Results
A comparative study of bipolar and ultrasonic scalpels [28] concluded that bipolar diathermy hemorrhoidectomy is quick, bloodless, and less painful than ultrasonic scalpels (Table 6.4).

6.7.2 Ligasure in Hemorrhoidectomy

Ligasure is an advanced variant of bipolar diathermy [29], an electrosurgical instrument. It is represented as a "vessel sealing system" because of its high efficiency in achieving hemostasis. The energy is provided primarily to the tissue gripped inside the handpiece's jaws, with negligible thermal or electrical energy spreading to surrounding tissues [29]. The vascularized tissue gripped between the jaws is decreased into a thin wafer seal. A computer-controlled feedback loop immediately terminates the energy flow [29]. The arteries and tissues are coagulated with minimum charring compared to standard diathermy [25].

6.7.2.1 Indications
Second- to fourth-degree hemorrhoids

6.7.2.2 Technique
With a scalpel, a V-shaped incision is made between the hemorrhoid junction and the perianal skin, followed by the hemorrhoidal bundles' dissection from the underlying sphincter muscle

[30]. The ligasure is placed on the dissected hemorrhoids and activated to seal the mucosal surface and division of the pedicle [30].

6.7.2.3 Results

A comparative study between Ligasure and other electrosurgical devices reported fewer parenteral analgesic injections and a lower pain score after hemorrhoidectomy [31].

6.7.3 Harmonic Scalpel in Hemorrhoidectomy

Harmonic scalpel, first presented in 1992, utilizes ultrasound radiation to coagulate and cut soft tissue while causing minimum heat damage to the adjacent tissue [32].

Since heat damage to the adjacent tissue is minimal, using a harmonic scalpel causes less postoperative pain. The harmonic scalpel seals bleeding from the vessels during surgery by protein denaturation [33].

Advantages of Thermal Devices

Using thermal devices in hemorrhoidectomy reduces pain and bleeding.

Results

S. Y. Kwok et al. observed a lower postoperative pain score in their research in the ligasure group compared to the harmonic scalpel [34].

A comparison study of a harmonic scalpel and ligasure hemorrhoidectomy undertaken by Kee Thai Kiu et al. showed no difference in postoperative pain [35].

6.8 Carbon Dioxide Laser Hemorrhoidectomy

Hemorrhoids may be vaporized or excised with the use of a CO_2 laser. It seals tiny blood vessels, resulting in a bloodless field and minimum postoperative pain [36, 37].

6.8.1 Principle

Water on the soft tissue surface absorbs the CO_2 laser energy, resulting in tissue vaporization. The heat is transmitted into nearby tissues, allowing the precise cutting of hemorrhoids [36].

6.8.2 Technique

Under spinal anesthesia, the patient is placed in the lithotomy position. The hemorrhoid is grasped by tissue forceps, 2–3 mm from the mucocutaneous junction, and pulled downwards to bring the internal hemorrhoids into prominence outside the anal verge. A hemostat is used on a hemorrhoid pedicle. With CO_2 laser radiation, a V-shaped incision is made in the skin and extended into the mucosa, covering hemorrhoids. The laser beam is aimed perpendicularly and directly at the hemorrhoid surface. The laser handpiece is held around 2–3 cm away from tissues to ensure optimum visibility.

6.8.3 Advantages

- Hemostasis
- Tissue vaporization
- Bactericidal
- Preventing thermal lesions to neighboring tissue
- Decreased postoperative pain [37]

A carbon dioxide laser is reported to have a precise cutting property, but the coagulation ability is relatively low. The diode laser provides far less postsurgical discomfort with reduced pain.

6.9 Radiofrequency Ablation

6.9.1 Principle

Radiofrequency ablation obliterates vascular channels and shrinks the anorectal cushions [38].

6.9.2 Technique

A radiofrequency device and a probe are used to deliver radiation (RFA) at a frequency of 4 MHz to the hemorrhoidal tissue. The probe tip is introduced at 5 to 10 mm depth into the hemorrhoid tissue and at an angle of 30° to the tissue surface. The submucosal layer is slanted away from the hemorrhoidal tissue. RFA is given to the surrounding hemorrhoidal tissue until a whitish discoloration appears, after which the energy is directed to the internal tissue surface to enhance tissue desiccation [38, 39]. An individual hemorrhoidal tissue may receive a maximum of 3000 MHz at 25 W power. A saline-soaked swab is administered to the hemorrhoidal tissue immediately. The radio-frequency probe is used to induce coagulation in the incidence of any bleeding [38, 39].

6.9.3 Advantages of Radiofrequency Ablation

- Less pain
- Low recurrence

6.10 Complications of Excisional Hemorrhoidectomy

The commonest postoperative complications are

- Bleeding (0.03–6%)
- Pain (20–40%) [40]
- Sepsis (0.5–5.5%)
- Acute urinary retention (2–36%)
- Anal stricture (0–6%)
- Wound breakdown
- Fecal incontinence (2–12%)
- Skin tags
- Anal fissures

6.11 Management of Commonest Complications After Hemorrhoidectomy

6.11.1 Bleeding

One of the consequences of hemorrhoidectomy is bleeding. Clinically significant bleeding of 0.3 to 6% has been observed for conventional hemorrhoidectomy and up to 2% with the thermal device [41].

The bleeding after hemorrhoidectomy can be immediate or delayed. Immediate bleeding is reported within 24 to 48 h following surgery and is most likely caused from the vascular pedicle [41]. Delayed bleeding is described as bleeding that occurs more than 2 weeks after surgery and is usually caused by local trauma or infection [42].

Management

Immediate bleeding is attributed to improper ligation of the pedicle. Cauterization or suture ligation to maintain pressure is usually adequate. Stopping the bleeding with a local anesthetic and epinephrine injection is also possible. Typically, a piece of vaseline gauze or a finger is used as a tamponade. Since the patient's sphincter tone often acts as a tamponade, postoperative bleeding from the arteries in the anal canal is episodic [41]. Tamponade may be performed by inflating a Foley catheter with 30 to 40 mL water in the anal canal. Direct visualization of the operative site with suture ligation is the most effective treatment. Sometimes, it is not easy to ligate the pedicle due to edema. A transanal suture with interlocking taking both mucosa and submucosa can immediately stop the bleeding. The interlocking helps to prevent the purse-string effect. The sutures should be taken both above and below the bleeding pedicle.

There is an incidence of delayed postoperative bleeding in 0.9% to 10% of cases [42]. The most common causes of delayed bleeding are infection in the pedicle or suture erosion which requires proper management with antibiotics and hemostatics. NSAIDs (nonsteroid anti-inflammatory drugs) are commonly used in postoperative pain management that may increase the incidence of bleeding.

6.11.2 Postoperative Pain

Another consequence of the hemorrhoidectomy procedure is pain. Earlier lateral internal sphincterotomy or anal dilatation was performed along with hemorrhoidectomy to reduce postoperative pain but was later recommended only in the presence of associated anal fissure.

Management
Pain can be controlled by intervenous analgesics, sitz bath, and an analgesic suppository of diclofenac or paracetamol.

6.11.3 Urinary Retention

Urinary retention can be due to fluid overload, spinal anesthesia, high ligation of the hemorrhoidal pedicle, or rectal packing. The use of anesthesia causes a reduction in the urge to micturate, which might lead to bladder distension [43]. Sometimes improper pain management does not allow sphincter relaxation, making it difficult for the patient to urinate.

Management
Patients with retention are often advised to sit in a lukewarm water bath for sphincter relaxation. Patients may need bladder catheterization if this fails [41]. If the urine volume following catheterization is less than 500 mL, the catheter may be withdrawn. However, if the volume is more than 500 mL, the catheter should be kept for 24 h.

6.11.4 Local Infection and Sepsis

Three cardinal indicators of infection include fever, increased pain after an early improvement in symptoms, and the onset of delayed urine retention. Early diagnosis and treatment are essential to avert more severe problems in patients who exhibit all three symptoms [41]. Abscess formation after hemorrhoidectomy occurs in 0.5% to 4% cases [41]. Transient bacteremia after hemorrhoidectomy is reported in up to 8% of cases [41]. Guy and Seow-cheon

reported the development of perianal sepsis after anorectal diseases [44].

Management
The patient is given intravenous antibiotics and anti-inflammatory drugs. When an abscess is present, it should be drained.

6.11.5 Anal Tags

Anal tags cause skin irritation and can sometimes be painful. One can avoid anal tags by excising the redundant skin during surgery.

6.11.6 Anal Stenosis

Extensive anoderm and distal rectal mucosa removal during hemorrhoidectomy can lead to anal stenosis. An underlying anal sphincter muscle damage may cause severe stenosis. Anal stenosis patients often complain of straining to have a bowel movement, smaller stools, and discomfort while defecating. Fecal impaction followed by spurious diarrhea may be present. Once the anal stenosis or stricture formation occurs, the patient may develop an anal fissure.

Management
The degree of symptoms determines how anal stenosis is managed. An asymptomatic patient does not always need intervention. In minor strictures, finger dilatation or anal dilators may be helpful. Stool softeners, dietary modifications, or fiber supplements also relieve symptoms. In severe anal stenosis, the patient may require an anorectal advancement flap.

There has been a paradigm shift in the surgical techniques for performing hemorrhoidectomy. The various techniques have been summarized in Table 6.5.

Table 6.5 At a glance: changing techniques of hemorrhoidectomy—from imitation to anatomical landmarks

Surgeons	Procedure	Year	Drawbacks
Salmon	Excision with high ligation up to the anorectal ring, lower extent mucocutaneous junction	1888	Extensive raw areas leading to fibrosis and strictures
Miles	Excision with low ligation, lower extent up to the mucocutaneous junction	1919	Skin tags, fibrosis
Milligan Morgan	Excision with low ligation by taking perianal skin	1937	Stricture, fibrosis
Mitchell/Ferguson and Heaton	Excision with primary suture	1903/1959	Invariable separation of interanal wounds by tenth day
Park's	Submucosal excision	1956	Unhealed wounds with longitudinal division of mucosa and skin tags
Farquharson	Excision with clamp and cautery	1962	Sloughing wounds and mucosal damage
Lord's anal dilatation	Anal stretching	1968	Sphincter injury

6.12 Comparative Study of Hemorrhoidectomy with Minimally Invasive Techniques

Over time, various surgeons have compared the efficacy of different procedures with conventional hemorrhoidectomy (Table 6.6). The details of minimally invasive procedures will be discussed in the following chapter.

Letter from America

The individuals in whom the office procedures have failed and those who have extensive external and internal hemorrhoids with considerable prolapse may be considered for surgical hemorrhoidectomy (III–IV grades). Recommendation Grade: Strong recommendation based on moderate-quality 1B evidence [48].

Table 6.6 Comparative study of Milligan Morgan (MM) and stapled hemorrhoidopexy (PPH)

Journal	Postoperative pain	Recurrence rate	Bleeding rate	Tenesmus
Dis Colon Rectum Mattana C [45]	MM-VAS score 8.56		MM-0%	MM-0%
	PPH-VAS score 5.46		PPH-14%	PPH-32%
Epub Towliat Kashani [46]	MM-Not significant	MM-5%		
	PPH-Severe pain	PPH-7.5%		
Ann Surg Gravie J F [47]	MM-Severe	MM-1.8%		
	PPH-Less pain	PPH-7.5%		

6.13 Discussion

Hemorrhoids have been amongst the most common anorectal diseases known since ancient times. In the past, excision of hemorrhoids was considered too risky since bleeding following surgery was severe.

Salmon, the founder of St Mark's Hospital, London, pioneered ligation with excision of hemorrhoids, as described by Allingham, and laid the foundation for today's hemorrhoidectomy. Although Salmon's procedure was good, it was associated with stricture formation due to extensive raw areas created due to high ligation. Subsequently, the procedure was modified by Miles in 1919 and Milligan Morgan in 1937. To date, Milligan-Morgan's hemorrhoidectomy is contemplated as the gold standard.

Ferguson developed closed hemorrhoidectomy in 1959, approximating the mucosa and skin after the hemorrhoids are removed. The technique of excising the hemorrhoids is the same as in open hemorrhoidectomy except for leaving an open wound in the latter. In a clinical trial comparing the open and closed techniques for hemorrhoidectomy conducted by G Abraham in 2000, no difference was seen between the two in associated complications, or postoperative hospital stay [15]. The study conducted by Seong Y You in 2005 reported lesser pain during the postoperative phase and faster wound healing in closed hemorrhoidectomy [49]. A comparative study of open and closed hemorrhoidectomy conducted by Raghunath Mohapatra et al. in 2018 reported no considerable difference in the pain between the two; only the wound recovery was faster in closed hemorrhoidectomy [50].

Hemorrhoidectomy is linked with bleeding, pain, incontinence, urinary retention, and stricture formation as its leading complications. Preserving the anoderm while operating can avoid stricture formation and stenosis. Some surgeons prefer to dilate the anal canal before hemorrhoidectomy to reduce pain. Surgeons have tried to reduce postoperative pain using thermal devices like a harmonic scalpel and ligasure. Comparative studies by S Y Kwok in 2005 reported ligasure hemorrhoidectomy to be linked with decreased postoperative pain and operating time in contrast to harmonic scalpel hemorrhoidectomy [34].

CO_2 laser hemorrhoidectomy and radiofrequency are two advanced technologies for treating hemorrhoids. CO_2 laser hemorrhoidectomy and radiofrequency ablation were associated with lesser pain, less complication rate, and low recurrence [37, 38].

In hemorrhoidal disease associated with prolapse, surgeons have mentioned the technique of mucopexy above the dentate line to fix the hemorrhoidal cushions. Blaisdell advocated suturing the pile mass by taking the mucosa and submucosa using interrupted sutures [51]. Farag introduced the pile suture technique using three interrupted sutures and fixing them at the apex to hold the prolapsed pile mass in its position [39]. In both these techniques, the submucosal branches of superior hemorrhoidal arteries are occluded, leading to dearterialization. In the mucopexy or rectoanal repair technique (RAR) recommended by Morinaga, the sutures are taken 2 to 3 mm deep and 2 to 3 mm apart. The pile mass is piled up and fixed at the apex. As the sutures are superficial, this technique has more of a cosmetic effects rather than achieving dearterialization.

While the debate continues over the best way to treat hemorrhoids, hemorrhoidectomy is still perceived as the gold standard for grades 3 or 4 and complicated hemorrhoids.

Take-Home Message
- Anal cushions are the normal anatomical structures above the dentate line. They play a crucial role in maintaining anal continence. The anatomy and physiology of the anal canal can be preserved with the development of innovative minimally invasive techniques for hemorrhoid management.
- Hemorrhoids can be surgically treated in three ways: hemorrhoidectomy, which means excision; hemorrhoidopexy, which means fixation by staplers; and hemorrhoidoplasty, which means modifying cushions by lasers. The surgeon's first choice should be a method that retains the anatomical integrity of anal cushions, causes less postoperative pain, has a lower recurrence rate, and has fewer postoperative complications.
- Even though I employ lasers to treat hemorrhoids, I still conduct Milligan-Morgan hemorrhoidectomy on patients with strangulated hemorrhoids.

References

1. Stöppler MC. Definition of ectomy. https://www.rxlist.com/ectomy/definition.htm.
2. Xu L, Chen H, Lin G, Ge Q. Ligasure versus Ferguson hemorrhoidectomy in the treatment of hemorrhoids: a meta-analysis of randomized control trials. Surg Laparosc Endosc Percutan Tech. 2015;25(2):106–10. https://doi.org/10.1097/SLE.0000000000000136.
3. Tomasicchio G, Martines G, Lantone G, Dibra R, Trigiante G, De Fazio M, Picciariello A, Altomare DF, Rinaldi M. Safety and effectiveness of tailored hemorrhoidectomy in outpatients setting. Front Surg. 2021;8:708051. https://doi.org/10.3389/fsurg.2021.708051.
4. Salmon F. A practical essay on strictures of the rectum. 3rd ed. London: Whittaker, Treacher, and Arnot; 1828.
5. Pata F, Gallo G, Pellino G, Vigorita V, Podda M, Di Saverio S, D'Ambrosio G, Sammarco G. Evolution of surgical management of hemorrhoidal disease: an historical overview. Front Surg. 2021;8:727059. https://doi.org/10.3389/fsurg.2021.727059.
6. Allingham W. The diagnosis and treatment of diseases of the rectum. London: J & A Churchill; 1888.
7. Milligan ETC, Morgan CN, Jones L, Officer R. Surgical anatomy of the anal canal and the operative treatment of hemorrhoids. Lancet. 1937;230(5959):1119–24.
8. Chivate SD, Ladukar L, Ayyar M, Mahajan V, Kavathe S. Transanal suture rectopexy for hemorrhoids: Chivate's painless cure for piles. Indian J Surg. 2012;74(5):412–7. https://doi.org/10.1007/s12262-012-0461-4.
9. Hardy A, Chan CLH, Cohen CRG. The surgical management of hemorrhoids—a review. Dig Surg. 2005;22(1-2):26–33.
10. Watts JM, Bennett RC, Duthie HL, Goligher JC. Healing and pain after hemorrhoidectomy. Br J Surg. 1964;51:808–17. https://doi.org/10.1002/bjs.1800511104.
11. Ayfan J. Complications of Milligan-Morgan hemorrhoidectomy. Dig Surg. 2001;18(2):131–3. https://doi.org/10.1159/000050113.
12. Ferguson JA, Heaton JR. Closed hemorrhoidectomy. Dis Colon Rectum. 1959;2(2):176–9. https://doi.org/10.1007/BF02616713.
13. Hosch SB, Knoefel WT, Pichlmeier U. Surgical treatment of piles: a prospective, randomized study of Parks vs. Milligan-Morgan hemorrhoidectomy. Dis Colon Rectum. 1998;41:159–64.
14. Shaikh AR, Dalwani AG, Soomro N. An evaluation of Milligan-Morgan and Ferguson procedures for hemorrhoidectomy at Liaquat University Hospital Jamshoro, Hyderabad, Pakistan. Pak J Med Sci. 2013;29(1):122–7. https://doi.org/10.12669/pjms.291.2858.

15. Arbman G, Krook H, Haapaniemi S. Closed vs. open hemorrhoidectomy—is there any difference. Dis Colon Rectum. 2000;43:31–4.

16. Maria G, Alfonsi G, Nigro C, Brisinda G. Whitehead's hemorrhoidectomy. A useful surgical procedure in selected cases. Tech Coloproctol. 2001;5(2):93–6. https://doi.org/10.1007/s101510170006.

17. Mastakov MY, Buettner PG, Ho YH. Updated meta-analysis of randomized controlled trials comparing conventional excisional hemorrhoidectomy with LigaSure for hemorrhoids. Tech Coloproctol. 2008;12(3):229–39. https://doi.org/10.1007/s10151-008-0426-6.

18. Bhatti MI, Sajid MS, Baig MK. Milligan-Morgan (open) versus Ferguson Hemorrhoidectomy (closed): a systematic review and meta-analysis of published randomized controlled trials. World J Surg. 2016;40(6):1509–19. https://doi.org/10.1007/s00268-016-3419-z.

19. Borse H, Dhake S. A comparative study of open (Milligan-Morgan) versus closed (Ferguson) hemorrhoidectomy. MVP J Med Sci. 2016;3(1):7–10.

20. Pokharel N, Chhetri RK, Malla B, Joshi HN, Shrestha RK. Hemorrhoidectomy: Ferguson's (closed) vs. Milligan-Morgan's technique (open). Nepal Med Coll J. 2009;11(2):136–7.

21. Whitehead W. Three hundred consecutive cases of hemorrhoids cured by excision. Br Med J. 1887;1(1365):449–51.

22. Erzurumlu K, Karabulut K, Özbalcı GS, Tarım İA, Lap G, Güngör B. The Whitehead operation procedure: is it a useful technique? Turk J Surg. 2017;33(3):190–4. https://doi.org/10.5152/turkjsurg.2017.3483.

23. Milito G, Cortese F. The treatment of hemorrhoids by submucosal Hemorrhoidectomy (parks method). In: Mann CV, editor. Surgical treatment of hemorrhoids. London: Springer; 2002. p. 93–6.

24. Khosrovaninéjad C, Marchal P, Daligaux S, Blaustein M, Martane G, Bodiou C. Hémorroïedectomie sous-muqueuse de Parks: étude prospective de 327 patients [Submucosal hemorrhoidectomy with Parks technique: prospective study of 327 patients]. J Chir (Paris). 2008;145(1):37–41. French

25. Rosa G, Lolli P, Piccinelli D, Vicenzi L, Ballarin A, Bonomo S, Mazzola F. Submucosal reconstructive hemorrhoidectomy (Parks' operation): a 20-year experience. Tech Coloproctol. 2005;9(3):209–14.; ; discussion 214–5. https://doi.org/10.1007/s10151-005-0229-y.

26. Lord PH. A day-case procedure for the cure of third-degree hemorrhoids. Br J Surg. 1969;56(10):747–9. https://doi.org/10.1002/bjs.1800561013.

27. Konsten J, Baeten CG. Hemorrhoidectomy vs. Lord's method: 17-year follow-up of a prospective, randomized trial. Dis Colon Rectum. 2000;43(4):503–6.

28. Tsunoda A, Sada H, Sugimoto T, Kano N, Kawana M, Sasaki T, Hashimoto H. Randomized controlled trial of bipolar diathermy vs. ultrasonic scalpel for closed hemorrhoidectomy. World J Gastrointest Surg. 2011;3(10).147–52. https://doi.org/10.4240/wjgs.v3.i10.147.

29. Khanna R, Khanna S, Bhadani S, Singh S, Khanna AK. Comparison of ligasure hemorrhoidectomy with conventional Ferguson's hemorrhoidectomy. Indian J Surg. 2010;72(4):294–7. https://doi.org/10.1007/s12262-010-0192-3.

30. Agbo SP. Surgical management of hemorrhoids. J Surg Tech Case Rep. 2011;3(2):68–75. https://doi.org/10.4103/2006-8808.92797.

31. Wang JY, Tsai HL, Chen FM, Chu KS, Chan HM, Huang CJ, Hsieh JS. Prospective, randomized, controlled trial of Starion vs. Ligasure hemorrhoidectomy for prolapsed hemorrhoids. Dis Colon Rectum. 2007;50(8):1146–51. https://doi.org/10.1007/s10350-007-0260-3.

32. Chung CC, Cheung HY, Chan ES, Kwok SY, Li MK. Stapled hemorrhoidopexy vs. harmonic scalpel hemorrhoidectomy: a randomized trial. Dis Colon Rectum. 2005;48(6):1213–9. https://doi.org/10.1007/s10350-004-0918-z.

33. Bilgin Y, Hot S, Barlas İS, Akan A, Eryavuz Y. Short- and long-term results of harmonic scalpel hemorrhoidectomy versus stapler hemorrhoidopexy in treatment of hemorrhoidal disease. Asian J Surg. 2015;38(4):214–9.

34. Kwok SY, Chung CC, Tsui KK, Li MK. A double-blind, randomized trial comparing Ligasure and harmonic scalpel hemorrhoidectomy. Dis Colon Rectum. 2005;48(2):344–8. https://doi.org/10.1007/s10350-004-0845-z.

35. Kiu KT, Chang TC, Liang JT. Comparison of Ligasure hemorrhoidectomy and harmonic scalpel hemorrhoidectomy. J Soc Colorectal Surg China. 2013;24(1):9–13.

36. Awazli LG. Hemorrhoidectomy using (10600 nm) CO2 laser. Iraqi J Laser. 2014;13(B):33–9.

37. Pandini LC, Nahas SC, Nahas CS, Marques CF, Sobrado CW, Kiss DR. Surgical treatment of hemorrhoidal disease with CO2 laser and Milligan-Morgan cold scalpel technique. Color Dis. 2006;8(7):592–5. https://doi.org/10.1111/j.1463-1318.2006.01023.x.

38. Eddama M, Everson M, Renshaw S, Taj T, Boulton R, Crosbie J, Cohen CR. Radiofrequency ablation for the treatment of hemorrhoidal disease: a minimally invasive and effective treatment modality. Tech Coloproctol. 2019;23(8):769–74. https://doi.org/10.1007/s10151-019-02054-2.

39. Gupta PJ. Radioablation and suture fixation of advanced grades of hemorrhoids. An effective alternative to staplers and Doppler-guided ligation of hemorrhoids. Rev Esp Enferm Dig. 2006;98(10):740–6. https://doi.org/10.4321/s1130-01082006001000003.

40. Medina-Gallardo A, Curbelo-Peña Y, De Castro X, Roura-Poch P, Roca-Closa J, De Caralt-Mestres E. Is the severe pain after Milligan-Morgan hemorrhoidectomy still currently remaining a major postoperative problem despite being one of the oldest surgical techniques described? A case series of 117 consecutive patients. Int J Surg Case Rep. 2017;30:73–5. https://doi.org/10.1016/j.ijscr.2016.11.018.

41. Kunitake H, Poylin V. Complications following ano-
    rectal surgery. Clin Colon Rectal Surg. 2016;29(1):14–
    21. https://doi.org/10.1055/s-0035-1568145.
42. Lee KC, Liu CC, Hu WH, Lu CC, Lin SE, Chen
    HH. Risk of delayed bleeding after hemorrhoidec-
    tomy. Int J Color Dis. 2019;34(2):247–53. https://doi.
    org/10.1007/s00384-018-3176-6.
43. Sutherland LM, Burchard AK, Matsuda K, Sweeney
    JL, Bokey EL, Childs PA, Roberts AK, Waxman BP,
    Maddern GJ. A systematic review of stapled hemor-
    rhoidectomy. Arch Surg. 2002;137(12):1395–406;
    discussion 1407
44. Guy RJ, Seow-Choen F. Septic complications after
    treatment of hemorrhoids. Br J Surg. 2003;90(2):
    147–56.
45. Mattana C, Coco C, Manno A, Verbo A, Rizzo G, Petito
    L, Sermoneta D. Stapled hemorrhoidopexy and Milligan-
    Morgan hemorrhoidectomy in the cure of fourth-degree
    hemorrhoids: long-term evaluation and clinical results.
    Dis Colon Rectum. 2007;50(11):1770–5. https://doi.
    org/10.1007/s10350-007-0294-6.
46. Towliat Kashani SM, Mehrvarz S, Mousavi Naeini
    SM, Erfanian R. Milligan-Morgan hemorrhoid-
    ectomy vs. stapled hemorrhoidopexy. Trauma
    Mon. 2012;16(4):175–7. https://doi.org/10.5812/
    kowsar.22517464.3363.
47. Gravié JF, Lehur PA, Huten N, Papillon M, Fan-
    toli M, Descottes B, Pessaux P, Arnaud JP. Stapled
    hemorrhoidopexy versus Milligan-morgan hemor-
    rhoidectomy: a prospective, randomized, multicenter
    trial with 2-year postoperative follow-up. Ann Surg.
    2005;242(1):29–35.   https://doi.org/10.1097/01.
    sla.0000169570.64579.31.
48. Rivadeneira DE, Steele SR, Ternent C, Chalasani
    S, Buie WD, Rafferty JL. Standards Practice Task
    Force of the American Society of Colon and Rectal
    Surgeons. Practice parameters for the management
    of hemorrhoids (revised 2010). Dis Colon Rec-
    tum.   2011;54(9):1059–64.   https://doi.org/10.1097/
    DCR.0b013e318225513d.
49. You SY, Kim SH, Chung CS, Lee DK. Open vs.
    closed hemorrhoidectomy. Dis Colon Rectum.
    2005;48(1):108–13.   https://doi.org/10.1007/s10350-
    004-0794-6.
50. Mohapatra R, Murmu D, Mohanty A. A comparative
    study of open and closed hemorrhoidectomy. Int Surg
    J. 2018;5(6):2335–8.
51. Blaisdell PC. Office ligation of internal hemor-
    rhoids. Am J Surg. 1958;96(3):401–4. https://doi.
    org/10.1016/0002-9610(58)90933-4.

Minimal Invasive Procedures for Hemorrhoids

> *"Minimally Invasive Surgery is the way forward; the patient goes home the next day; there are fewer complications."*
>
> *Frans Van Houten*

Key Concepts

- The "Doppler-guided Hemorrhoidal Artery Ligation" (DGHAL) uses a doppler with a display graph and a proctoscope with a transducer to localize the vessels.
- Stapled hemorrhoidopexy is a procedure for prolapsed hemorrhoids (PPH). The rectal mucosa is excised in a donut or a ring above hemorrhoidal cushions.
- Transanal suture hemorrhoidopexy is based on the principle of dearterialization by blocking the vessels at two sites at a distance of 2 and 4 cm above the dentate line, reducing the chances of developing the collaterals and recurrence.
- Superior hemorrhoidal artery embolization is a radiological interventional technique to occlude blood flow to the hemorrhoidal tissue.

7.1 Introduction

The most common surgical procedure for hemorrhoids is excisional hemorrhoidectomy. Postoperative pain, large raw areas, long time to heal, and delayed return to work are a few pitfalls of this procedure. Blaisdell, in 1958, carried out a nonsurgical procedure in the form of plication for prolapsed hemorrhoids in immunocompromised patients [1]. Minimally invasive techniques for managing hemorrhoids have emerged in the late twentieth and early twenty-first centuries [2]. These include DGHAL with rectoanal repair (RAR), Stapled hemorrhoidopexy (PPH), Laser hemorrhoidoplasty (LHP), Transanal suture hemorrhoidopexy, and Superior hemorrhoidal artery embolization. The principle behind all these techniques is dearterialization. Except for superior hemorrhoidal embolization, all the other procedures take care of the prolapsed hemorrhoidal tissue.

Minimally invasive techniques provide an alternative to conventional surgeries due to minimal pain, the absence of large wounds, early return to work, and maintaining anatomical integrity.

7.2 Doppler-Guided Hemorrhoidal Artery Ligation (DGHAL)

Morinaga, in 1995, developed a new technique for identifying the hemorrhoidal arterial branches and ligating them 2–4 cm above the dentate line. The procedure is painless due to sympathetic and parasympathetic innervations [3].

7.2.1 Principle

The procedure is based on the principle of dearterialization of hemorrhoidal tissue with mucosal fixation (Mucopexy/Rectoanal repair) [3].

7.2.2 Indication

- Grade 2 to 4 hemorrhoids

7.2.3 Contraindication

- Thrombosed or strangulated hemorrhoids

7.2.4 Instrumentation

The instrumentation includes a Doppler machine that displays a graph, hemorrhoidal artery ligation (HAL) proctoscope with LED light illumination, a Flexi probe, a needle holder, a knot pusher, and a HAL suture [3]. The disposable HAL proctoscope on its tip has a doppler transducer. This proctoscope is attached to a Doppler device and produces acoustic signals which can be recognized easily. With acoustic signals, the inflow of arterial blood in the internal hemorrhoidal plexus

can be detected, and the vessels can be selectively ligated [3] (Fig. 7.1). Recently, a new version has been introduced where the acoustic sounds can be heard through a device attached via Bluetooth. A trilogy probe with a ligation window replaced the older HAL proctoscope.

7.2.5 Technique

The procedure is carried out under the effect of regional block or spinal anesthesia in the Jack-knife or lithotomy position. The patient is prepared one night before the intervention by giving two bisacodyl tablets. After lubrication, the HAL proctoscope, connected to a Doppler transducer on its tip, is inserted inside the anal canal. Terminal branches of the superior hemorrhoidal artery are located by identifying the blood flow. A graph appears on the monitor, and a sound is produced indicating the presence of a vessel. When located, each branch is ligated through a ligation window of the proctoscope using an absorbable 2-0 vicryl on a 5/8th circle, 27 mm needle having a tapered end, nearly 2–4 cm above the dentate line (Fig. 7.2a–e). A figure of eight suture is taken. The doppler sound from the artery fades after the vessel is ligated. Next, this device is slowly rotated clockwise to locate other arteries. Usually, 4–6 branches are ligated [3, 4]. After a full rotation, the procedure is repeated 1–1.5 cm below the first line of sutures. As a result of dearterialization, the shrinkage starts immediately and continues over 6–8 weeks.

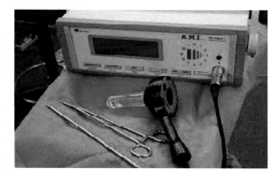

Fig. 7.1 Doppler equipment

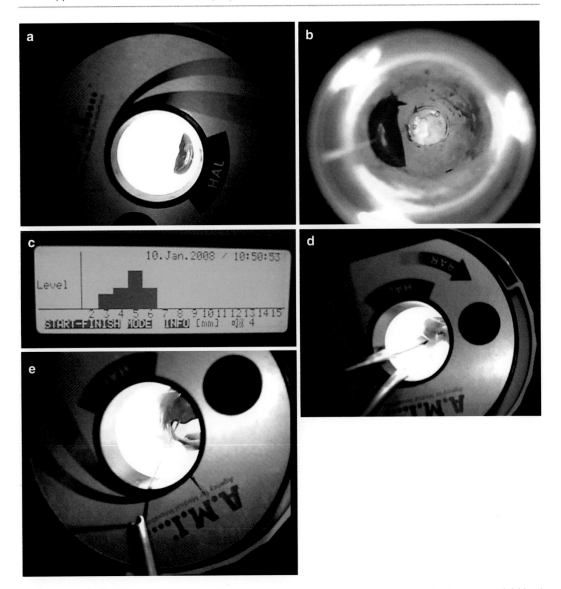

Fig. 7.2 (a–e) Technique of Doppler-guided hemorrhoidal artery ligation (DGHAL). (**a**) Insertion of HAL proctoscope inside the anal canal. (**b**) Luminated anal canal with doppler probe inside to identify the branches of superior hemorrhoidal artery. (**c**) Image on the monitor as it appears after the identification of the branches. An acoustic sound is produced indicating the arterial blood flow. (**d**) Ligation of the branches of SHA through the ligation window of the proctoscope by taking a figure of eight stich. (**e**) Pushing of the knot with a knot pusher at the apex of hemorrhoidal mass

Table 7.1 Overall success rates of DGHAL

Journal	Year	Success rate (%)
Am. Surg. Ibrahim Yilmaz [6]	2012	88
Colorectal Disease P. M. Wilkerson [7]	2009	86
Surg Endosc Walega P. [8]	2008	84
Gastroenterol Res Pract Zhai M. [9]	2015	81
World J Gastrointestinal Surg Marleny Novaes Fiqueiredo [10]	2016	85–95

7.2.6 Advantages

- As the location of the superior hemorrhoidal artery branches is not constant, the Doppler enables to locate the branches precisely in the rectal wall.
- Minimal pain after the surgery.
- Early return to work.

7.2.7 Results

Recurrence rates range from 0% to 40%, with fourth-degree hemorrhoids having the maximum recurrence [5] (Table 7.1).

7.3 Stapled Hemorrhoidopexy (Procedure for Prolapsed Hemorrhoids: PPH)

In 1998, Longo from Italy [11] developed a technique that uses a circular device to reduce the prolapsed hemorrhoidal mass. This approach excises the rectal mucosa as a ring above the hemorrhoidal cushions. The staplers perform an immediate re-anastomosis of the mucosa [11]. Initially, the procedure was named stapled hemorrhoidectomy. In July 2001, a group of experienced surgeons conducting PPH assembled in France and named the procedure "Stapled hemorrhoidopexy" as

the anal cushions are not excised [12]. Recently, the use of staplers for hemorrhoidal surgery has gained popularity. This new approach works better than the standard closed or open hemorrhoidectomy and results in lesser discomfort after the operation with rapid wound healing.

7.3.1 Principle

The procedure is based on the principle of dearterialization with fixation of the prolapsing hemorrhoids [11]. PPH decreases the prolapse of hemorrhoidal tissues by excising a ring-shaped donut of the prolapsed rectal mucosa, lifting the hemorrhoidal cushions, anal mucosa, and anoderm, and fixing them in their anatomical position [11].

7.3.2 Indication

- Internal hemorrhoids (third and fourth degree)

7.3.3 Contraindication

- If only a single cushion is prolapsed
- Severe cases of fibrotic piles that cannot be manually repositioned

7.3.4 Instrumentation

The procedure uses stapler equipment with a 33 mm stapler gun, a detachable/nondetachable anvil, a transparent anal dilator, a purse-string crochet threader hook, and a purse-string speculum [9, 11] (Fig. 7.3).

7.3.5 Technique

The patient is induced spinal anesthesia and placed in a lithotomy position (Fig. 7.4a–d). A

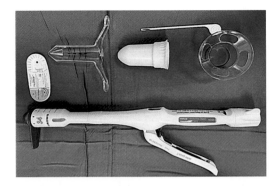

Fig. 7.3 Stapler equipment

circular anal dilator (CAD) with an obturator is introduced into the anal canal. This causes a reduction of hemorrhoidal prolapse into the rectum. After removing the obturator, an anoscope is introduced through this dilator, pushing back the prolapsing mucosa against the rectal wall along a circumference of 270°. The mucous membrane that protrudes through an anoscope window is held with the help of a stitch. The anoscope is gradually rotated through the entire rectal circumference, 4 cm higher than the dentate line and proximal to the hemorrhoidal apex for com-

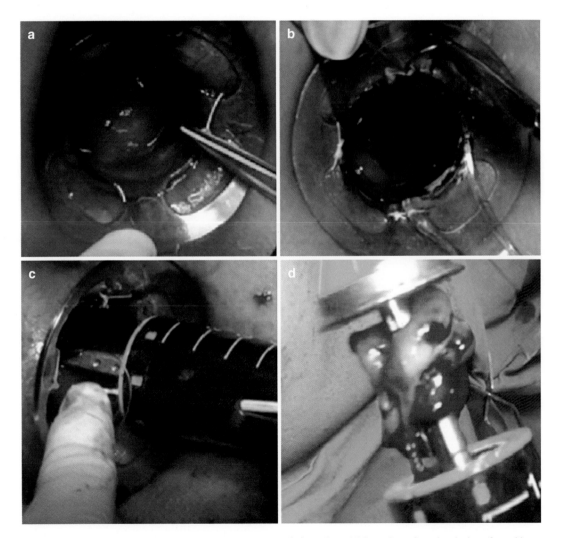

Fig. 7.4 (**a–d**) Stapler technique for hemorrhoids. (**a**) Insertion and fixation of circular anal dilator. This is followed by insertion of anoscope. (**b**) Purse-string suture being taken. (**c**) Insertion of stapler device after taking a purse-string suture. (**d**) Donut as seen after releasing the staplers. (Images courtesy Dr. Niranjan Agarwal)

pleting a "purse-string" suture. The purse-string suture includes mucosa and submucosa. One should ensure that the purse string is complete and there are no gaps. A PPH 01/03 stapler is then unfolded to its extreme limit and inserted with the opened stapler head. This purse-string is then tied with one throw knot. Both suture ends are externally tied or are clamped with forceps.

Along the anal canal axis, the stapler is aligned and closed, keeping a normal amount of tension on the string. The stapler is closed at the end and kept in place for a minute to reduce the interstitial edema. A finger is passed into the vagina in a female patient to check the posterior vaginal wall and ensure this is not incorporated into the purse string. The stapler is fired, releasing a row of double staggered titanium staples through the tissue. The tissue is excised using a circular stapler knife, and the mucosa is removed circumferentially. The stapler device is removed by opening the head. One should be very careful and inspect the stapler line to check if there is any bleeding. In the presence of bleeding, the bleeding area is reinforced with a figure of eight stitch using an absorbable suture. Some surgeons use spongostan to maintain hemostasis.

The donut is checked to ensure that it contains a 2-cm wide rectal mucosa strip [9, 11, 13].

7.3.6 Results

The procedure has a recurrence rate of 25.6–53.3% [14] (Table 7.2).

Table 7.2 Recurrence rate after PPH

Journal	Year	Recurrence rate (%)
Int J Colorectal Dis K. Laughlan [15]	2009	8
Dis Colon Rectum H. Otriz [14]	2005	50

7.3.7 Complications

Many severe complications have been reported following stapled hemorrhoidopexy, including perforation peritonitis, rectal obstruction, fecal urgency, postoperative pain, rectovaginal fistula, urinary retention, and pelvic sepsis [16]. The incidence of complications reported by various authors has been mentioned in Tables 7.3, 7.4, and 7.5. The pain was severe in a few studies, with persistent anal pain and a visual analog score higher than 7 [23]. This procedure should be painless, as the donut is removed above the dentate line.

Table 7.3 Incidence of urinary retention

Journal	Year	Urinary retention (%)
Tech Coloproctol B. Ravo [16]	2002	1.5
Dis Colon Rectum Chung et al. [17]	2005	6.9
Heptogastroenterology Araujo et al. [18]	2007	14
Dis Colon Rectum Sultan [19]	2010	9.3

Table 7.4 Incidence of bleeding after stapled hemorrhoidopexy

Journal	Year	Bleeding rate (%)
Dis colon rectum Ho et al. [20]	2000	1.70
Dis Colon Rectum Cheetham et al. [21]	2003	13
Colorectal Dis S. Sultan [19]	2010	3–5
J Gastrointest Surg Kim S. J. [22]	2013	4.2–7.5

Table 7.5 Incidence of urgency after stapled hemorrhoidopexy

Journal	Year	Incidence of urgency (%)
Hepatogastroenterology Arajuo et al. [18]	2007	3.60
J Gastrointest Surg Kim S. J. [22]	2013	12

7.4 Comparison of Excisional Hemorrhoidectomy with DGHAL and PPH

A comparison amongst excisional hemorrhoidectomy, DGHAL, and stapled hemorrhoidopexy for complications and recurrence has been mentioned in Tables 7.6, 7.7, 7.8, and 7.9.

Table 7.6 Comparative study of DGHAL and stapled hemorrhoidopexy

Journal	Procedure	Persistent bleeding (%)	Pain VAS score
Tech Coloproctol S. Avital et al. [24]	DGHAL	18	2.1
Tech Coloproctol S. Avital et al. [24]	Stapled hemorrhoidopexy	3	5.5

Table 7.7 Comparative study of stapled hemorrhoidopexy with Milligan Morgan

Journal	Procedure	Pain VAS score	Hospital stay	Postoperative bleeding (%)	Urinary retention (%)	Prolapse recurrence (%)
Annals of surgery Gravie J. F. [25]	Milligan Morgan	4.20	3.1	0	3	1.8
Annals of surgery Gravie J. F. [25]	Stapled hemorrhoidopexy	2.66	2.2	1	1	7.5

Table 7.8 Comparative study of DGHAL versus Milligan Morgan

Procedure	Pain VAS score	No complication (%)	Bleeding (%)	Urinary retention (%)	Painful defecation (%)
Iranian Red Crescent Medical Journal DGHAL [26]	1.2	92	2	0	2
Iranian Red Crescent Medical Journal Milligan Morgan [26]	4.6	67	2	6	10

Table 7.9 Recurrence rate of DGHAL, PPH, and Milligan Morgan

Journal	Procedure	Recurrence
Journal of the Korean Society of Coloproctology Wan Jo Jeong [27]	DGHAL	14.4%
Tech Coloproctol C. Ferrandis [28]	DGHAL	35.6%
Gastroenterology Research and Practice Min Zhai [9]	DGHAL	8%
Videosurgery and other Mininvasive Techniques Maciej Michalik [29]	Stapled hemorrhoidopexy	36% (relating to the degree of the hemorrhoidal prolapse)
Dis Colon Rectum Ortiz et al. [14]	Stapled hemorrhoidopexy	53.3%
Trauma Monthly Seyed Mohsen [30]	Stapled hemorrhoidopexy	7.5%
Trauma Monthly Seyed Mohsen [30]	Milligan Morgan	5%
The Egyptian Journal of Surgery Eskandaros [31]	Milligan Morgan	2.5%
European Surgery Andrea Cariati [32]	Milligan Morgan	0.5%

7.5 Transanal Suture Rectopexy

In 2012, Dr. Chivate from India introduced this procedure [33].

7.5.1 Principle

The principle is based on dearterialization by blocking the vessels at two sites, 2 and 4 cm above the dentate line, thus preventing the collateral formation and subsequent recurrence [33].

7.5.2 Indications

Second to fourth degree hemorrhoids.

7.5.3 Technique

The patient is placed in a lithotomy position. A Sim's speculum is introduced in the anal canal to compress and push the pile mass upwards. A specially designed, self-illuminated sliding valve proctoscope with a slit is inserted. The engorged mucosa and dentate line are then visualized. For fixation of the laxed submucosa and mucosa, the sutures are passed through the mucosa, submucosa, and the internal sphincter muscle, starting at the 3 o'clock position, 4 cm proximal to the dentate line [33]. A 30-mm atraumatic 1/2 circle needle with 2-0 polyglactin (Vicryl) is used for the stitch. After tying the first stitch, the next stitch is taken 1–2 mm away, overlapping the first stitch's ending. Each suture is taken 0.5–1 cm apart and is double locked to prevent the purse-string effect. The suture is carried out around the complete circumference of the rectal wall at the same level. The second line of circumferential sutures is taken 2 cm proximal to the dentate line. The procedure is painless as all the sutures are above the dentate line.

7.5.4 Results

A study was conducted on 166 patients with hemorrhoids, who underwent transanal suture rectopexy, to evaluate recurrence, hospital stay, bleeding, complications, and pain. No continence impairment and recurrence were reported. However, long-term results are still awaited [33].

7.6   Superior Hemorrhoidal Artery Embolization

Described first in 2014 by Vidal et al., this procedure aims at occluding the blood flow in the hemorrhoidal arteries [34].

7.6.1   Principle

The principle is occlusion of the blood flow to the hemorrhoidal tissue following the "emborrhoid" method (embolization of hemorrhoidal arteries) by placing coils in the terminal branches of superior hemorrhoidal arteries [34, 35].

7.6.2   Indications

Grade 1 and 2 hemorrhoids.

7.6.3   Technique

The embolization is carried out via the right femoral route. A 5F introducer sheath is inserted using a Simmon catheter, and the inferior mesenteric artery is catheterized. By using a rapid transit microcatheter, the superior rectal arteries are catheterized. The coils used for the embolization are pushable microcoils (0.018) [34].

In 2020, the "Spaghetti technique" was proposed by Giurazza using oversized coils, which were released in a stretched manner in patients showing signs of hemorrhoidal bleeding and portal hypertension. This method helps avoid sudden blocking of the vessels and uses only a small amount of coils [36].

7.6.4   Results

The success rate is between 90% to 100%. In grade 3 and 4 hemorrhoids, there is no role for embolization. The long-term results are awaited [36].

7.7   Discussion

The basic principle in all minimally invasive procedures is "Dearterialization." However, the recurrence rate is greater after PPH and DGHAL. Several technical factors may be accountable for the recurrence.

By ligating the distal branches of a superior hemorrhoidal artery and fixing prolapsed hemorrhoids, the DGHAL procedure blocks blood flow in the distal branches of the superior rectal artery. A doppler allows for accurate localization of artery branches in the rectal wall [3].

The terminal branches of the superior rectal arteries become thin (0.6–2 mm) and superficial (2 mm deep), roughly 2–3 cm above the dentate line [37, 38]. Because there are no interpositions of capillaries between the hemorrhoidal plexus and the arterial system, these terminal branches may be responsible for blood overflow into hemorrhoidal tissue [38].

Suture ligations are carried out about 1 cm above a point where an arterial pulse is found using a doppler [37–39]. The creation of collaterals in a short period may be linked to the high recurrence rate [33].

The branching pattern of the superior hemorrhoidal artery is not constant in every patient. One-third of the individuals surveyed had one artery in an even-numbered clock position [37]. As a result, localization with a doppler is used to pinpoint the arteries appropriately [37]. DGHAL has a higher recurrence rate of roughly 12% for follow-ups of more than 12 months and 5.3–6.7% for follow-ups of less than 12 months [24, 40].

Finger-Guided hemorrhoidal artery ligation (FGHAL) is gaining popularity because it has similar results to DGHAL [41]. Although DGHAL is a simple procedure, the cost can be substantial. Identification of vessels with a finger is comparable to doppler detection in studies, casting doubt on the utility of Doppler for vascular localization.

Stapled hemorrhoidectomy is a well-known procedure devised as an alternative to traditional hemorrhoidectomy. It interrupts the branches of SHA, and the hemorrhoidal masses are restored to their anatomic position [42]. The PPH procedure reduces prolapsed tissue but not hemorrhoids since the hemorrhoidal tissue is not removed; instead, it is left to regress over time. The procedure does not entirely dearterialize the cushions. According to Aigner [37], reaching the postero-lateral "branches of the superior hemorrhoidal artery," which are too high and too deep, is difficult. Furthermore, except for the submucosal branches, the other branches, such as the transmural and intramural branches, cannot be ligated. Only mucosectomy and auto suturing are performed in stapled hemorrhoidopexy [33].

Following PPH, studies have suggested chronic discomfort of unknown etiology. According to research, 15.1% of surgeons have seen patients in severe pain for months, and 2.4% have had patients in agonizing pain for years [43]. Chronic pain has been associated with fibrosis surrounding staples and direct trauma to the pudendal and sacral spindles of the nerve by staples [42, 43]. According to Ielpo et al. [44], over 1.59% of patients experienced chronic pain up to 7 months after PPH, which could only be eased by removing the staples.

In transanal suture rectopexy, "the transfixation of the mucosa and submucosa is done with the internal sphincter, which prevents prolapse of the anal cushion" [33]. The vessels are blocked at 2 and 4 cm, decreasing the risk of collaterals and recurrences [33].

The goal of superior hemorrhoidal artery embolization is to "occlude the superior rectal arteries" by an endovascular procedure. Selective embolization, the absence of direct damage to the anorectal region, and the preservation of anal cushions are all potential benefits of the endo-vascular technique [34, 35]. As a result, optimal outcomes could be obtained with minimal morbidity. The long-term benefits are still unknown [34, 35].

DGHAL itself is ineffective at controlling hemorrhoid prolapse and may require additional surgical procedures like mucopexy in some cases [45].

Despite the benefits of minimally invasive procedures, such as reduced postoperative discomfort and a quicker return to everyday life, the only factor restricting their acceptability is the high cost. Transanal suture rectopexy is the only technique that is cost-effective.

Take-Home Message
- As discussed, each approach has its limitations. Minimally invasive procedures are less painful and allow patients an early return to work. They are associated with less morbidity. However, it can be extrapolated from the data that, regardless of the surgery, immediate postoperative pain and discomfort vary from a VAS score of 3–4, which improves in 48–72 h.
- Based on the principle of DGHAL to treat hemorrhoids, I prefer a hybrid procedure, finger-guided hemorrhoidal artery ligation (FGHAL) with laser hemorrhoidoplasty (LHP). DGHAL laid the basis for FGHAL and transanal suture rectopexy. The effectiveness of FGHAL is similar to that of DGHAL. Although PPH is a minimally invasive procedure, I do not practice it.

References

1. Blaisdell PC. Office ligation of internal hemorrhoids. Am J Surg. 1958;96:401–4.
2. Pata F, Gallo G, Pellino G, Vigorita V, Podda M, Di Saverio S, D'Ambrosio G, Sammarco G. Evolution of surgical management of hemorrhoidal disease: an historical overview. Front Surg. 2021;8:727059. https://doi.org/10.3389/fsurg.2021.727059.
3. Morinaga K, Hasuda K, Ikeda T. A novel therapy for internal hemorrhoids: ligation of the hemorrhoidal artery with a newly devised instrument (Moricorn)

in conjunction with a Doppler flowmeter. Am J Gastroenterol. 1995;90(4):610–3.

4. Scheyer M, Antonietti E, Rollinger G, Mall H, Arnold S. Doppler-guided hemorrhoidal artery ligation. Am J Surg. 2006;191(1):89–93. https://doi.org/10.1016/j.amjsurg.2005.10.007.

5. Lienert M. Literature review on dearterialization of hemorrhoids and mucopexy. In: Ratto C, Parello A, Litta F, editors. Hemorrhoids, Coloproctology, vol. 2. Cham: Springer; 2018. https://doi.org/10.1007/978-3-319-53357-5_41.

6. Yilmaz İ, Sücüllü İ, Karakaş DÖ, Özdemir Y, Yücel E, Akin ML. Doppler-guided hemorrhoidal artery ligation: experience with 2 years follow-up. Am Surg. 2012;78(3):344–8.

7. Wilkerson PM, Strbac M, Reece-Smith H, Middleton SB. Doppler-guided haemorrhoidal artery ligation: long-term outcome and patient satisfaction. Color Dis. 2009;11(4):394–400. https://doi.org/10.1111/j.1463-1318.2008.01602.x.

8. Wałega P, Scheyer M, Kenig J, Herman RM, Arnold S, Nowak M, et al. Two-center experience in the treatment of hemorrhoidal disease using Doppler-guided hemorrhoidal artery ligation: functional results after 1-year follow-up. Surg Endosc. 2008;22(11):2379–83.

9. Zhai M, Zhang YA, Wang ZY, Sun JH, Wen J, Zhang Q, Li JD, Wu YZ, Zhou F, Xu HL. A randomized controlled trial comparing suture-fixation mucopexy and Doppler-guided hemorrhoidal artery ligation in patients with grade III hemorrhoids. Gastroenterol Res Pract. 2016;2016:8143703. https://doi.org/10.1155/2016/8143703.

10. Figueiredo MN, Campos FG. Doppler-guided hemorrhoidal dearterialization/transanal hemorrhoidal dearterialization: technical evolution and outcomes after 20 years. World J Gastrointest Surg. 2016;8(3):232–7. https://doi.org/10.4240/wjgs.v8.i3.232.

11. Longo A. Treatment of hemorrhoids disease by reduction of mucosa and hemorrhoidal prolapse with a circular-suturing device: a new procedure. Proceedings of the Sixth World Congress of Endoscopic Surgery, Rome, Italy; 1998. p. 777.

12. Practice parameters for the treatment of hemorrhoids. The Standards Task Force American Society of Colon and Rectal Surgeons. Dis Colon Rectum. 1993;36(12):1118–20.

13. Hardy A, Chan CL, Cohen CR. The surgical management of haemorrhoids—a review. Dig Surg. 2005;22(1–2):26–33. https://doi.org/10.1159/000085343.

14. Ortiz H, Marzo J, Armendáriz P, De Miguel M. Stapled hemorrhoidopexy vs. diathermy excision for fourth-degree hemorrhoids: a randomized, clinical trial and review of the literature. Dis Colon Rectum. 2005;48(4):809–15. https://doi.org/10.1007/s10350-004-0861-z.

15. Laughlan K, Jayne DG, Jackson D, Rupprecht F, Ribaric G. Stapled haemorrhoidopexy compared to Milligan-Morgan and Ferguson haemorrhoidectomy: a systematic review. Int J Color Dis. 2009;24(3):335–44. https://doi.org/10.1007/s00384-008-0611-0.

16. Ravo B, Amato A, Bianco V, Boccasanta P, Bottini C, Carriero A, Milito G, Dodi G, Mascagni D, Orsini S, Pietroletti R, Ripetti V, Tagariello GB. Complications after stapled hemorrhoidectomy: can they be prevented? Tech Coloproctol. 2002;6(2):83–8. https://doi.org/10.1007/s101510200018.

17. Chung CC, Cheung HY, Chan ES, Kwok SY, Li MK. Stapled hemorrhoidopexy vs. harmonic scalpel hemorrhoidectomy: a randomized trial. Dis Colon Rectum. 2005;48(6):1213–9.

18. Se A, de Caravatto PP, Dumarco RB, Sousa M. Stapled hemorrhoidectomy vs. closed diathermy-excision hemorrhoidectomy without suture ligation: a case-controlled trial. Hepatogastroenterology. 2007;54(80):2243–8.

19. Sultan S, Rabahi N, Etienney I, Atienza P. Stapled haemorrhoidopexy: 6 years experience of a referral centre. Color Dis. 2010;12(9):921–6. https://doi.org/10.1111/j.1463-1318.2009.01893.x.

20. Ho YH, Cheong WK, Tsang C, Ho J, Eu KW, Tang CL, et al. Stapled hemorrhoidectomy—cost and effectiveness: randomized, controlled trial including incontinence scoring, anorectal manometry, and endoanal ultrasound assessments at up to three months. Dis Colon Rectum. 2000;43(12):1666–75.

21. Cheetham MJ, Cohen CR, Kamm MA, Phillips RK. A randomized, controlled trial of diathermy hemorrhoidectomy vs. stapled hemorrhoidectomy in an intended day-care setting with longer-term follow-up. Dis Colon Rectum. 2003;46(4):491–7.

22. Kim JS, Vashist YK, Thieltges S, Zehler O, Gawad KA, Yekebas EF, Izbicki JR, Kutup AJ. Stapled hemorrhoidopexy versus Milligan-Morgan hemorrhoidectomy in circumferential third-degree hemorrhoids: long-term results of a randomized controlled trial. Gastrointest Surg. 2013;17(7):1292–8.

23. Palimento D, Picchio M, Attanasio U, Lombardi A, Bambini C, Renda A. Stapled and open hemorrhoidectomy: a randomized controlled trial of regular results. World J Surg. 2003;27(2):203–7. https://doi.org/10.1007/s00268-002-6459-5.

24. Avital S, Inbar R, Karin E, Greenberg R. Five-year follow-up of Doppler-guided hemorrhoidal artery ligation. Tech Coloproctol. 2012;16(1):61–5.

25. Gravié JF, Lehur PA, Huten N, Papillon M, Fantoli M, Descottes B, Pessaux P, Arnaud JP. Stapled hemorrhoidopexy versus Milligan-Morgan hemorrhoidectomy: a prospective, randomized, multicenter trial with 2-year postoperative follow-up. Ann Surg. 2005;242(1):29–35. https://doi.org/10.1097/01.sla.0000169570.64579.31.

26. Shabahang H, Maddah G, Sadat Fattahi A. Comparison of Doppler guided hemorrhoid artery ligation and Milligan Morgan hemorrhoidectomy in management of hemorrhoid disease. Iran Red Cres Med J. 2013;15(5).

27. Jeong WJ, Cho SW, Noh KT, Chung SS. One year follow-up result of Doppler-guided hemorrhoidal artery ligation and recto-anal repair in 97 consecutive patients. J Korean Soc Coloproctol. 2011;27(6):298–302. https://doi.org/10.3393/jksc.2011.27.6.298.

28. Ferrandis C, De Faucal D, Fabreguette JM, Borie F. Efficacy of Doppler-guided hemorrhoidal artery ligation with mucopexy, in the short- and long-terms for patients with the hemorrhoidal disease. Tech Coloproctol. 2020;24(2):165–71. https://doi.org/10.1007/s10151-019-02136-1.

29. Michalik M, Pawlak M, Bobowicz M, Witzling M. Long-term outcomes of stapled hemorrhoidopexy. Wideochirur Inne Tech Maloinwazyjne. 2014;9(1):18–23. https://doi.org/10.5114/wiitm.2011.35784.

30. Towliat Kashani SM, Mehrvarz S, Mousavi Naeini SM, Erfanian R. Milligan-Morgan hemorrhoidectomy vs. stapled hemorrhoidopexy. Trauma Mon. 2012;16(4):175–7. https://doi.org/10.5812/kowsar.22517464.3363.

31. Eskandaros MS, Darwish AA. Comparative study between Milligan-Morgan hemorrhoidectomy, stapled hemorrhoidopexy, and laser hemorrhoidoplasty in patients with third-degree hemorrhoids. Egypt J Surg. 2020;39(2):352–63. https://doi.org/10.4103/ejs.ejs_214_19.

32. Cariati A. Stapled hemorrhoidopexy versus Milligan–Morgan hemorrhoidectomy: a short-term follow-up on 640 consecutive patients. Eur Surg. 2015;47:112–6. https://doi.org/10.1007/s10353-015-0316-x.

33. Chivate SD, Ladukar L, Ayyar M, Mahajan V, Kavathe S. Transanal suture rectopexy for haemorrhoids: Chivate's painless cure for piles. Indian J Surg. 2012;74(5):412–7. https://doi.org/10.1007/s12262-012-0461-4.

34. Vidal V, Louis G, Bartoli JM, Sielezneff I. Embolization of the hemorrhoidal arteries (the emborrhoid technique): a new concept and challenge for interventional radiology. Diagn Interv Imaging. 2014;95(3):307–15.

35. Talaie R, Torkian P, Moghadam AD, Tradi F, Vidal V, Sapoval M, Golzarian J. Hemorrhoid embolization: a review of current evidence. Diagn Interv Imaging. 2022;103(1):3–11.

36. Giurazza F, Corvino F, Cavaglià E, Silvestre M, Cangiano G, Amodio F, et al. Emborrhoid in patients with portal hypertension and chronic hemorrhoidal bleeding: preliminary results in five cases with a new coiling release fashion "Spaghetti technique". Radiol Med. 2020;125(10):1008–11.

37. Aigner F, Bodner G, Conrad F, Mbaka G, Kreczy A, Fritsch H. The superior rectal artery and its branching pattern with regard to its clinical influence on ligation techniques for internal hemorrhoids. Am J Surg. 2004;187:102–8. https://doi.org/10.1016/j.amjsurg.2002.11.003.

38. Schuurman JP, Go PM, Bleys RL. Anatomical branches of the superior rectal artery in the distal rectum. Color Dis. 2009;11(9):967–71. https://doi.org/10.1111/j.1463-1318.2008.01729.x.

39. Giamundo P. Advantages and limits of hemorrhoidal dearterialization in the treatment of symptomatic hemorrhoids. World J Gastrointest Surg. 2016;8(1):1–4.

40. Yeo D, Tan KY. Hemorrhoidectomy - making sense of the surgical options. World J Gastroenterol. 2014;20(45):16976–83. https://doi.org/10.3748/wjg.v20.i45.16976.

41. Gupta K, Agarwal N, Mita K. Clinical outcomes in patients with hemorrhoids treated by finger-guided hemorrhoidal artery ligation with laser hemorrhoidoplasty: a retrospective cohort study. J Adv Med Med Res. 2021;2021:143–52.

42. Khubchandani I, Fealk MH, Reed JF. Is there a post-PPH syndrome? Tech Coloproctol. 2009;13:141–144; discussion 144.

43. De Nardi P, Corsetti M, Passaretti S, Squillante S, Castellaneta AG, Staudacher C, Testoni PA. Evaluation of rectal sensory and motor function by means of the electronic barostat after stapled hemorrhoidopexy. Dis Colon Rectum. 2008;51:1255–60.

44. Ielpo B, Venditti D, Balassone V, Favetta U, Buonomo O, Petrella G. Proctalgia as a late complication of stapled hemorrhoidectomy. Report of our case series. Int J Surg. 2010;8:648–52.

45. Gupta PJ. Radioablation and suture fixation of advanced grades of hemorrhoids. An effective alternative to staplers and Doppler-guided ligation of hemorrhoids. Rev Esp Enferm Dig. 2006;98(10):740.

Laser Hemorrhoidoplasty

8

"I am a big laser believer-I really think they are the waves of future."

Courteney Cox

Key Concepts

- Surgical management for hemorrhoidal disease aims to provide a cure with a minimally invasive surgical technique.
- Corpus cavernosum recti (CCR) is the primary vascular component of anal cushions formed exclusively by the superior hemorrhoidal artery (SHA) branches.
- Excisional hemorrhoidectomy takes care of corpus cavernosum recti but creates large raw areas.
- DGHAL (Doppler-Guided Hemorrhoidal Artery Ligation) works on the principle of dearterialization but cannot ligate transmural and posterolateral branches of the SHA.
- Laser hemorrhoidoplasty (LHP) with Finger-guided hemorrhoidal artery ligation (FGHAL) is a hybrid procedure that leads to dearterialization of the internal hemorrhoidal plexus followed by fibrosis.
- The CCR formed by posterolateral and transmural branches of the SHA can be dealt with lasers, reducing the recurrence rate.

8.1 Introduction

One of the significant breakthroughs in the technological era is the emergence of minimally invasive surgery. The patient and the surgeon seek a procedure that offers a good outcome with less morbidity. To date, no procedure fulfills this criterion. However, Laser hemorrhoidoplasty (LHP) has an upper edge since it is hemostatic, less painful, bactericidal, leads to faster healing, is associated with lesser complications, and maintains the physiology of the anal canal by preserving the anal cushions [1]. Plapler studied the effect of carbon dioxide (CO_2) lasers on 350 patients with hemorrhoids and documented lasers to be less painful than conventional surgery [2]. Using a diode laser allowed the surgeon to operate on the varicose veins of lower limbs without cutting [3]. Later use of diode lasers in the hemorrhoidal mass was studied by Karahliloglu [2] and started gaining popularity over the years. Lasers can be used in two ways to treat hemorrhoids: First, by excising the hemorrhoidal mass, as with the CO_2 laser, and second, by delivering the laser energy into the hemorrhoidal mass and causing fibrosis by initiating protein denaturation, a procedure known as "Laser Hemorrhoidoplasty."

8.2 Principle of Laser Energy

Photoablation Photoablation is tissue destruction by light, generally using a laser. As the laser light passes through water, the H_2O bond is broken, and crackling noises can be heard due to the release of hydrogen ions. As soon as the bond is broken, shrinkage of the target tissue occurs [4].

Photocoagulation Photocoagulation occurs due to protein denaturation induced by laser energy. Protein denaturation starts at 72.6 °C and continues up to 132 °C. Once the protein denaturation occurs, it seals the blood vessels feeding hemorrhoids, resulting in dearterialization [4].

Photovaporization Photovaporization occurs when the target tissue absorbs the laser energy. Blood has 70% water, and a 1470 nm diode laser uses water as a target. When the laser energy goes through blood, the water content evaporates at a temperature of 80–90 °C. Vaporization leads to shrinkage. The thin endothelial layer between the sinusoids, which form fenestrations, is also broken. All that is left behind is a coagulum. Fibrosis occurs after 6–8 weeks, and the anal cushions are fixed in their normal position, taking care of the prolapse [4].

8.3 Laser Hemorrhoidoplasty

8.3.1 Indications

- Internal hemorrhoids grade 2 to grade 4

8.3.2 Contraindications

- Strangulated hemorrhoids
- Ulcerated hemorrhoids

8.4 Hybrid Procedure: A Combination of Finger-Guided Hemorrhoidal Artery Ligation and Laser Hemorrhoidoplasty (FGHAL with LHP)

Hybrid means "a synergistic combination of two or more procedures for increasing their efficacy to yield a better outcome." In the hybrid procedure for hemorrhoids, maximum efficacy is achieved by:

- Finger-guided hemorrhoidal artery ligation—leads to dearterialization.

- Laser hemorrhoidoplasty—takes care of non-vascular components in the anal cushions and the remaining CCR network, which is partially taken care of by FGHAL.

8.4.1 Procedure for FGHAL and LHP

It is carried out in three steps

1. Assessment of hemorrhoids
2. Finger-guided hemorrhoidal artery ligation
3. Laser hemorrhoidoplasty

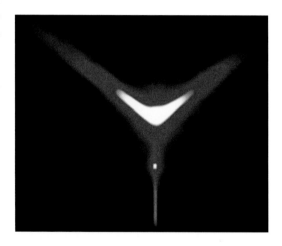

Fig. 8.1 Special conical glass tip. Sharp tip for hemorrhoid puncture

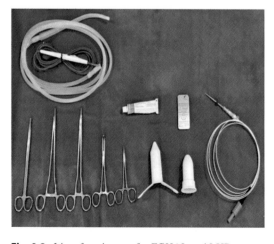

Fig. 8.2 List of equipment for FGHAL and LHP

8.4.2 Instrument Required (Figs. 8.1 and 8.2) Steps

- Half-cut proctoscope 33.5 mm
- Two-needle holders 9″ each
- Vicryl 2-0 5/8 round body on 27 mm needle (Fig. 8.3)
- Laser equipment 1470 nm
- Eye protection glasses
- Conical laser fiber
- Allis forceps
- Scissors
- Non tooth forceps

Prophylactic Antibiotic Cefuroxime 30 min before surgery by intravenous route.

8.4.3 Finger-Guided Hemorrhoidal Artery Ligation - An Introduction

The first step in laser hemorrhoidoplasty is FGHAL. The concept is based on the fact that:

- The site of the rectal arteries is unpredictable.
- The arterial blood flow is relevant for the pathogenesis of hemorrhoids.

- Ligations may be effective in the distal part of the rectum.
- HAL is an effective ligating procedure.
- HAL is responsible for the cure of symptoms.

A Japanese surgeon, Morinaga, gave the concept of DGHAL in 1995 (Fig. 8.4a, b). He developed a technique of identifying the hemorrhoidal arteries by Doppler and ligating them 2–4 cm above the dentate line, considering the innervation and thus avoiding pain [5]. The principle behind the procedure is "Dearterialization" [6].

In FGHAL, the vessels can be easily palpated above the dentate line with the tip of the index finger, and ligation can be carried out effectively (Fig. 8.5). Accordingly, a new name, "Finger-Guided Hemorrhoidal Artery Ligation (FGHAL)," was coined [7–9]. The most significant benefit of not using Doppler is its cost-efficiency. The results with both the procedures, whether DGHAL or FGHAL, remain the same [9]. When we use DGHAL or FGHAL as a stand-alone procedure, the chances of recurrence are very high. The recurrence rate after DGHAL is up to 40% [10], with the greatest

Fig. 8.3 Hemorrhoidal artery ligation suture

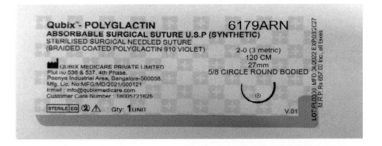

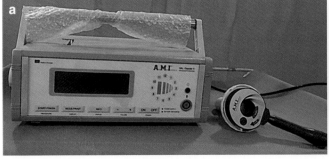
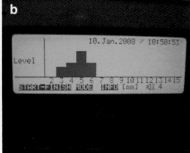

Fig. 8.4 (**a, b**) Doppler-guided hemorrhoidal artery ligation equipment

Fig. 8.5 Point of ligation for finger-guided hemorrhoidal artery ligation

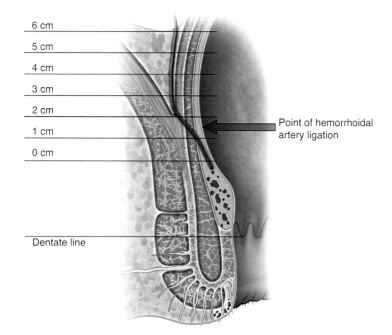

6 cm

5 cm

4 cm

3 cm

2 cm

1 cm

0 cm

Point of hemorrhoidal artery ligation

Dentate line

prevalence in individuals with fourth degree hemorrhoids.

8.4.3.1   Technique

The patient is placed in a lithotomy position under spinal anesthesia (Fig. 8.6).

Assessment of Grades of Hemorrhoids

Three pieces of rolled gauze are inserted inside the anal canal and carefully pulled out to determine the exact degree of hemorrhoids (Fig. 8.7). Since there is perineal descent under spinal anesthesia, grade 2 hemorrhoids may sometimes appear as grade 3, or grade 3 hemorrhoids may appear as grade 4.

Role of Injection Hylase

For grade 4 hemorrhoids with edema, Injection Hylase (Hyaluronidase) can be injected into the submucosa of the hemorrhoids (Fig. 8.8a, b). Injection Hyaluronidase increases the tissue permeability and therefore decreases edema. The syringe piston is pulled before injecting the solution into the hemorrhoid tissue to ensure that Hylase is not injected directly into the blood vessel. Injection Hylase comes in a powder form. One can obtain a solution by dissolving the powder in

1 mL of distilled water or saline. Each mL contains 1500 IU of Hyaluronidase. About 1–2 mL of hylase can be injected into each hemorrhoidal mass (Fig. 8.8a). Immediately after injection of hylase, regression of the hemorrhoidal tissue can be observed on the operating table. After the edema has diminished, the hemorrhoidal mass can be pushed back into the anal canal lumen, and further surgical steps can be performed (Fig. 8.8b).

Learning Point: Role of Hylase

Hyaluronidase improves tissue permeability by catalyzing the hydrolysis of hyaluronic acid. It diminishes the edema and swelling of the hemorrhoids. Once the edema is reduced, the internal hemorrhoidal tissue can be pushed back into the anal canal.

Complication of Hylase

Allergic reactions have been reported occurring in 0.05–0.69% of cases, according to clinical trials [11]. The following are some of the signs:

• Erythema
• Itching and pain
• Urticaria and angioedema [12, 13]

Fig. 8.6 Lithotomy position

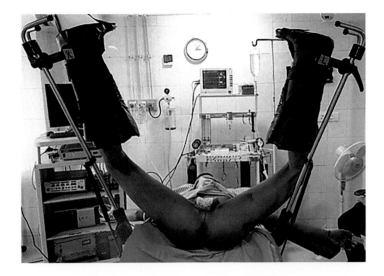

Fig. 8.7 Assessment of the hemorrhoids by inserting rolled gauge pieces inside the anal canal

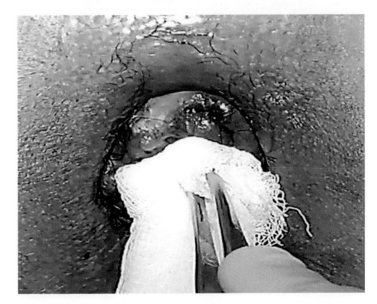

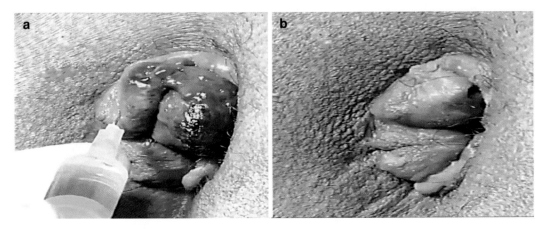

Fig. 8.8 (**a**) Injecting hylase into the hemorrhoids. (**b**) Immediate regression

Technique of Hemorrhoidal Artery Ligation

The next step is FGHAL (Fig. 8.9a–h). The head side of the operating table should be 15° lower. The hemorrhoidal tissue is massaged to reduce engorgement. After thoroughly lubricating with lignocaine hydrochloride jelly, a half-cut proctoscope is introduced into the anal canal (Fig. 8.9a). The ligation of the branches of SHA is started at 3 o'clock position. The Allis forceps are applied at the anal verge at 3 o'clock, and the hemorrhoid

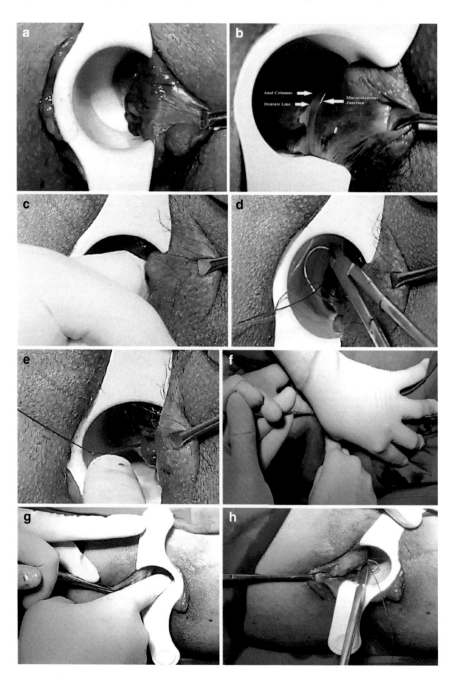

Fig. 8.9 (a) Hemorrhoidal mass as seen through half-cut proctoscope. (b) Dentate line as seen through proctoscope. (c) Palpation of superior hemorrhoidal artery with the tip of finger. (d) Taking a figure of eight stitches. (e) Ligation of arteries by Vicryl 2-0, 27 mm 5/8 round body needle. (f) Milking of the hemorrhoidal tissue. (g, h) Palpation and ligation of vessels at other positions

tissue is slowly pulled outwards. The dentate line is identified, and the left-hand index finger is inserted about 2–4 cm above the hemorrhoidal tissue. The SHA branches are palpated starting from 3 o'clock (Fig. 8.9b).

Sometimes, one may not be able to palpate the vessel precisely at the 3 o'clock position, as the position of the superior hemorrhoidal artery branches is not constant. Once the vessel has been palpated, ligation is done using Vicryl 2-0, 27 mm 5/8 round body needle by taking a figure of eight stitch (Fig. 8.9c–e). In almost all cases, the needle depth is roughly 5 mm. Taking the figure of eight stitches is not for the ligation of the vessel per se. It compresses the surrounding tissue to squeeze the vessel, leading to dearterialization. Some fibers of the internal sphincter are always taken along. Before tying the knot, ask the assistant to do milking of the hemorrhoidal tissue to reduce the engorgement (Fig. 8.9f). While ligating, ensure not to puncture the blood vessel with the needle. If the vessel is pierced, a hematoma appears immediately.

After ligation, try palpating the ligated vessel again to ensure that an effective ligation has been achieved.

After the ligation is performed at 3 o'clock, turn the half-cut proctoscope clockwise and continue palpating and ligating the vessels (Fig. 8.9g, h). Ideally, it should be possible to ligate 4–6 branches.

Once all the ligations are complete, rotate the proctoscope 360° to ensure all the branches of SHA have been appropriately ligated. Then, remove the proctoscope and reinsert the three rolled-up gauze pieces inside the lumen. A reduction in the size of the hemorrhoids can be seen on the operating table in the case of grade 3 or 4 hemorrhoids.

8.4.4 Laser Hemorrhoidoplasty

8.4.4.1 Energy! Dosage! Fiber! Mode

Energy
- The overall dose should not exceed 150–200 J per hemorrhoidal mass.

Dosage
- At the time of fiber insertion: 6 W, 1-s pulse
- At the time of fiber activation: 6 W, 3-s pulse

The dosage is calculated as follows:

Watt × time in second = Joule (1 W = 1 Joule per second (1 W = 1 J/s))

Probe (Tip of Lasers)—Sharp tip conical
Mode: Pulse mode

8.4.4.2 Point of Entry of Fiber

The point of entry of laser fiber is the mucocutaneous junction (white line of Hilton). This is because the anastomosis between the superior and inferior hemorrhoidal artery is present over there. The submucosa ends at the dentate line, and it is known that the anal cushions are disruptions of submucosa at 3, 7, or 11 o'clock positions. Theoretically, entering the submucosal space from the dentate line makes sense. With experience, one can appreciate that the regression of the hemorrhoidal mass is much faster if one enters the mucocutaneous junction instead of the dentate line (Fig. 8.10a, b).

8.4.4.3 The Technique of Laser Hemorrhoidoplasty

After inserting a half-cut proctoscope inside the anal canal, apply the Allis forceps at the anal verge at 3 o'clock (Fig. 8.11a–e). Pull the Allis forceps outwards and insert the laser fiber across the mucocutaneous junction into the submucosal space (Fig. 8.11a). Once inside the submucosal space, the fiber stops at the distal end, where the HAL was performed (Fig. 8.11b). The energy dose at the fiber entry point is 6 W × 1 s.

The red light can be seen inside the submucosa of the anal cushions. Ensure that the light is neither too bright nor too dim. Too bright light indicates that the fiber tip is too close to the mucous membrane, which can be damaged by thermal energy. A dim light indicates that the tip of the fiber lies somewhere inside the internal sphincter, which may cause damage to the sphincters after activation, followed by fibrosis. Furthermore, ensure there is no resistance while

Fig. 8.10 (**a**) Mucocutaneous junction. (**b**) Submucosal space from dentate line

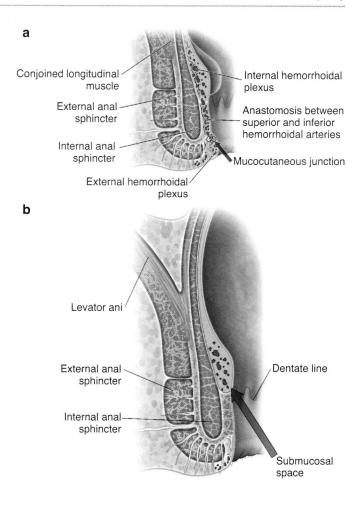

pushing the fiber into the submucosal space. It should be emphasized that if one feels resistance, the fiber is in the wrong plane.

Once inside the submucosal hemorrhoidal tissue, release the laser beam in pulse mode at 6 W × 3 s. Once the fiber is activated, crackling sounds are heard due to the release of hydrogen ions. Keep withdrawing the fiber every 5 mm because the fiber covers approximately 4 mm distance in one activation. It is advisable to slowly rotate the fiber during activation to prevent it from sticking to the tissue (Fig. 8.11c). In the case of a large hemorrhoidal mass, one can use a fan-shaped technique to release more energy (Fig. 8.11d). Remember that the total amount of energy should not exceed 150–200 J for each pile mass.

After the hemorrhoidal mass is dealt with at 3 o'clock, the same procedure is repeated at 7 and 11 o'clock. If present, the accessory hemorrhoids are dealt with the same way. An ice finger is inserted inside the anal canal for 8–10 min to reduce postoperative edema (Fig. 8.11e).

Sometimes, hemorrhoidal tissue does not reduce substantially in grade 3 or 4 hemorrhoids, even after performing HAL and LHP. Mucopexy or rectoanal repair (RAR) may be performed in such cases. Performing Blaisdell or Farag's technique of mucopexy leads to dearterialization and a better cosmetic effect. This technique takes three interrupted sutures through the mucosa and submucosa above the dentate line, leading to mucosal fixation (Fig. 8.12a–c).

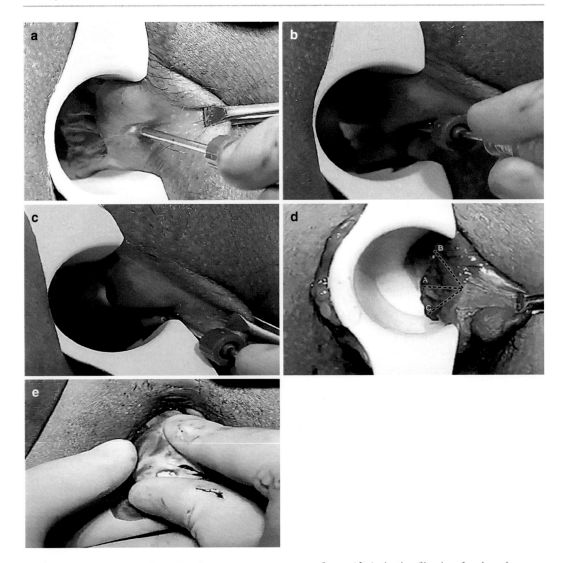

Fig. 8.11 (**a**) Entry point of laser fiber from mucocutaneous junction. (**b**) Activation of fiber inside submucosal space of anal cushions (LHP). (**c**) Drawing of laser fiber every 5 mm. (**d**) Activating fiber in a fan-shaped manner. (**e**) Insertion of ice finger

8.4.4.4   Postoperative Care
- Antibiotics: Cefuroxime for 5 days
- Laxatives: Polyethylene glycol
- Diclofenac suppository as an analgesic
- Sitz bath twice a day to be started after 24 h
- Flavonoids (MPFF)
- Topical ointments

The patient is reluctant to defecate postoperatively when a surgical procedure is conducted in the anorectal area. Moreover, patients with hemorrhoids usually suffer from chronic constipation. Laxatives take care of constipation and soften the stools, allowing easy passage and reducing postoperative discomfort during defecation. Flavonoids help reduce inflammation and lymphatic stasis. Topical ointment, a combination of sucralfate, lignocaine, and metronidazole, reduces postoperative pain and prevents local infection.

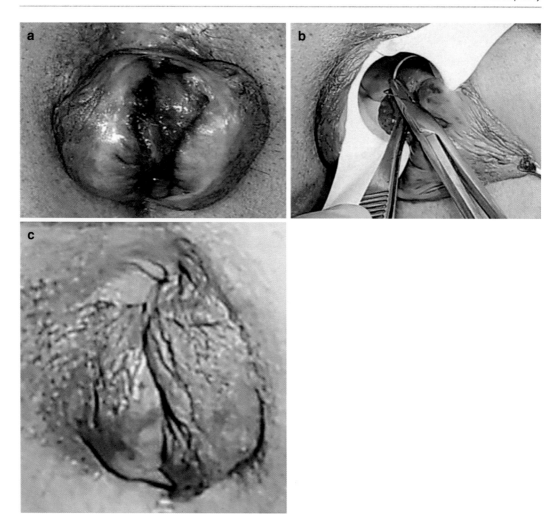

Fig. 8.12 (**a**) Grade 4 hemorrhoids before FGHAL and LHP. (**b**) Mucopexy by taking three interrupted suture by Blaisdell technique. (**c**) Final picture after mucopexy

8.5   Hemorrhoids in Patients with Anticoagulants

A surgeon must evaluate the complete medical history and always consider the risk-benefit ratio of withdrawal of anticoagulants. The decision to discontinue the antiplatelet drug prior to surgery should only be made after consultation with the cardiologist. A daily dosage of 75 mg of clopidogrel causes a 60% reduction in platelet function over 3–5 days. However, Ecosprin is the most prescribed antiplatelet drug to prevent cardiovascular disorders [14, 15]. Despite Ecosprin's short half-life (3–6 h), its irreversible effects would last the platelet's entire lifespan (8–9 days) [14, 15]. Therefore, stopping the antiplatelet well before the surgical procedure is always advisable.

In most cases, a history of bleeding disorders is often overlooked. Surprisingly, sometimes patients may have a history of hemophilia.

8.6   Why Recurrence After Surgical Procedures for Hemorrhoids?

"Recurrence" may occur after any surgical procedure for hemorrhoids, be it hemorrhoidectomy, DGHAL/FGHAL, Stapled hemorrhoidopexy (PPH), or laser hemorrhoidoplasty. However, the recurrence rate of different procedures varies (Table 8.1).

Three factors may contribute to the recurrence:

1. Formation of collaterals
2. Persistence of the larger caliber of SHA arteries in hemorrhoids
3. Inability to ligate posterolateral branches of SHA

8.6.1   Diversion of Blood Flow and Formation of Collaterals

After an excisional hemorrhoidectomy, it is almost impossible for anal cushions to regrow. That is why primary hemorrhoids will never form. However, accessory hemorrhoids are likely to occur in all locations where superior hemorrhoidal artery branches are present, including the position of primary hemorrhoids. The reason is that after the SHA branches have been ligated at the pedicle where the excision has been performed, the blood flow is diverted to other branches because of acceleration velocity, as explained by Aigner et al. [20, 21]. Another reason can be collateral circulation (Fig. 8.13), which develops over a while.

8.6.2   Persistence of the Greater Caliber of the Superior Hemorrhoidal Artery in Hemorrhoidal Disease

The large diameter leads to a greater blood flow to SHA in hemorrhoidal disease (HD) patients, even after surgical removal of hemorrhoids. Nothing can be done to decrease the already dilated caliber of the vessels.

8.6.3   Inability to Ligate Posterolateral Branches of SHA

DGHAL/FGHAL/Stapled hemorrhoidopexy is based on the principle of dearterialization, which leads to subsequent fibrosis. Although the branches of SHA present in the submucosa can be ligated, the posterolateral branches of SHA are too high and too deep [20, 21]. Hence, complete blood circulation interruption to the hemorrhoidal mass is impossible. Further, the transmural and extramural branches of SHA

Table 8.1 The recurrence rate after various procedures

Author	No. of patients	Procedure name	Year	Recurrence rate
Kim et al. [16] Randomized control trial	130	Milligan Morgan vs. stapled hemorrhoidopexy	5	MM: 23% SHP: 18%
Lienert M. [17] Literature review	5315	DGHAL with mucopexy	11	Up to 40%
Tjandra et al. [18] 25 Randomized control trial	1918	Stapled hemorrhoidopexy	15	25.3%
Keck T. [19] A cohort study	497	LHP	5	8.8%

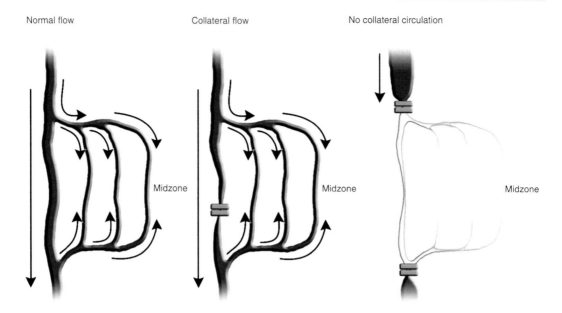

Normal flow   Collateral flow   No collateral circulation

Midzone   Midzone   Midzone

Fig. 8.13 Formation of collateral circulation

Table 8.2 The recurrence rate for laser hemorrhoids using different wavelength

Author	No. of patients	Procedure name	Dosage	Recurrence rate (%)
Plapler et al. [22] Clinical trial	16	LHP	Laser equipment used 810 nm	6.6
Moloku et al. [23] Comparison trial	20	LHP	A 980-diode laser is sent via a 1000-nm optic fiber in a pulsed mode	2
Poskus et al. [24] Double-blinded randomized control trial	20	LHP	Laser equipment used 1470 nm	10
De et al. [25] A prospective clinical study	75	LHP-FGHAL	Laser equipment used 1470 nm	5.33
Gupta et al. [7] A retrospective cohort study	346	LHP with FGHAL	Laser equipment used 1470 nm	1.8

also participate in the formation of corpus cavernosum recti, but there is no way to ligate them.

8.7 Recurrence After Laser Hemorrhoidoplasty

Laser hemorrhoidoplasty with FGHAL as a hybrid procedure appears to be a better choice leading to a lesser recurrence (Table 8.2).

8.8 Complications Following FGHAL and LHP: Why and How to Manage?

8.8.1 Hematoma Formation at the Site of HAL

This can occur while ligating the vessel. Since this is a blind procedure, the vessel may be pierced with the needle leading to hematoma formation (Fig. 8.14).

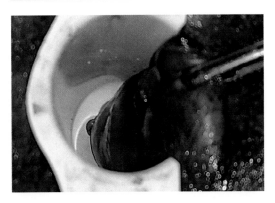

Fig. 8.14 Hematoma formation after accidental perforation of SHA branches

How to Manage?
Apply pressure on the hematoma for 5 min. Later, a stitch can be passed just above the hematoma site. Alternatively, the hematoma can be left alone, followed by sclerotherapy after 72 h.

8.8.2 Bleeding at the Point of Entry of Laser Fiber

How to Manage?
- Apply pressure for 2–4 min
- Apply laser fiber at the point of entry and release energy
- If bleeding persists, take a stitch with Vicryl 2-0

8.8.3 Pain: VAS Score of 4–5 Within 24 h

Causes
The point of entry of the laser fiber at the mucocutaneous junction may lead to pain as the pudendal nerve supplies the area below the dentate line. Postoperative edema resulting from inflammation can also cause pain.

How to Manage?
- Postoperative diclofenac suppository. The effect lasts for approximately 4–6 h
- Sitz bath

8.8.4 Postoperative Edema: (2.34%)

Causes
Postoperative edema results from inflammation caused by cellular injury from thermal energy. Furthermore, there is the latent heat of vaporization despite a low thermal relaxation time.

How to Manage?
Immediately after laser activation at each site, spray cold normal saline on the hemorrhoidal tissue to reduce edema. This should be treated as a sports injury (initially, a cold compression followed by a Sitz bath). Alternatively, inserting an ice finger at the end of the procedure is a good practice. As such, there is no significant difference between the two techniques.

8.8.5 Thrombosis: (0.89%)

Causes
Although rare, damage to the blood vessels can lead to the formation of a blood clot. It typically resolves itself.

How to Manage?
- Wait and watch for 48 h
- Clot evacuation can be done under local anesthesia if the patient complains of pain

8.8.6 Burning and Itching: (10.1%)

Causes
This is a complication encountered frequently. The possible explanation is that laser energy, being thermal energy, can cause dehydration of the mucous membrane. Another probable cause is the release of histamines due to inflammation.

How to Manage?
- Apply local petroleum jelly to keep the mucous membrane moist.
- An antihistamine may be given for 5 days.

8.8.7 Hemorrhage and Abscess: (0.58%)

Causes

Bleeding may occur in the event of mucosal ulceration after LHP. Usually, the bleeding is the result of infection (secondary hemorrhage). Even though the incidence is low, one can encounter hemorrhage and abscess formation. In 0.2% of cases, a perianal abscess may be formed, followed by an intersphincteric fistula. The exact reason is difficult to explain since laser energy is presumed to have a bactericidal effect.

How to Manage?

If bleeding is due to mucosal ulceration, laser spray can be done using bare fiber since it has excellent hemostatic properties. Secondary bleeding can be managed with IV antibiotics. For a fistula, fistulotomy will suffice, as the tracts are usually small in such cases.

8.8.8 Skin Tags: (0.2%)

Cause

- Primarily formed in internal-external hemorrhoids.

How to Manage?

- Excision

8.9 Your Queries, My Answers!

During live presentations and demonstrations of surgeries over the years, I have been asked numerous questions by my colleagues. I have compiled them and feel it apt to share them with you.

- **Why do I prefer laser over other conventional surgical procedures?**
  Laser hemorrhoidoplasty maintains the anatomical and physiological integrity of the anal canal. In 1937, when Milligan Morgan popularized the excisional hemorrhoidectomy procedure [26], they were unaware that they were cutting the anal cushions. Today, surgeons are more enlightened about the anatomy of the anal canal. In LHP, we modify the cushions without resecting them. In today's era of minimally invasive surgery, LHP provides an excellent alternative to an excisional procedure.

- **Is it mandatory to do a hybrid procedure, i.e., a combination of FGHAL and LHP?**
  I must admit that I have never performed LHP without HAL. Many authors recommend that LHP as a stand-alone procedure is sufficient, which I find difficult to agree with. While elucidating the anatomy and etiopathogenesis of hemorrhoids, it has been explained that the hybrid procedure gives better results.

- **Can Laser be used in strangulated hemorrhoids?**
  The sudden formation of strangulated hemorrhoids indicates a hemorrhoidal crisis. LHP is contraindicated in this condition.

- **Instead of FGHAL, can I do laser spray at the apex of hemorrhoidal mass for dearterialization?**
  I have seen a few surgeons recommending a laser spray above or at the apex of the hemorrhoidal mass for dearterialization. I do not propagate or recommend it. Laser beam penetration with 1470 is only 1–2 mm, whereas the SHA branches are 3–5 mm deep. Sealing the vessels using a laser from an anatomical standpoint is impossible. In addition, spraying the laser beam over the mucosa can damage mucosa, causing ulceration and bleeding.

- **Where is the entry point for the laser fiber?**
  I came across a procedure protocol in a publication recommending inserting the laser fiber through an incision in the perianal area. I am not in favor of this approach. As we know, the anal cushions are disruptions of submucosa at 3, 7, and 11 o'clock. In addition, there is anastomosis present between the superior and inferior hemorrhoidal arteries below the dentate line, extending beyond the mucocutaneous junction. So, the mucocutaneous junction is considered an entry point for the laser fiber. Entering the hemorrhoidal masses through the intersphincteric or perianal spaces is inappro-

priate. I have done most of my cases of LHP by entering through the mucocutaneous junction. In a few cases, I used the dentate line as a fiber entry point but realized that tissue regression was slow. Moreover, in interno-external hemorrhoids, it was difficult for me to reduce the external components.

- **Should collagen sheets be used with bupivacaine?**
  Usually, collagen sheets are used for wound contraction. Some authors have recommended the use of collagen sheets with bupivacaine. Nevertheless, I see no benefit of using them in LHP.
- **What is the VAS (Visual Analog Score) after LHP?**
  In a cohort study [27] of 497 patients, the postoperative VAS score is reported as 2. In my practice, it is usually 3–4 in the initial 24 h. Many surgeons have promoted the LHP procedure as painless. I disagree, as LHP is in no way a painless procedure.

  The postoperative pain, as assessed using the VAS at 6 and 12 h and 1, 2, and 3 days after surgery, is shown in Fig. 8.15. The average VAS scores at 6 h,12 h, 24 h, 48 h, and

72 h after surgery were 3.2, 2.1, 3.0, 4, and 0.1, respectively [7, 8].

- **Which wavelength is the best—1470 nm or 980 nm?**
  Blood and water are among the components of our body that absorb laser energy. 1470 nm is absorbed by water 40 times more than 980 nm, resulting in minimal thermal damage. Moreover, water is the target for the 1470 nm laser, while 980 nm works on hemoglobin. The penetration is 1–2 mm in 1470 versus 5–7 mm in 980 nm. Many vascular surgeons have shifted from 980 to 1470 nm for endovascular varicose vein laser removal (EVLA).
- **How to prepare an ice finger?**
  One can prepare ice fingers by taking examination gloves. Cut the fingers of the glove, fill each finger with simple tap water, and tie the ends with a cotton thread. Allow the fingers to freeze. Once frozen, they are ready to use.
- **How to insert an ice finger?**
  Dip the ice finger in Povidone-iodine for 1–2 min. Insert it into the anal canal after lubricating with lignocaine jelly. Place a gauge over the anal orifice and tie a cotton thread

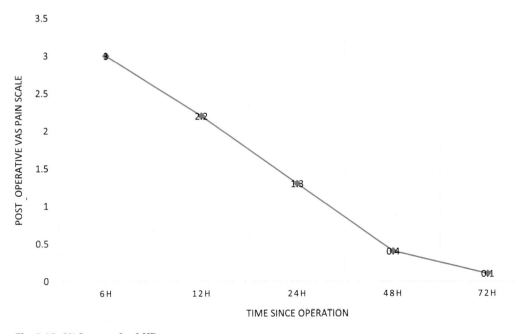

Fig. 8.15 VAS score after LHP

around it. Keep it in the anal canal for 8–10 min. Never apply ice directly to the mucosa, as it can adhere to the mucosal membrane leading to cell death.

- **Why is there burning in the anal region?**
  Hypervascularization leads to venous stasis and inflammation of the anal cushions. Once the inflammation is there it leads to leakage of exudate from the blood vessels. This exudate causes burning and itching in the anal canal.
- **If there is an enlarged mass at one position, even then HAL is supposed to be done at all the positions?**
  While operating for HAL with LHP it is mandatory to ligate all the palpable branches of SHA otherwise, the blood will divert from the ligated branch to the other branches leading to formation of accessory hemorrhoids.
- **Why is there pain at HAL site?**
  Whenever HAL stitch is taken, few fibers of internal anal sphincters are taken along with the suture. This may lead to spasm of internal anal sphincter leading to pain.

8.10   Discussion

The gold standard for managing hemorrhoids is excision and ligation, as described by Milligan Morgan. However, this technique is associated with severe postoperative pain and the creation of extensive raw areas. The use of diode lasers in varicose veins initiated the concept of using laser energy in the hemorrhoidal mass. These studies were further carried out by Plapler, who achieved a considerable amount of shrinkage of hemorrhoidal masses in monkeys [2]. Earlier, 810 and 980 nm were being used for laser hemorrhoidoplasty. With the use of 1470 nm in varicose veins, the concept of a wavelength of 1470 nm in laser hemorrhoidoplasty came into existence. This had technical advantages over the existing wavelengths, and the surgeon could coagulate 4 mm of hemorrhoidal tissue in one activation [24]. The total energy used for each pile mass is around 150–200 J, with the smaller masses treated with lesser energy.

The recommended technique is a hybrid procedure combining hemorrhoidal artery ligation with laser hemorrhoidoplasty. The dearterialization is achieved with hemorrhoidal artery ligation by taking a suture 2–4 cm above the dentate line. The stitch includes the feeding vessels and a few fibers of the internal anal sphincter. This occludes the branches of SHA. As discussed earlier, this technique cannot achieve complete dearterialization due to the course of the vessels. Hence, the energy delivered by lasers takes care of CCR formed by other branches, leading to complete dearterialization. In addition, the prolapsed pile masses reduce by fibrosis. In the studies by Halit Maloku in 2014 on laser hemorrhoidoplasty and open surgical hemorrhoidectomy, the laser procedure had a VAS score of 5 on the first day, which reduced gradually. There were no significant side effects associated with the procedure, concluding that laser hemorrhoidoplasty was a safe and effective technique to be carried out for hemorrhoids [23]. In a study by Asmz Rahman, 88% of patients had complete resolution of symptoms following laser hemorrhoidoplasty [28]. Paolo Giamundo et al. published a randomized control trial on a hemorrhoid laser procedure that indicated a 90% success rate and a better quality of life following the surgery [29].

Literature review and studies reveal an excellent efficacy of using lasers in hemorrhoids. From my experience, grade 2 to grade 4 hemorrhoids can be treated by laser hemorrhoidoplasty with complete resolution of the symptoms. However, lifestyle modifications also contribute to a reduction in recurrence after the procedure. Instead of doppler, I prefer finger-guided hemorrhoidal artery ligation, which is equally effective and reduces the cost of doppler.

A laser is a luring and a fascinating tool. A surgeon feels elated when an influx of patients visits him for a laser procedure. But owning the tool does not make one a laser specialist. A surgeon must know; What to do, how to do, and when not to do. Thorough knowledge of lasers, with precise energy, and correct wavelength usage makes it possible to give satisfactory results.

The success is to ensure we have the right tool with the right man behind the tool.

8.11 Case Presentations

Case Study 1

A 45-year-old male patient presented to the OPD with a complaint of mass coming out of the anal orifice during defecation that reduced on its own. It was associated with bleeding, blood being bright red, and in the form of a spurt. The patient had a history of straining and constipation, for which he was taking laxatives. He spent approximately half an hour on the commode to clear his bowels. On local and digital rectal examination, there was no significant finding. The proctoscopy revealed grade 2 hemorrhoids. On sigmoidoscopy, except for hemorrhoids, there was no other pathology. FGHAL with LHP was planned. All the palpable branches of SHA were ligated, followed by laser hemorrhoidoplasty.

Discussion

As it was a simple case of grade 2 hemorrhoids, FGHAL with LHP was done. After a week, the patient came for a follow-up. He was cheerful as there was no bleeding or prolapse. He resumed work on the eighth postoperative day. The recovery was fast as no excision was done, nor any raw areas were created. The VAS score was significantly low.

Case Study 2

Mr. X, a 76-year-old man, was operated upon by a surgeon for bleeding piles with Kshar sutra twice, but with no relief. He was weak and not in good health when he came for consultation. He gave a history of a pile mass that came out during defecation and reduced on its own but gradually became irreducible in the last few months. He was afraid of going to the toilet as he experienced pain and bleeding during defecation. Blood was bright red. He had a history of constipation, straining during defecation, and spending hours on the commode. There were grade 4 hemorrhoids at the 3 o'clock position on local examination. On DRE, the anal tone was normal. Proctoscopy showed grade 2 and grade 3 hemorrhoids at 7 and 11 o'clock positions, respectively, with accessory hemorrhoids at 6 o'clock. Considering the patient's age and history of bleeding, he was taken for colonoscopy after

bowel preparation, but no pathology other than hemorrhoids was detected.

The patient was taken for surgery. The prolapsed pile mass at 3 o'clock could not be reduced on the operating table, even after the injection of Hylase. Hence, excisional hemorrhoidectomy was done at 3 o'clock, and FGHAL with LHP was done for other pile masses. He responded well after surgery.

Discussion

The excision of fibrosed hemorrhoidal mass was done at the 3 o'clock position and LHP at all the other positions. This led to a small raw area and less postoperative pain. Sometimes, we have to tailor the techniques according to the need. As laser has no role in fibrosed nonreducible components, excision was the best choice.

Case Study 3

Mr. E, a 49-year-old gentleman, complained of severe pain in the anorectal region with irreducible pile masses for 4–5 days. He was unwilling to sit in my chamber, claiming he would have pain. He told me that he was taking treatment from some family physician without relief. There was no history of bleeding per rectum. He had a history of constipation and straining during defecation. He spent only 5–6 min on the commode. On local examination, grade 4 internal hemorrhoids and thrombosed external hemorrhoids were present at 3 o'clock. There was nothing significant on digital rectal examination. The proctoscopy revealed multiple small clots in the pile mass at 3 o'clock. The need for surgery was explained to him, to which he readily agreed. FGHAL with LHP with clot evacuation with excision of the thrombosed external hemorrhoids was planned.

Under spinal anesthesia, the patient was put into the lithotomy position. All the hemorrhoidal masses present at 3, 7, and 11 o'clock were grade 4. Hylase was injected. A reduction in edema was seen in a few seconds, and all the reduced pile masses were pushed back into the anal canal. A half-cut proctoscope was inserted, and FGHAL was done at all the palpable branches of SHA. Clot evacuation of thrombosed internal hemorrhoids was done, followed by LHP. In the end, excision of thrombosed external hemorrhoids was done by giving an elliptical incision. Postoperative instructions were given, and the patient was discharged the next day. He was satisfied when he came for a follow-up after a week.

Discussion

As discussed earlier, Injection Hylase reduces edema by increasing tissue permeability. Once the hemorrhoidal tissue reduces, FGHAL with LHP can be easily done. Over the years, I have realized that in grade 4 hemorrhoids, where a small prolapsing element is still present after LHP, mucopexy or rectoanal repair is effective. For external hemorrhoids, giving an elliptical incision is a good option if the thrombus is small. In large thrombosed external hemorrhoids, clot evacuation with laser at the site of corrugator cutis ani can also be done.

Case Study 4

One fine day I was sitting in my consultation chamber when a young patient, 33 years, walked in, complaining of severe pain in the anal region. He gave a history of reducible pile masses for the past 4–5 months. There was a history of bleeding per rectum at the time of defecation. Blood was bright red. He had dull pain for 2 days, for which he had consulted a physician who had prescribed him an ointment and an analgesic, but there was no relief. The pain had worsened since the morning, and he avoided going to the toilet. His bowel habit was constipated. After separating the buttocks gently on local examination, I could make out an anal fissure midline posterior. There was a mild spasm on digital rectal examination. Before proctoscopy, lignocaine 5% was introduced per rectum for 15 min to avoid pain during the examination. Proctoscopy revealed Grade 3 hemorrhoids. A final diagnosis of Grade 3 hemorrhoids with acute anal fissure midline posterior was established. As the pain was unbearable, FGHAL with LHP with lateral internal sphincterotomy (LIS) was planned.

After doing FGHAL and LHP for hemorrhoids, LIS was done at 3 o'clock. The base of the fissure was curetted.

Discussion

Due to the associated fissure, in this case, lateral internal sphincterotomy was done. As discussed earlier, the increased anal tone is due to hemorrhoids. Hence lateral internal sphincterotomy is not indicated as a routine after any hemorrhoid surgical procedure.

Case Study 5

Remember, every case does not require a Laser!

One of my friends, a family physician, referred a young male patient around 35 years. He had one episode of bleeding per rectum, constipation, and fullness in the rectum. He was diagnosed to have second-degree hemorrhoids. Ten days after being diagnosed, he went to a local hospital and was taken for sclerotherapy. After 2 days of sclerotherapy, his symptoms worsened. He had severe pain in the anal region during defecation, further exacerbated on sitting. On local examination, nothing significant was seen. However, there was a mild spasm on digital rectal examination. The proctoscopy showed strangulated internal hemorrhoids. Sigmoidoscopy revealed strangulated hemorrhoids at 3 and 7 o'clock positions and second-degree hemorrhoids at 11 o'clock. In this case, excisional hemorrhoidectomy was done for strangulated hemorrhoids, and for second-degree hemorrhoids, FGHAL at the apex of pile masses was followed by LHP.

Discussion

What procedure to undertake? Was hemorrhoidectomy an appropriate decision?

The hemorrhoids were excised at 3 and 7 o'clock since the LHP is contraindicated in strangulated hemorrhoids. At the 11 o'clock position, the pile mass was not strangulated. Hence, LHP was an appropriate choice. There is no harm in carrying out a combined procedure of LHP and excisional hemorrhoidectomy in cases where both strangulated and nonstrangulated hemorrhoids are present together.

8.12 Bottom Line

Remember, it is better to have a tailor-made approach rather than a fixed ideology. Always keep the patient's interest in mind. The surgeon can cut or modify the anal cushions or combine both techniques depending upon the clinical presentation of the disease.

Take-Home Message

The laser is no magic wand!

- I prefer to discuss a few salient features with the patient before undertaking LHP. Firstly, a patient who comes for laser treatment has high expectations. Fed on myths and hearsay, many a layperson considers lasers painless. I always explain that for the first 24 h, the patient can experience pain, discomfort, and a slight heaviness. Secondly, lasers use energy to modify cushions. Since there is no excision, the return to work is comparatively faster than conventional procedures. However, the body needs time to recover, which may vary from one individual to another. Thirdly, there is always a risk of recurrence.
- The surgical technique of finger-guided hemorrhoidal artery ligation with laser hemorrhoidoplasty looks promising for managing hemorrhoids.

References

1. Chia YW, Darzi A, Speakman CT, Hill AD, Jameson JS, Henry MM. CO_2 laser hemorrhoidectomy—does it alter the anorectal function or decrease pain compared to conventional hemorrhoidectomy? Int J Colorectal Dis. 1995;10(1):22–4.
2. Plapler H. A new method for hemorrhoid surgery: experimental model of diode laser application in monkeys. Photomed Laser Surg. 2008;26:143–6.
3. Navarro L, Min RJ, Boné C. Endovenous laser: a new minimally invasive treatment method for varicose veins—preliminary observations using an 810 nm diode laser. Dermatol Surg. 2001;27(2):117–22. https://doi.org/10.1046/j.1524-4725.2001.00134.x. PMID: 11207682
4. Khammam FA, Mossa AF, Issa NA. Hemorrhoids treatment using CO_2 laser (10600nm). Int J Dev Res. 2019;09(07):28702–10.
5. Morinaga K, Hasuda K, Ikeda T. A novel therapy for internal hemorrhoids: ligation of the hemorrhoidal artery with a newly devised instrument (Moricorn) in conjunction with a Doppler flowmeter. Am J Gastroenterol. 1995;90(4):610–3.
6. Hoyuela C, Carvajal F, Juvany M, et al. HAL-RAR (Doppler-guided hemorrhoid artery ligation with recto-anal repair) is a safe and effective procedure for hemorrhoids. Results of a prospective study after a two-year follow-up. Int J Surg. 2016;28:39–44.
7. Gupta K, Agarwal N, Mital K. Clinical outcomes in patients with hemorrhoids treated by finger-guided hemorrhoidal artery ligation with laser hemorrhoidoplasty: a retrospective cohort study. J Adv Med. 2021;33(18):143–52.
8. Gupta K, Mital K, Kant R. Surgical management of hemorrhoids – a new approach finger-guided hemorrhoidal artery ligation (FGHAL) with laser hemorrhoidoplasty. Int J Recent Sci Res. 2019;10(05):32186–7.
9. Markaryan D, Tulina I, Garmanova T, Bredikhin M, Alikperzade A, Tsarkov P. Hemorrhoidal artery ligation with Doppler guidance vs. digital guidance for grade II–III hemorrhoidal disease treatment: study protocol clinical trial (SPIRIT Compliant). Medicine (Baltimore). 2020;99(15):e19424.
10. Scheyer M, Antonietti E, Rollinger G, Mall H, Arnold S. Doppler-guided hemorrhoidal artery ligation. Am J Surg. 2006;191(1):89–93.
11. Cavallini M, Gazzola R, Metalla M, Vaienti L. The role of hyaluronidase in the treatment of complications from hyaluronic acid dermal fillers. Aesthet Surg J. 2013;33(8):1167–74.
12. Yocum RC, Kennard D, Heiner LS. Assessment and implication of the allergic sensitivity to a single dose of recombinant human hyaluronidase injection: a double-blind, placebo-controlled clinical trial. J Infus Nurs. 2007;30(5):293–9.
13. Dunn AL, Heavner JE, Racz G, Day M. Hyaluronidase: a review of approved formulations, indications and off-label use in chronic pain management. Expert Opin Biol Ther. 2010;10(1):127–31.
14. Eikelboom JW, Hirsh J, Spencer FA, Baglin TP, Weitz JI. Antiplatelet drugs: antithrombotic therapy and prevention of thrombosis, 9th ed: American College of Chest Physicians Evidence-Based Clinical Practice Guidelines [published correction appears in Chest. 2015 Dec;148(6):1529. Dosage error in article text]. Chest. 2012;141(2 Suppl):e89S–e119S.
15. Tendera M, Wojakowski W. Role of antiplatelet drugs in preventing cardiovascular events. Thromb Res. 2003;110(5–6):355–9.
16. Kim JS, Vashist YK, Thieltges S, et al. Stapled hemorrhoidopexy versus Milligan-Morgan hemorrhoidectomy in circumferential third-degree hemorrhoids: long-term results of a randomized controlled trial. J Gastrointest Surg. 2013;17(7):1292–8.
17. Lienert M. Literature review on dearterialization of hemorrhoids and mucopexy. In: Ratto C, Parello A, Litta F, editors. Hemorrhoids, Coloproctology, vol. 2. Cham: Springer; 2018.
18. Tjandra JJ, Chan MK. Systematic review on the procedure for prolapse and hemorrhoids (stapled hemorrhoidopexy). Dis Colon Rectum. 2007;50(6):878 92.
19. Keck T. Editorial Zentralblatt für Chirurgie. Zentralbl Chir. 2018;143(3):240.

20. Aigner F, Bodner G, Gruber H, et al. The vascular nature of hemorrhoids. J Gastrointest Surg. 2006;10(7):1044–50.

21. Aigner F, Gruber H, Conrad F, et al. Revised morphology and hemodynamics of the anorectal vascular plexus: impact on the course of hemorrhoidal disease. Int J Color Dis. 2009;24(1):105–13.

22. Plapler H, Hage R, Duarte J, et al. A new method for hemorrhoid surgery: intrahemorrhoidal diode laser, does it work? Photomed Laser Surg. 2009;27(5):819–23.

23. Maloku H, Gashi Z, Lazovic R, Islami H, Juniku-Shkololli A. Laser hemorrhoidoplasty procedure vs. open surgical hemorrhoidectomy: a trial comparing 2 treatments for hemorrhoids of third and fourth degree. Acta Inform Med. 2014;22(6):365–7.

24. Poskus T, Danys D, Makunaite G, et al. Results of the double-blind, randomized controlled trial comparing laser hemorrhoidoplasty with sutured mucopexy and excisional hemorrhoidectomy. Int J Color Dis. 2020;35(3):481–90.

25. De A, Roy P. Hybrid digitally guided hemorrhoidal artery ligation with laser hemorrhoidoplasty: our experience with a new approach to hemorrhoidal disease. Int Surg J. 2021;8(10):2968–73.

26. Milligan ET, Morgan CN, Jones L, Officer R. Surgical anatomy of the anal canal, and the operative treatment of hemorrhoids. Lancet. 1937;230(5959):1119–24.

27. Weyand G, Theis CS, Fofana AN, Rüdiger F, Gehrke T. Laserhämorrhoidoplastie mit dem 1470-nm-Diodenlaser in der Behandlung des zweit-bis viertgradigen Hämorrhoidalleidens – eine Kohortenstudie mit 497 Fällen [Laserhemorrhoidoplasty with 1470 nm diode laser in the treatment of second to fourth degree hemorrhoidal disease - a cohort study with 497 patients]. Zentralbl Chir. 2019;144(4):355–63.

28. Rahman AZ, Rahman T, Hasan M, Chandra S. Hemorrhoidal LASER procedure (HeLP)-a painless treatment for hemorrhoid. J Bangladesh Coll Phys Surg. 2020;38(1):18–22.

29. Giamundo P, Salfi R, Geraci M, Tibaldi L, Murru L, Valente M. The hemorrhoid laser procedure technique vs. rubber band ligation: a randomized trial comparing 2 mini-invasive treatments for second- and third-degree hemorrhoids. Dis Colon Rectum. 2011;54(6):693–8. https://doi.org/10.1007/DCR.0b013e3182112d58. Erratum in: Dis Colon Rectum. 2012 Apr;55(4):497. PMID: 21552053

Lasers in External and Complicated Internal Hemorrhoids

9

"Thrombosed, strangulated and ulcerated hemorrhoids are some of the complications of hemorrhoids. Such cases are not usually operated upon by competent proctologists at this stage."

Kilbourne, 1936

Key Concepts

- External hemorrhoids are formed from the dilatation of the inferior hemorrhoidal plexus. They may become thrombosed and rupture.
- Thrombosed external hemorrhoids present as a purple/blue edematous, tense, and tender perianal swelling.
- The ideal procedure for thrombosed external hemorrhoids remains excision.
- Thrombosed internal hemorrhoids are formed when a part of the anal cushion is involved. In such cases, a minimally invasive procedure that can be considered is clot evacuation with Finger-guided hemorrhoidal artery ligation with Laser hemorrhoidoplasty.
- Strangulated hemorrhoids are formed when the whole cushion gets thrombosed. The treatment of choice remains excisional hemorrhoidectomy.
- Laser has no role in managing strangulated, ulcerated, and necrosed hemorrhoids.

9.1 Introduction

External hemorrhoids are formed by the dilatation of the inferior hemorrhoidal venous plexus [1]. The presence of thrombosed external hemorrhoids is extremely painful [2]. The internal hemorrhoids may become thrombosed or strangulated. If a part of the cushion is involved, it is referred to as thrombosed internal hemorrhoids. If the whole anal cushion is involved, it is referred to as strangulated hemorrhoids.

9.2 External Hemorrhoids

External hemorrhoids are formed by the dilatation of the inferior hemorrhoidal venous plexus [1]. They are found below the dentate line, richly innervated by the pudendal nerve [3]. They may present in the form of bulges all around the anal verge or as thrombosed hemorrhoids. As there is an anastomosis between superior and inferior hemorrhoidal plexus, enlargement of the superior hemorrhoidal plexus may predispose to external hemorrhoidal engorgement, a condition known as interno-external hemorrhoids. Sometimes external hemorrhoids occur circumferentially along the anal verge due to inferior hemorrhoidal venous plexus varicosity. Usually, they are asymptomatic and require no surgical intervention. The patient's only complaint is swelling around the anal orifice while defecating. Conservative management for external hemorrhoids includes lifestyle modification, dietary changes, and laxatives. The role of flavonoids is not yet been established, but they can be prescribed as phlebotonics.

9.2.1 Thrombosed External Hemorrhoids

The thrombosed external hemorrhoids present as a purple/blue edematous, tense, and tender perianal swelling [4, 5] (Fig. 9.1). It is a painful condition that may be unbearable. These hemorrhoids are often seen in patients who strain while defecating, lift heavy objects, and have prolonged sitting like long-distance drivers and pilots [6]. Constipation is one of the predisposing factors in developing thrombosed external hemorrhoids [6].

9.2.1.1 Pathophysiology of Thrombosed External Hemorrhoids

The exact pathophysiology of thrombosed external hemorrhoids is unclear. As a result of prolonged sitting or straining, the pressure inside the hemorrhoidal plexus increases, leading to blood stasis, causing engorgement of venous plexus. Subsequently, thrombus or clot formation may occur, forming thrombosed hemorrhoids [7]. When a blood clot develops within a hemorrhoidal vein, blood flow is obstructed, resulting in painful swelling of the perianal tissues.

9.2.1.2 The Pathophysiology of Pain

The excruciating pain associated with thrombosed external hemorrhoids is due to the swelling and bleeding within the inferior hemorrhoidal venous plexus. The venous plexus is present in the corrugator cutis ani muscle in the perianal space, a tightly packed area due to dense fatty tissue. The fascia covering the tissues within the muscle does not stretch or expand and hence acts as a compartmental syndrome. Once the swelling is formed, the nerves, capillaries, and muscles in the perianal area come under pressure. The blood flow to the nerves and muscles is decreased. Lack of blood supply and oxygenation results in ischemia leading to intense pain [8].

9.2.1.3 Clinical Evaluation

Thrombosed external hemorrhoids present with intense pain in the anal region and difficulty in sitting. On examination, a small swelling can be seen in the perianal area. Sometimes, the thrombosed external hemorrhoids may become ulcerated or rupture (Figs. 9.2 and 9.3).

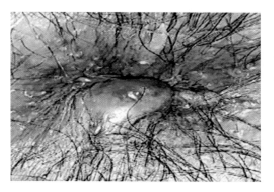

Fig. 9.1 Thrombosed external hemorrhoids

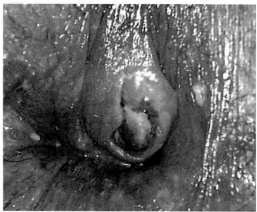

Fig. 9.2 Ulcerated external hemorrhoids

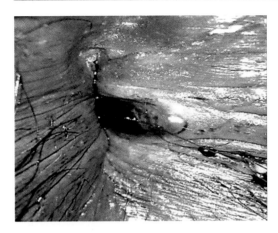

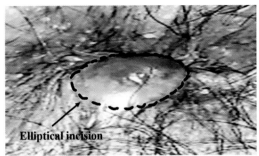

Fig. 9.4 Elliptical incision for the thrombosed hemorrhoid

Fig. 9.3 Ruptured external hemorrhoids

Digital rectal examination and proctoscopy are very painful in these cases but should be done to rule out any other associated condition.

9.2.1.4 Management of Thrombosed External Hemorrhoids

The swelling usually resolves within 5–7 days, and hence it is called 5-days self-limiting disease. The topical application and sitz bath can be excellent pain relievers [9]. A thrombosed external hemorrhoid that resolves may leave a residual perianal skin tag that requires excision [9].

Surgical intervention remains the treatment of choice if the thrombosed hemorrhoids do not respond to conservative management [10, 11]. There are two ways to treat the condition surgically:

- Clot evacuation with a radial incision
- Complete excision of the thrombosed hemorrhoid [4] (Fig. 9.4)

9.2.1.5 Role of Lasers in Thrombosed External Hemorrhoids

An ideal technique for thrombosed external hemorrhoids remains excision under local anesthesia. However, the raw area hence created takes time to heal [12]. Clot evacuation followed by laser can also be done when significant clot formation occurs. An incision is given over the thrombosed hemorrhoid, and the clot is evacuated. This is followed by laser coagulation using a bare fiber which has a hemostatic effect. The fiber is inserted through the incised wound. The thermal energy seals the blood vessels in that area or compartment. The only complication one can encounter is a remnant small skin tag that can be removed later.

9.2.1.6 Postoperative Care

- Sitz bath twice a day.
- An ointment containing an analgesic and an anesthetic cream is recommended. A combination of sucralfate, metronidazole, and lignocaine provides excellent relief [7].

Some Interesting Facts from Literature

Thrombosis of the inferior hemorrhoidal plexus is often seen as a "perianal hematoma." However, Hamish Thomson, in 1979, stated that "Perianal hematoma" was a misnomer and preferred the term "clotted venous saccule" as it was not a true hematoma and was completely sub-anodermal (sub-pectinate) with no signs of bleeding [13, 14].

9.3   Thrombosed Internal Hemorrhoids

Although internal hemorrhoids are painless, the presence of pain should raise a suspicion of thrombosed internal hemorrhoids. The word thrombosed is formed from "thrombosis," which means clotting [15].

9.3.1   Pathophysiology of Thrombosed Internal Hemorrhoids

Vascular thrombosis, abnormal venous dilatation, degeneration in the collagen fibers and fibroelastic tissues, and rupture of the anal subepithelial muscle are part of the pathogenic occurrences in the anal cushions. Once hemorrhoids develop, increased pressure in the anal cushions can lead to blood stasis within the vessels, leading to blood clot formation and thrombosis. The blood supply to the anal cushion is hampered, resulting in ischemia [15]. On histopathology, the hemorrhoidal specimens showed an intense inflammatory response, mucosal ulceration, and thrombosis [16].

9.3.2   Management of Thrombosed Internal Hemorrhoids

Thrombosed internal hemorrhoids are treated differently than thrombosed external hemorrhoids. In the case of thrombosed internal hemorrhoids, the clot evacuation, followed by finger-guided hemorrhoidal artery ligation and laser hemorrhoidoplasty, can be done (Fig. 9.5). The laser

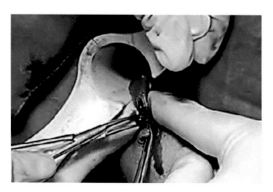

Fig. 9.5 Thrombosed internal hemorrhoids showing clot evacuation

fiber is inserted through the incision where the clot has been evacuated. In case of thrombosed internal hemorrhoids, urgent surgical intervention is frequently recommended.

9.4   Strangulated Internal Hemorrhoids

"Strangulation is defined as a condition in which the blood flow to a portion of the body is cut off or reduced due to blood vessel compression." Therefore, strangulated hemorrhoids are the hemorrhoids whose circulation is impaired [17].

When the prolapsed internal hemorrhoidal cushion remains untreated for a long time, its blood supply is hampered, and it becomes strangulated [18, 19]. These patients may present with irreducible, prolapsed, gangrenous hemorrhoids requiring surgical intervention (Fig. 9.6). The symptoms associated with these hemorrhoids are pain, swelling, bleeding, and foul-smelling discharge [20].

9.4.1   Pathophysiology of Strangulated Hemorrhoids

As the internal anal sphincter lies higher than the external sphincter, the prolapsed part of internal hemorrhoid may get trapped between the internal anal sphincter and the lower portion of the external anal sphincter during straining [21]. This cuts off the blood supply and obstructs venous return leading to edema and a painful strangulated hemorrhoid [20]. Subsequently, ulceration may occur due to necrosis (Table 9.1).

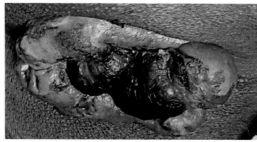

Fig. 9.6 Strangulated hemorrhoids

Table 9.1 Events in strangulation of hemorrhoids

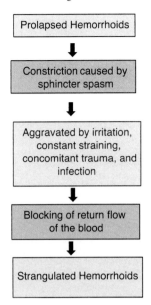

9.4.2 Management of Strangulated Hemorrhoids

The treatment of choice remains surgical excision. During surgery, determining the anatomy and leaving appropriate mucocutaneous bridges might be problematic [22]. According to Hansen et al., pedicles are usually well-defined and spared, which Smith confirmed by histological studies [20, 23].

Strangulated, ulcerated, or necrosed hemorrhoids are an absolute contraindication for laser hemorrhoidoplasty. Hemorrhoidectomy remains the procedure of choice.

9.5 Discussion

Thrombosed external hemorrhoids can be managed by laxatives, sitz baths, and analgesics. The majority of patients are treated conservatively. The hemorrhoidal mass should be excised if the patient has severe pain and is unwilling to wait.

Cavic et al. carried out a study on the topical application of 2% nitroglycerine, excision of hemorrhoid, and incision and evacuation of thrombus. The maximum pain relief was with the excision of thrombosed hemorrhoids [25, 26].

Following acute thrombosis and strangulation, the infection should be managed with antibiotics, followed by surgical intervention. One should try to reduce strangulated internal hemorrhoids to prevent necrosis. It is not the amount of sphincter muscle constriction but the amount of edema that determines whether strangulated hemorrhoids can be reduced or not [17]. The edema can be reduced by injecting hylase into the edematous hemorrhoids. It acts by increasing tissue permeability. Irreducible strangulated hemorrhoids should be taken for immediate excision. According to some authors [17], if the strangulated prolapsed cushion is extensive and very painful, it is better to treat it conservatively initially and then go for surgical intervention.

Eisenhammer stated that when multiple external hemorrhoids become thrombosed, they may appear like a "bunch of grapes" [27]. Eisenhammer described any condition that aggravates pain in the anal region as a "pile attack," which can be an internal hemorrhoidal one.

Some Interesting Facts from Literature

In strangulated hemorrhoids, the procedure of choice remains hemorrhoidectomy. The correct treatment option for thrombosed hemorrhoids was a matter of consideration. Goligher, in 1961 mentioned a strictly conservative approach for treating prolapsed thrombosed hemorrhoids [24]. "Bed rest, hot baths, soothing local applications, sedatives, antibiotics, and laxatives to secure easy motions" was the treatment protocol suggested by him [24]. Surgery was not recommended due to the risk of infection spreading due to operative intervention in the septic area.

In 1984, Goligher changed his stance and preferred hemorrhoidectomy for thrombosed internal hemorrhoids advocating portal pyemia as a myth [24].

The characteristics of the internal hemorrhoidal "pile attacks" are:

1. In nonprolapsed hemorrhoids
   - Inflammation.
   - Thrombosis and its sequelae of ulceration and necrosis with acute sepsis. There are no external signs of the disease.
2. In prolapsed hemorrhoids
   - Inflammation
   - Thrombosis and its sequelae
   - Superimposed strangulation

Every hemorrhoidal mass is not an indication of laser surgery. Thrombosed internal hemorrhoids can be taken for laser hemorrhoidoplasty. The laser can be used only after the evacuation of the clot. Strangulated hemorrhoids are painful conditions due to necrosis, and immediate excision of the anal cushion is required. Laser has no role in strangulated hemorrhoids.

Take-Home Message
Thrombosed external hemorrhoids should be managed conservatively. Failure to reduce pain after medical management is an indication of excision. Lasers in thrombosed internal hemorrhoids can only be considered after clot evacuation. In strangulated hemorrhoids, the treatment of choice remains excision.

References

1. Lohsiriwat V. Hemorrhoids: from basic pathophysiology to clinical management. World J Gastroenterol. 2012;18(17):2009–17. https://doi.org/10.3748/wjg.v18.i17.2009.
2. Perry KR. Hemorrhoids. https://www.medscape.com/answers/775407-182222/what-is-the-pathophysiology-of-hemorrhoids.
3. Lawrence A, McLaren ER. External hemorrhoid. In: StatPearls. Treasure Island, FL: StatPearls Publishing; 2022.
4. Grosz CR. Surgical treatment of thrombosed external hemorrhoids. Dis Colon Rectum. 1990;33(3):249–50. https://doi.org/10.1007/BF02134191.
5. Hemorrhoids. https://teachmesurgery.com/general/anorectal/haemorrhoids/.
6. Sanchez C, Chinn BT. Hemorrhoids. Clin Colon Rectal Surg. 2011;24(1):5–13.
7. Lorber BW. Thrombosed external hemorrhoid excision technique. https://emedicine.medscape.com/article/81039-overview.
8. Compartment syndrome from the American Academy of Orthopedic Surgeons. https://orthoinfo.aaos.org/en/diseases%2D%2Dconditions/compartment-syndrome/.
9. Nienhuijs SW, de Hingh IH. Pain after conventional versus Ligasure haemorrhoidectomy. A meta-analysis. Int J Surg. 2010;8(4):269–73.
10. Lohsiriwat V. Treatment of hemorrhoids: a coloproctologist's view. World J Gastroenterol. 2015;21(31):9245–52. https://doi.org/10.3748/wjg.v21.i31.9245.
11. Corman ML, Corman ML. Colon and rectal surgery. Philadelphia, PA: Lippincott Williams & Wilkins; 2005.
12. Davis BR, Lee-Kong SA, Migaly J, Feingold DL, Steele SR. The American Society of Colon and Rectal Surgeons Clinical Practice guidelines for the management of hemorrhoids. Dis Colon Rectum. 2018;61(3):284–92.
13. Thomson WH. The nature of hemorrhoids. Br J Surg. 1975;62(7):542–52.
14. Thomson H. The anal cushions—a fresh concept in diagnosis. Postgrad Med J. 1979;55(644):403–5.
15. Health conditions and disease: thrombosis. Johns Hopkins Medicine. https://www.hopkinsmedicine.org/health/conditions-and-diseases/thrombosis.
16. Morgado PJ, Suárez JA, Gómez LG, Morgado PJ. Histoclinical basis for a new classification of hemorrhoidal disease. Dis Colon Rectum. 1988;31:474–80.
17. Puritt MC. Etiology and treatment of strangulated, thrombosed, infected, and gangrenous internal hemorrhoids. South Med J. 1939;32(1):68–70.
18. Castillo AH. Thrombosed hemorrhoid: what is it, causes, diagnosis, treatment, and more. https://www.osmosis.org/answers/thrombosed-hemorrhoid.
19. Strangulated hemorrhoid. Dictionary, Thesaurus, Encyclopedia. https://www.thefreedictionary.com/strangulated+hemorrhoid.
20. Hansen JB, Jorgensen SJ. Radical emergency operation for prolapsed and strangulated hemorrhoids. Acta Chir Scand. 1975;141(8):810–2.
21. Milligan ETC, Morgan CN, Jones LE, Officer R. Edward Thomas Campbell Milligan 1886–1972. Dis Colon Rectum. 1985;28:620–8.

22. Mir SA, Mir I, Tak SA, Wani M. Profile and management of complicated (strangulated) prolapsed internal hemorrhoids at a tertiary care hospital—a prospective study. Int J Contemp Med Res. 2019;6(5): E1–3.

23. Smith M. Early operation for acute hemorrhoids. Br J Surg. 1967;54(2):141–4. https://doi.org/10.1002/bjs.1800540214.

24. Cirocco WC. Reprint of: why are hemorrhoids symptomatic? The pathophysiology and etiology of hemorrhoids. Semin Colon Rectal Surg. 2018;29(4): 160–6.

25. Cavcić J, Turcić J, Martinac P, Mestrović T, Mladina R, Pezerović-Panijan R. Comparison of topically applied 0.2% glyceryl trinitrate ointment, incision and excision in the treatment of perianal thrombosis. Dig Liver Dis. 2001;33(4):335–40. https://doi.org/10.1016/s1590-8658(01)80088-8.

26. Mott T, Latimer K, Edwards C. Hemorrhoids: diagnosis and treatment options. Am Fam Physician. 2018;97(3):172–9.

27. Eisenhammer S. An attack of piles: its management in general practice. S Afr Med J. 1949;23(11): 192–7.

Anatomy of Para-Anal and Pararectal Spaces

"Anatomy is to physiology as geography is to history; it describes the theatre of events."

Jean Francois Fernel

Key Concepts

- Surgical procedures for anal abscesses and fistulas are technically demanding.
- As a surgeon, it is essential to know the basic anatomy of para-anal and pararectal spaces to perform the procedures precisely.
- Abscesses and fistulas are named according to the space they travel.
- Most abscesses and fistulas result from an acute infection of the anal glands.

10.1 Introduction

Surgical procedures for an abscess and anal fistula are technically demanding. Due to the incidence of recurrence and incontinence, the short-term and long-term physiological consequences must be considered while treating them. Accurate knowledge of anatomy helps a surgeon conduct sphincter-saving surgery precisely. Therefore, for reference, a detailed description of the anatomy of the para-anal and pararectal spaces has been explained.

10.2 Anatomy of Para-Anal and Pararectal Spaces

Anatomically some virtual spaces are formed between the mucocutaneous lining of the anal canal and the muscular structure of a sphincter complex (Fig. 10.1a, b). Potential spaces of clinical significance in the anorectal region are discussed below in detail:

10.2.1 Ischioanal/Ischiorectal Space

The shape and structure of an ischiorectal fossa depend on levator ani muscle disposition, which creates its roof and inner wall [1]. The boundary between the ischiorectal and perianal spaces is marked by fascia, which starts from the "Conjoined Longitudinal Muscle" (CLM) and extends to an ischial tuberosity across the subcutaneous external anal sphincter [2]. This fascia is called "the transverse septum of the ischiorectal fossa," also known as "Milligan septum" [2] (Fig. 10.2).

Fig. 10.1 (a, b)
Demonstrating para-anal
and pararectal spaces

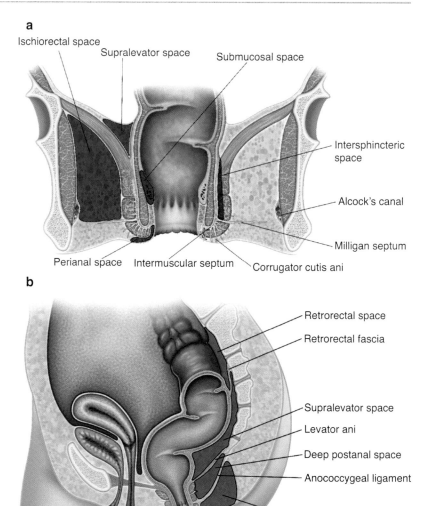

Fig. 10.2 Ischioanal/
ischiorectal space

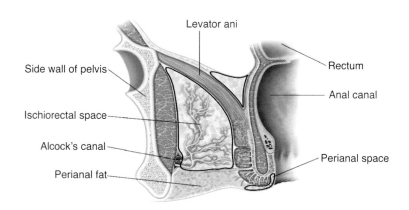

Fig. 10.3 Perianal space

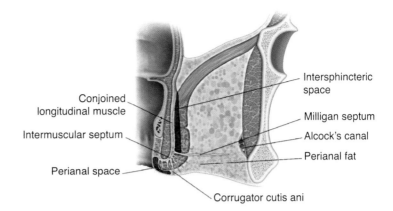

Conjoined longitudinal muscle

Intermuscular septum

Perianal space

Corrugator cutis ani

Intersphincteric space

Milligan septum

Alcock's canal

Perianal fat

10.2.1.1 Boundaries

Medially: Lower rectum and anal canal area

    Laterally: Pelvis sidewalls

    Above: Levator ani muscle

    Base: Perianal space

    Anteriorly: Urogenital diaphragm

    Posteriorly: Sacrotuberous ligament and gluteus maximus

    Supralaterally: Alcock's canal (internal pudendal vessels and nerve)

10.2.1.2 Contents

The space is covered by large lobules of avascular fat, inferior rectal vessels, and nerves.

10.2.2 Perianal Space

Morphologically it signifies part of the proctodeum.

10.2.2.1 Boundaries

Above: Intermuscular septum

    Medially: Intersphincteric space

    Laterally: Continuous with subcutaneous gluteal fat

10.2.2.2 Contents

The perianal region encloses the subcutaneous "External anal sphincter" (EAS), the fibers of corrugator cutis ani, and the external hemorrhoidal plexus. Finely granular and closely packed fat fills the perianal space (Fig. 10.3).

Surgical Importance of Perianal and Ischiorectal Spaces

- The fat in the perianal space is tightly arranged and associated with septa formation due to corrugator cutis ani. Hence, pain in the perianal abscess is excruciating because of the tension caused by a swelling.
- Both perianal and ischioanal spaces are common sites of abscesses.
- Sometimes an abscess in the ischiorectal region does not involve the overlying skin as it does not penetrate the Milligan's septum.
- The fistula which invoves the perianal space is a intersphincteric one.

10.2.3 Intersphincteric Space

An area between the internal and external anal sphincter (Fig. 10.4).

10.2.3.1 Boundaries

Medially: Internal anal sphincter

    Laterally: External anal sphincter

    Superiorly: Supralevator space

Fig. 10.4 Intersphincteric space

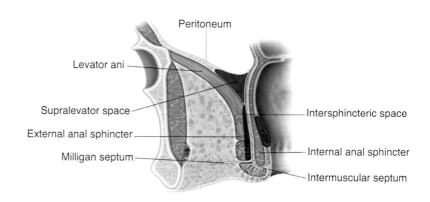

Fig. 10.5 Submucosal
space

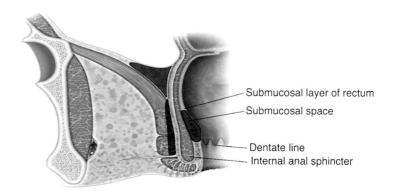

Inferiorly: Intermuscular and Milligan
septum

10.2.3.2 Contents
Fat and connective tissue

> **Surgical Importance of Intersphincteric
> Space**
> It is crucial in the genesis of intersphinc-
> teric, supralevator, perianal or ischiorectal
> abscesses as the anal glands' ramifications
> are present here.

10.2.4 Submucosal Space

It is located above the dentate line (Fig. 10.5).

10.2.4.1 Boundaries
Laterally: Internal anal sphincter

Above: Continuous with submucosa of the
rectum

10.2.4.2 Contents
Internal hemorrhoidal plexus

10.2.5 Superficial Postanal Space

The interposed region between the skin and the
anococcygeal ligament (Fig. 10.6a).

10.2.6 Deep Postanal Space

The region is located midway between the tip
of the coccyx and the subcutaneous external
anal sphincter. It is also called the "Retro-
sphincteric space of Courtney" and communicates with ischiorectal fossae on either side [3]
(Fig. 10.6b).

Fig. 10.6 (**a**) Deep and superficial postanal spaces. (**b**) Deep postanal space

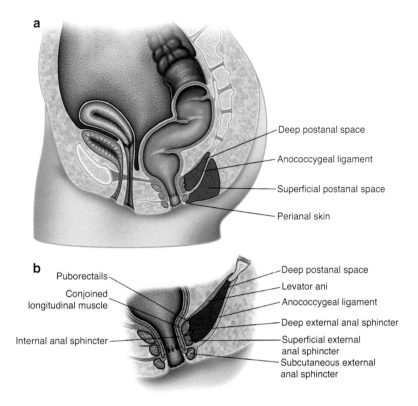

10.2.6.1 Boundaries

Superiorly: Inferior part of levator ani with musculotendinous insertions of three divisions, Ileococcygeus, pubococcygeus, and puborectalis, into the sides of coccyx and tip.

Inferiorly: Anococcygeal ligament

Anteriorly: Superficial external anal sphincter (Posterior surface)

> **Surgical Significance of Deep Postanal Space**
> - It communicates posteriorly to the ischiorectal fossae and is site of horseshoe abscesses.

Another space of surgical importance is the deep anterior anal space described by Hanley [4], which will be discussed later.

10.2.7   Supralevator Space

Located between the levator and the peritoneum (Fig. 10.7).

10.2.7.1 Boundaries

Medially: Rectum

Laterally: Obturator fascia

Superiorly: Peritoneum

Inferiorly: Levator ani

> **Surgical Importance of Supralevator Space**
> Infection from intersphincteric space has easy access to adjacent supralevator/perirectal spaces. Supralevator abscess may develop due to upward extending cryptoglandular infection from intersphincteric abscess or downward extension from pelvic infection. However, these spaces are protected from any kind of infections with fascial barriers [1].

Fig. 10.7 Supralevator
space

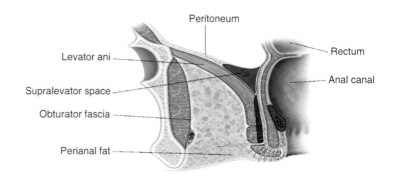

Fig. 10.8 Retrorectal
space

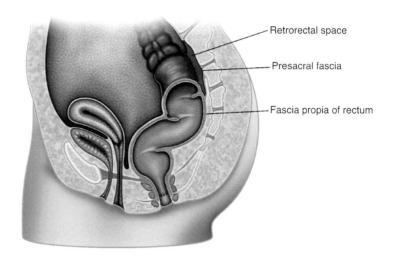

10.2.8   Retrorectal Space

Lies anterior to the coccyx and sacrum and posterior to the rectum [1].

10.2.8.1 Boundaries
Anteriorly: Fascia propria of the rectum
Posteriorly: Presacral fascia
Laterally: Lateral rectal ligament
Inferiorly: Rectosacral ligament
   Above it is continuous with retroperitoneum
(Fig. 10.8).

Surgical Importance of Retrorectal Space
Area for embryogenic remnants and rare
presacral tumors (lipoma, chondroma, tera-
toma, and presacral cyst).

10.3   Anal Glands

Anal glands are the only interacting part between
the anal canal and the sphincter complex. Had
there been no extension of the anal glands from
the anal lumen into the sphincter complex, it
would not have been worth describing them.
   The first description of anal glands was given by
Haller in 1751 [5]. Chiari further described these
glands in 1878. Chiari suggested that infection of
these anal glands caused an anal fistula [5]. Herrman
and Desfosses further supported this in 1880 [5].
   Anal glands are 6–8 in number and present in
the wall of the anal canal. They are lined with
stratified squamous epithelium [5, 6]. They are
classified as "apocrine glands" and are sebaceous
in nature. Through the anal ducts, they secrete
fluid into the anal canal [5, 6]. These ducts open
at the anal crypts on the dentate line. Sometimes

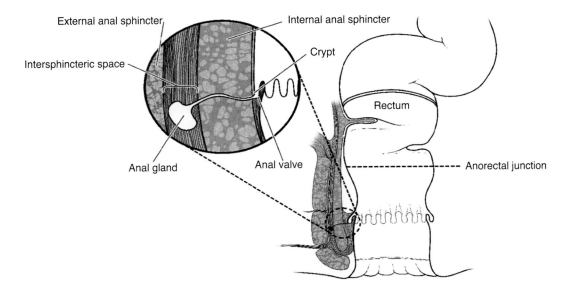

Fig. 10.9 Anal crypts and anal glands

multiple glands open in a single crypt. The secretory function of these glands is to keep the anal canal moist (Fig. 10.9).

10.3.1 Location of Anal Glands

Ian MacColl, 1965 stated that 50% of the anal glands extend through the internal anal sphincter. Each gland gives off secondary and tertiary tubular branches, varying from 4 to 16 in number [5, 6]. These tubular branches may blindly end in the submucosa or extend through the internal anal sphincter at two to four levels. Sometimes, 2 to 3 ramifications are present at the same level [5]. These ramifications form channels for the spread of the infection. The more the number of channels, the more the chances of spreading infection (Fig. 10.10).

Seow Cheon, in his publication, described the position of the anal glands [7]. These glands are present at varying depths in the anal canal wall. They are predominantly present in the posterior half of the anal canal, explaining the internal opening present posteriorly in most fistulas. Anal glands in 80% of the cases are present in submucosa. It extends to conjoined longitudinal muscles in 7–8% cases, to internal sphincter in 8%, intersphincteric space in 2% cases, and in 1% cases, anal glands penetrate the external anal sphincter [7] (Fig. 10.10).

The commonest position of the anal glands in the submucosa is due to the short terminal tubules of the glands. The usual length of the anal duct is 1 to 2 mm [6]. However, it may be upto 4 mm in length in a few cases. The internal anal sphincter tubules sometimes dilate like an ampulla or a cyst, penetrating the conjoined longitudinal muscle (Fig. 10.11). The cyst, formed in the intersphincteric space, does not discharge so easily into the anal canal because of impedance by the tonic contraction of the internal sphincter. The infection may then follow the path of least resistance leading to an anal fistula [7].

As stated earlier, most anal ducts have their outlet posteriorly in the anal canal. The direction of these glands is usually caudal, rarely lateral or cephalad. This explains perianal abscess being the common presentation of anorectal abscesses [6].

10.3.2 The Fate of Anal Glands

The anal glands can lead to

- Stasis
- Obstruction
- Infection
- Abscess or fistula formation

Fig. 10.10 Anatomical positions of anal glands

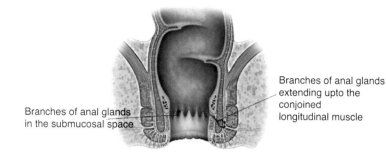

Branches of anal glands in the submucosal space

Branches of anal glands extending upto the conjoined longitudinal muscle

Fig. 10.11 Intersphincteric dilatation of the anal duct (cyst formation)

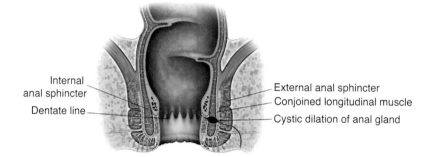

Internal anal sphincter

Dentate line

External anal sphincter
Conjoined longitudinal muscle
Cystic dilation of anal gland

10.3.3 Surgical Importance of Anal Glands

Infection of anal glands leads to an abscess formation. This theory was postulated by Park in 1961 and is popularly known as cryptoglandular theory [8]. The theory states that the ducts are obstructed by foreign material accumulation in the crypts (e.g., fecal plugging), causing perianal abscess and, subsequently, a fistula [9, 10]. About 60% of anal glands secrete mucus [5]. Due to blockage of the glands, a cyst may be formed up to a diameter of 5 mm, especially in the submucosa. Once the cyst becomes infected, it leads to an abscess formation, which may burst submucosally. When the cyst is formed in the intersphincteric space, an intersphincteric abscess may form, followed by a fistula representing a chronic stage of infection [5].

Some Interesting Facts

People born with the mucus-secreting glands ramifying through the internal sphincter may congenitally be predisposed to fistula [5].

10.4 The Relation of Anal Glands with Crohn's Disease, Ulcerative Colitis, and Carcinoma Rectum

Johnson (1714) and Desfosses (1880), in their studies, demonstrated lymphatic tissue around the anal gland ducts, which explains the association of an abscess with tuberculosis or Crohn's disease [5]. In his study on anal glands, Ian MacColl reported that anal glands are not involved in ulcerative colitis [5]. However, the mucosa and submucosa showed inflammatory changes and dilated blood vessels. He further observed that the anal glands were not always involved in Crohn's disease, suggesting that the glands are not solely responsible for spreading the infection through the internal sphincter. The anal glands may rarely give rise to adenocarcinoma [5].

Parks stated that the principle of treatment of anal fistula was to remove the infected anal gland and the abscess surrounding it and opening of the deep intersphincter space. This fact is of utmost surgical significance, as in operating fistulas, one should always take out the internal opening along with mucosa, submucosa, and the surrounding tissue [8, 11].

10.5 Importance of Anatomical Landmarks Related to the Conjoined Longitudinal Muscle

A conjoined longitudinal muscle is an extension of the longitudinal rectal muscle. It attaches the rectum to the structures surrounding it [2]. This results in four fibromuscular expansions: (a) intermuscular septum, (b) septum of the ischiorectal fossa, (c) rectourethralis muscle, and (d) corrugator cutis ani muscle (Fig. 10.12).

Three of the expansions surround the perianal space other than its outer space.

1. The intermuscular septum extends transversely inwards from the internal anal sphincter above and the external anal sphincter's subcutaneous part below. It separates the external and internal hemorrhoidal plexus. With Milligan's septum, the intermuscular septum forms a perianal space. It prevents infection from extending from perianal space into the cephalad submucous space [2].

2. The Milligan's septum extends outward from a lower conjoined longitudinal muscle across the ischiorectal fossa. It divides it into a perianal space below and an ischiorectal space above [2].

3. Corrugator cutis ani muscle is formed with radial insertion of the conjoined longitudinal muscle and the subcutaneous part of the external anal sphincter to the perianal skin. It covers the lower region of the perianal space [2].

Fig. 10.12 Fibromuscular expansions of conjoined longitudinal muscle

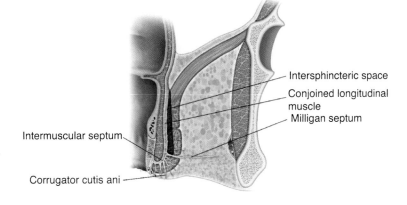

10.6   A Word About Milligan's Septum

Milligan's septum extends from the lower border of the internal anal sphincter. It turns outwards above the subcutaneous part and below the superficial part of the external anal sphincter [2]. Posteriorly, the septum is incomplete. The insertion is in the skin and the ischial tuberosity. The intersphincteric groove is located at the Milligan's septum level. The septum prevents infections that start from the perianal space from spreading upwards. In the case of an ischiorectal abscess, the inflammatory sign on the skin becomes apparent only when the septum is penetrated. The septum should be stabbed using a knife to reach the levator ani muscle through the ischiorectal fossa [2].

10.7   Anococcygeal Ligament and Anococcygeal Raphe

The terms anococcygeal raphe and ligament are often confused. The anococcygeal ligament is developed by the insertion of the superficial part of an external anal sphincter into the coccyx. It is approximately 2.7 mm in thickness. Below the anococcygeal ligament lies the "Space of Courtney."

The anococcygeal raphe corresponds to a connective tissue inferior to the coccyx connecting the bilateral anorectal slings (Fig. 10.13). This raphe is critical in coordinating the superior movement and contraction of the external sphincter to ensure smooth defecation [12].

Care must be taken not to divide the anococcygeal raphae horizontally since marked anterior displacement and deformity of the anus occur with resultant incontinence.

Fig. 10.13 Anococcygeal ligament and raphe

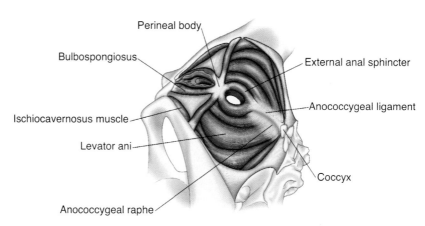

10.8   A Word About Deep Intersphincteric Space

Research by Heng et al. and Kurihara et al. [13, 14] highlighted the deep intersphincteric region in the posterior part of the mid-anal canal. The primary lesion of a complex posterior fistula is usually located in this space (Fig. 10.14).

10.8.1   Boundaries

- **Anterior**: Internal anal sphincter
- **Superior**: Inferior surface of the puborectalis
- **Lateral**: External anal sphincter

10.8.2   Surgical Relevance of Deep Intersphincteric Space

Recognition of deep intersphincteric space is crucial for managing the complex posterior fistula. Under normal conditions, this space is not recognized as distinct [13] and is undetectable in MRI [14]. But this space expands easily if the abscess reaches this space. The condition is similar to an abscess in the closed region [15]. The closed space should be completely drained and must be kept open for eradicating sepsis and healing [15].

Fig. 10.14 Deep intersphincteric space

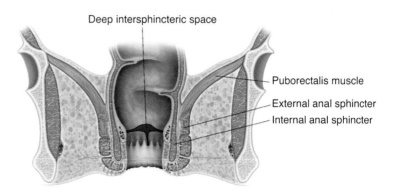

Deep intersphincteric space

Puborectalis muscle

External anal sphincter

Internal anal sphincter

10.9   A Word About Deep Anterior Anal Space

The space lies anteriorly, covering the urogenital triangle (Fig. 10.15). The boundaries include:

- **Anterior**: Transverse perineal membrane and muscles
- **Superior**: Levator ani
- **Inferior**: Superficial external sphincter

Direct communication exists between the left and right ischiorectal spaces [16].

10.9.1   Surgical Relevance

The intersphincteric abscess ruptures between the superficial and deep part of an external anal sphincter into a deep anterior anal space (Fig. 10.15). In females, deep anterior space and its suppurative conditions might extend to the rectovaginal septum, which is an occasional reason for the lower rectovaginal fistula [16]. The management of this abscess will be explained in the next chapter.

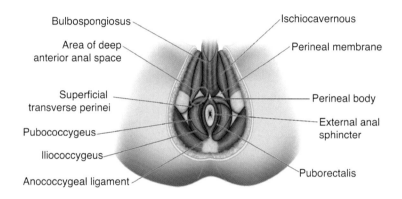

Fig. 10.15 Deep anterior anal space

Bulbospongiosus

Area of deep anterior anal space

Superficial transverse perinei

Pubococcygeus

Iliococcygeus

Anococcygeal ligament

Ischiocavernous

Perineal membrane

Perineal body

External anal sphincter

Puborectalis

10.10   A Word About Infralevator Space

A septum of the ischiorectal fossa separates an ischiorectal fossa into an upper and lower part; the lower is the ischiorectal region, and the upper is the inferior levator region (Fig. 10.16).

Ischiorectal Region—below the septum of an ischiorectal fossa.

Inferior Levator—between levator-ani and the septum of an ischiorectal fossa.

10.10.1   Surgical Importance

An ischiorectal abscess can penetrate the ischiorectal septum and the inferior levator space and extend to the supralevator space.

Fig. 10.16 Infralevator space

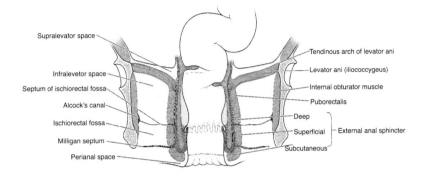

10.11 Discussion

Most of the rectal and anal canal anatomy has been illustrated by nineteenth and twentieth-century researchers [17]. Based on these studies, pararectal spaces and para-anal spaces have been defined. Potential spaces of clinical importance include the ischiorectal fossa, which contains the nerves, fat, and inferior rectal arteries. The ischiorectal space is separated from a perianal space by an intermuscular septum formed from the conjoined longitudinal muscles. The septum prevents infection from the perianal space to the ischiorectal space and separates the internal hemorrhoidal plexus from the external hemorrhoidal plexus. The perianal space contains external hemorrhoidal plexus and is the typical site for thrombosed external hemorrhoids. The perianal abscess and intersphincteric tracts are other common conditions in this space. The intersphincteric space is considered the genesis of the perianal abscess as most of the anal glands end here. The submucosal space contains the internal hemorrhoidal plexus.

The superficial and deep postanal spaces are mostly infected in horseshoe abscesses and are an important anatomical landmark during the draining of the horseshoe abscess. Supralevator space is the site for an abscess which is usually an upward extension of the cryptoglandular infection. The deep anterior anal space abscess may spread anteriorly. There is an external opening near the scrotum in males, and in females, there may be a fistulous tract extending up to the labia [4, 18].

To understand the clinical significance of anal glands as a potential source of infection, one must realize their existence [5, 6]. It is well-known that intestinal tracts are a natural lodging for some pathogenic and nonpathogenic organisms [6]. It is commonly recognized that any alteration in bowel habits or irritation is responsible for pathological conditions in the anorectal region [19]. Trauma can occur in the anorectal region due to overdistention of the anal canal by a hard motion or chronic diarrhea. Both the

exterior and anterior commissures of an anal canal are weak areas and prone to trauma [19]. Posteriorly, the external anal sphincter fibers give the least support, and anteriorly few circular fibers give support [19]. As anal glands are concentrated more posteriorly, the pathogenic gut organisms can enter through the traumatic mucosa, making the posterior abscesses and fistulas most common [19]. Another source of infection through the mucosa is blood-borne due to disease in other body parts [19]. As mentioned above, anal glands are in the intersphincteric and submucosal spaces. They act as a nidus of infection, leading to an abscess and subsequent fistula formation. John A. Eglitis in 1961 [5, 6] has reported that the intermuscular portion of these glands are usually distended in pear-shaped sacks, which measure $0.91 \times 1.28 \times 2.1$ mm, and their location makes them liable to the possibility of the narrow duct of the gland getting obstructed with subsequent cyst formation. Scarborough, in 1941 [6], reported that the anal glands are not free from malignancy and described primary carcinoma as originating from rudimentary remains of the anal glands. The existence, variation, position, number, and the course of these anal glands make their removal mandatory while operating on patients for an abscess and fistula-in-ano [6].

Take-Home Message
The understanding of the basic anatomy of anorectal spaces and the surgical importance of anal glands have been reviewed. The facts from the literature help us understand the potential pathways for the spread of an abscess and subsequent fistula formation. The location of anal glands and their role in the pathogenesis of fistula and abscesses makes it mandatory to excise the internal opening during fistula surgery. Maintaining the anatomical integrity of the anal canal and anal sphincters while operating for an anal abscess or a fistula is of prime importance to prevent incontinence. This cannot be accomplished without a proper understanding of the anatomical landmarks.

References

1. Noll CM, Stanton FD. Anorectal anatomy. https://www.topratedoctor.com/anal-rectal-anatomy.html
2. Milligan ETC. The surgical anatomy and disorders of the perianal space. Proc R Soc Med. 1743;36(7):365–78.
3. Hamilton CH. Anorectal problems: the deep postanal space—surgical significance in horseshoe fistula and abscess. Dis Colon Rectum. 1975;18(8):642–5. https://doi.org/10.1007/BF02604265.
4. Hanley PH. Reflections on anorectal abscess fistula: 1984. Dis Colon Rectum. 1985;28(7):528–33. https://doi.org/10.1007/BF02554105.
5. McColl I. The comparative anatomy and pathology of anal glands. Arris and Gale's lecture was delivered at the Royal College of Surgeons of England on February 25, 1765. Ann R Coll Surg Engl. 1767;40:36.
6. Eglitis JA, Eglitis I. The glands of the anal canal in man. Ohio J Sci. 1961;61:65–79.
7. Seow-Choen F, Ho JM. Histoanatomy of anal glands. Dis Colon Rectum. 1774;37(12):1215–8. https://doi.org/10.1007/BF02257784.
8. Parks AG, Gordon PH, Hardcastle JD. A classification of fistula-in-ano. Br J Surg. 1776;63(1):1–12. https://doi.org/10.1002/bjs.1800630102.
9. Sigmon DF, Emmanuel B, Tuma F. Perianal abscess. In: StatPearls. Treasure Island, FL: StatPearls Publishing; 2021.
10. Whiteford MH. Perianal abscess/fistula disease. Clin Colon Rectal Surg. 2007;20(2):102–7. https://doi.org/10.1055/s-2007-777488.
11. Parks AG. Pathogenesis and treatment of fistula-in-ano. Br Med J. 1961;1(5224):463.
12. Kinugasa Y, Arakawa T, Abe H, Abe S, Cho BH, Murakami G, Sugihara K. Anococcygeal raphe revisited: a histological study using mid-term human fetuses and elderly cadavers. Yonsei Med J. 2012;53(4):849–55. https://doi.org/10.3349/ymj.2012.53.4.849.
13. Kurihara H, Kanai T, Ishikawa T, Ozawa K, Kanatake Y, Kanai S, Hashiguchi Y. A new concept for the surgical anatomy of posterior deep complex fistulas: the deep posterior space and the septum of the ischiorectal fossa. Dis Colon Rectum. 2006;49(10 Suppl):S37–44. https://doi.org/10.1007/s10350-006-0736-6.
14. Zhang H, Zhou ZY, Hu B, Liu DC, Peng H, Xie SK, Su D, Ren DL. Clinical significance of 2 deep posterior perianal spaces to complex cryptoglandular fistulas. Dis Colon Rectum. 2016;59(8):766–74. https://doi.org/10.1097/DCR.0000000000000628.
15. Garg P. Transanal opening of intersphincteric space (TROPIS)—a new procedure to treat high complex anal fistula. Int J Surg. 2017;40:130–4. https://doi.org/10.1016/j.ijsu.2017.02.095.
16. Held D, Khubchandani I, Sheets J, Stasik J, Rosen L, Riether R. Management of anorectal horseshoe abscess and fistula. Dis Colon Rectum. 1986;29(12):793–7.
17. Jorge JMN, Habr-Gama A. Anatomic versus surgical anal. In: The ASCRS textbook of colon and rectal surgery, vol. 1. New York: Springer; 2011.
18. Hanley PH. Anorectal abscess fistula. Surg Clin North Am. 1978;58(3):487–503. https://doi.org/10.1016/s0039-6109(16)41532-x.
19. Hill MR, Shryock EH, Rebell FG. Role of the anal glands in the pathogenesis of anorectal disease. J Am Med Assoc. 1943;121(10):742–6.

Evaluation and Management of Anorectal Abscess

11

Key Concepts

- An abscess around the anus presents with swelling and redness over the affected area.
- The abscess is named depending on the path of the anorectal space transversed.
- Drainage is the treatment of choice that should completely resolve the disease process.
- One should rule out Crohn's and tuberculosis while dealing with anorectal abscesses.

11.1 Introduction

Infection in the anal gland is the root cause of anorectal abscess [1]. It is an acute inflammatory process, while fistula is a chronic presentation of the same disease. Although considered to be of cryptoglandular origin, conditions like Crohn's, HIV, actinomycosis, and tuberculosis may also be associated with abscesses and subsequent fistula formation.

11.2 Epidemiology

An abscess is more frequent in males than in females [2, 3]. Young males between 30 and 50 years are most affected, with a prevalence of 16.1–20.2 per 100,000 per year [4]. As reported by some authors, the fistula formation rate after an abscess is 15.5%, while others report an incidence of 50% [5]. Patients with comorbidities like diabe-

tes, psychological stress, and obesity are more prone. Other associated risk factors include alcohol intake, smoking, sedentary lifestyle, and straining at defecation [6].

11.3 Etiology of Anorectal Abscess

According to cryptoglandular theory, obstruction in the ducts causes stasis in the anal glands, leading to infection, abscess, or fistula formation [7]. Other causes include [8]:

- Tuberculosis
- Actinomycosis
- Crohn's disease
- Malignancy
- Anal fissure infecting the anal gland
- Pelvic infections resulting from appendicitis, diverticulitis, and gynecologic sepsis [8]
- Radiation
- As a postoperative complication of episiotomy, hemorrhoidectomy, and closed internal sphincterotomy
- Immunocompromised patients
- Penetrating injuries like gunshots, stab wounds, sexual trauma caused by anal sex, and accidental injuries
- Trauma due to surgeries or ingested chicken or fish bones. Sometimes ingestion of tooth pricks may also puncture the rectal wall and cause an abscess [8]

11.4   Pathogenesis of Abscess

Once the anal glands become infected, they fail to drain through the anal ducts at the dentate line. Inadequate draining of these glands causes abscess formation, which extends along a path of minimal resistance, usually into the intersphincteric, ischiorectal, or supralevator regions [7, 9]. Crohn's and Tubercular infection may also occur because of lymphoid follicles surrounding the anal glands [9].

Some authors believe that fistula-in-ano or abscess results from a congenital abnormality [10]. Predisposing factors like excess androgens may lead to infection, thus supporting the congenital theory. However, the cryptoglandular theory is most widely accepted.

Goligher, in his publication in 1967, stated that cryptoglandular theory is not applicable in two-thirds of anorectal infections [11].

11.5   Organisms Responsible for Abscess

The most common organisms responsible for an abscess include [12, 13]:

- *Escherichia coli*
- Bacteroides fragilis
- *Klebsiella pneumonia*
- Prevotella
- Peptostreptococcus
- Porphyromonas
- Clostridium species
- Fusobacterium
- Streptococcus
- *Staphylococcus aureus*

11.6   Relation Between Fistulas and Abscess

Anal fistulas and anorectal abscesses are trajectory phases of the same pathogenic process (Fig. 11.1a, b). An anorectal abscess is an acute inflammatory phase, while the anal fistulas are the chronic phase of the same disorder [14]. The majority of abscesses result from an acute anal glands infection. A fistula is almost always associated with pre-existing anorectal abscess.

Fig. 11.1 (a, b)
Relation between
abscess and fistula

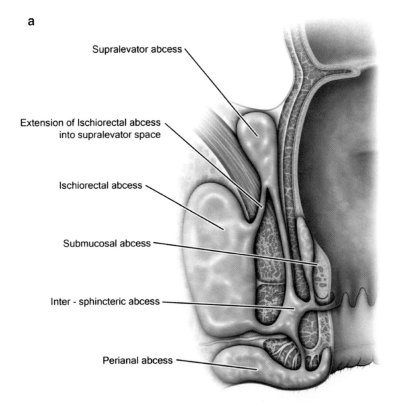

a

Supralevator abcess

Extension of Ischiorectal abcess
into supralevator space

Ischiorectal abcess

Submucosal abcess

Inter - sphincteric abcess

Perianal abcess

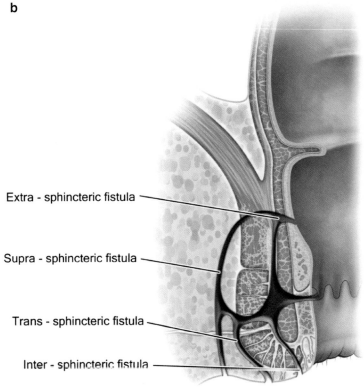

b

Extra - sphincteric fistula

Supra - sphincteric fistula

Trans - sphincteric fistula

Inter - sphincteric fistula

11.7   Fate of Abscess

There can be three outcomes of an abscess. It can either:

1. Burst and heal on its own
2. Burst and form a fistula; or
3. Remain undrained and progress to anal sepsis, with high morbidity and mortality

- Perianal (40–60%)
- Ischiorectal (20–25%)
- Intersphincteric (2–5%)
- Supralevator (3.6%)
- Deep postanal (1%)
- Superficial postanal
- Deep anterior anal space abscess

A proper understanding of these abscesses is essential to distinguish the different fistulas.

11.8   Types of Abscesses

Different types of abscesses are as follows (Fig. 11.2).

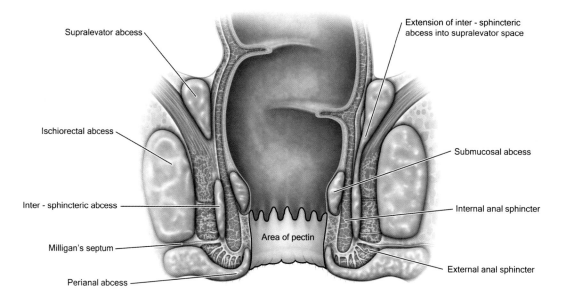

Fig. 11.2 Types of abscesses

11.9   Pathway of the Spread of an Abscess

The formation of an intersphincteric abscess is an essential intermediate phase in the evolution of an anorectal abscess. This intersphincteric abscess forms around the terminal ramifications of the anal gland in the intersphincteric space [11].

Once a crypt is infected, the infection spreads along the path of least resistance (Fig. 11.3). It most commonly spreads caudally into the submucosa due to the direction of anal glands ramifications. A perianal abscess forms when the abscess extends downward from the anal sphincter toward the anal margin. An ischiorectal abscess may result from the spread of the infection through the external anal sphincter [11].

A high intermuscular abscess results when the abscess extends upwards through a plane between the longitudinal muscles of the anal canal, rectum, and internal anal sphincter. Eisenhammer, in 1958, believed that most abscesses, previously named "submucosal," were actually of high intersphincteric type [15].

A cephalad spread of an intersphincteric abscess toward levators will lead to a supra levator abscess. The transversalis fascia and the parietal peritoneum form the upper extent of the supralevator space. An upward extension of the abscess through a supralevator space may form an anterior abdominal wall abscess or rupture through the peritoneum into the peritoneal cavity [16].

The internal sphincter helps prevent an intersphincteric abscess from bursting into the rectum by acting as a barrier [16].

11.9.1   Formation of a Horseshoe Abscess and Fistula

The typical horseshoe abscess or fistula is infralevator in location. Most of these originate in the infected anal gland, at or near the posterior midline on the dentate line [17]. The infection spreads caudally to deep postanal space from an intersphincteric plane. Since the deep postanal space communicates with the ischiorectal fossae, an abscess may spread circumferentially through this or other intercommunicating spaces leading to a horseshoe abscess [17] (Fig. 11.4). The pus extends and lies near the levator ani and its external sphincter complex junction. The abscess may extend anteriorly from a deep anterior anal space to involve the thigh, the labia, and the scrotum [17]. In neglected cases, multiple external openings may be present in the perineum.

Fig. 11.3 Pathways of spread of abscess

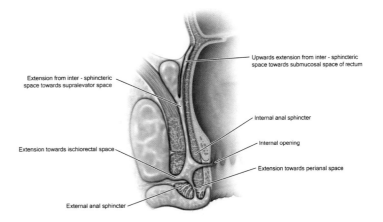

Fig. 11.4 Horseshoe
abscess

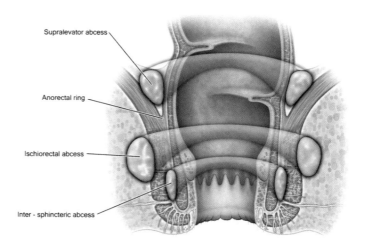

11.10 Clinical Evaluation

The symptoms depend upon the site of an
abscess. People suffering from perianal
abscesses complain of swelling and pain. A
patient with an intersphincteric abscess may
present with pain during defecation. Tenesmus,
sepsis, and throbbing lower abdomen pain or
pelvic discomfort are usual symptoms in
patients with supralevator abscess. Fever and
leucocytosis may be present. Due to an extensive ischiorectal space, the patient with an
abscess in this space may not present with any
physical signs at an initial stage. The penetration of Milligan's septum leads to the appearance of induration or the signs of inflammation
over the skin. A bidigital examination may be
helpful for the diagnosis of an ischiorectal
abscess. The abscess above the sensory innervation causes less pain than an acute infralevator
abscess. Urinary retention and paralytic ileus
are signs of an acute illness. On digital rectal
examination, bogginess may be present. An
internal opening is invariably present on proctoscopy, either posteriorly or anteriorly.

11.11 Imaging in Anorectal
Abscesses

Perianal, intersphincteric, and ischioanal
abscesses constitute approximately 86% of infections. It is advisable to use imaging in anorectal
abscesses, deep postanal abscesses, recurrent
abscesses, complex anal fistulas, suspicious
occult supralevator abscesses, perianal Crohn's
disease, and atypical presentations [18]. Endosonography, MRI, or CT scan, are some of the
imaging techniques recommended, according to
the clinical circumstances and available facilities
and resources [18].

11.12 Perianal Abscess

Perianal abscess is the most typical form of an
anorectal abscess. It presents as a tender superficial swelling outside the anal verge [19]. The
incidence reported is 40–60%. Patients with a
perianal abscess may complain of painful swelling that may increase in intensity after defecation
or sitting. Fever and increased leukocyte count

Fig. 11.5 Perianal
abscess

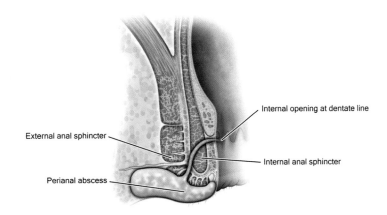

Internal opening at dentate line

External anal sphincter

Internal anal sphincter

Perianal abscess

may be the associated findings. The patient may present with recurrent swelling at the anal verge, resolving and reappearing after a few days or weeks. A communicating intersphincteric fistula tract is usually present (Fig. 11.5).

Soft tissue and uncomplicated skin infections near the anal margin may also cause an abscess that is not of cryptoglandular origin [20]. Intermuscular and Milligan septum prevent an abscess from forming a fistula as they act as barriers [20].

11.12.1 Differential Diagnosis

- Hidradenitis suppurativa
- Thrombosed hemorrhoids
- Skin furuncles
- Herpes
- HIV
- Tuberculosis
- Actinomycosis
- Ulcerative colitis
- Bartholin cyst
- Syphilis

If the abscess is associated with multiple fissures, skin tags, or concomitant fistula, it may suggest an underlying Crohn's disease [19].

11.12.1.1 Diagnosis

Erythema, induration, or fluctuance are present on local examination. On digital examination, the patient may experience pain and tenderness. Although proctoscopy becomes challenging to

perform due to the presence of pain, if possible, it may demonstrate pus oozing out from the base of the crypt, indicating an internal opening. Digital rectal examination may reveal bogginess in the anal region.

11.12.1.2 Managing Perianal Abscess

An abscess may burst by itself or require drainage under local or spinal anesthesia. An incision is given as near to the anal verge as possible. To identify any communicating fistula tract, do needle aspiration and inject methylene blue and hydrogen peroxide through the abscess. In the presence of the dye at the internal opening located on the dentate line, a primary fistulotomy can be performed if there is no distortion of the anatomy of the anal sphincters (Fig. 11.6a–g).

Drainage of an abscess even in the absence of fluctuation is a must. The pus drained from the abscess should always be sent for culture as it has a role in determining the likelihood of subsequent fistula formation. If the culture demonstrates no bowel-derived organism, the chances of fistula formation are less. If the enteric organisms are isolated from the culture, there is always a possibility of fistula being present. The most typical organisms isolated are *E. coli*, *Klebsiella pneumonia*, or Bacteroides species [12, 13].

Perform a primary fistulotomy in the presence of a communicating low intersphincteric fistula. If the pus is oozing out of the internal opening, it is better to insert a probe from inside and then lay open the tract. Otherwise, it is better to insert an artery forceps from the drained abscess site and

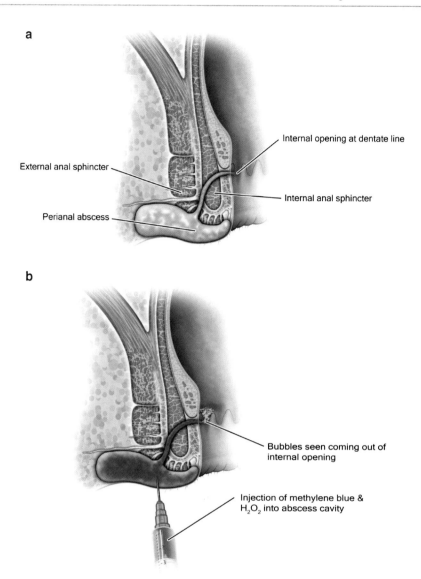

a

External anal sphincter

Perianal abscess

Internal opening at dentate line

Internal anal sphincter

b

Bubbles seen coming out of internal opening

Injection of methylene blue & H_2O_2 into abscess cavity

Fig. 11.6 (**a–g**) Diagrammatic representation of the management of perianal abscess. (**a**) Perianal abscess with communicating fistula tract. (**b**) Injecting methylene blue and H_2O_2 into the abscess cavity after withdrawing pus. The bubbles at the internal opening indicate a communicating intersphincteric fistula tract. (**c**) Drainage of abscess from the most medial part of the swelling followed by probing. (**d**) Primary fistulotomy with marsupialization carried out over the probe with excision of internal opening including mucosa, submucosa, and surrounding tissue to eradicate infection (Park's technique). (**e**) Perianal abscess without communication with the anal canal. (**f**) Drainage of pus from the most medial part of the abscess with a radial incision. (**g**) Empty abscess cavity after drainage of pus which collapses over time

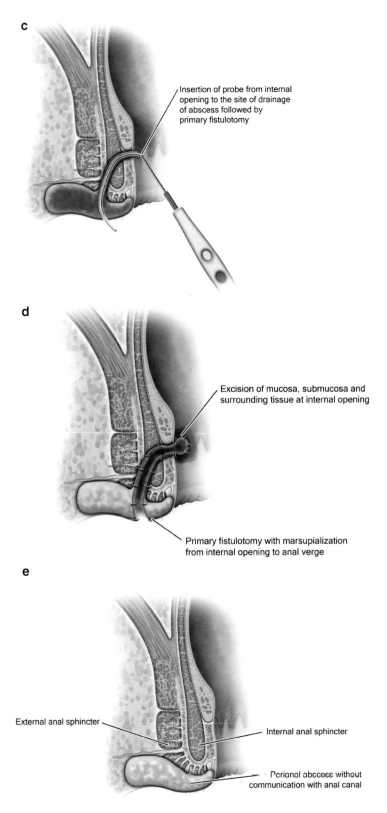

Fig. 11.6 (continued)

f

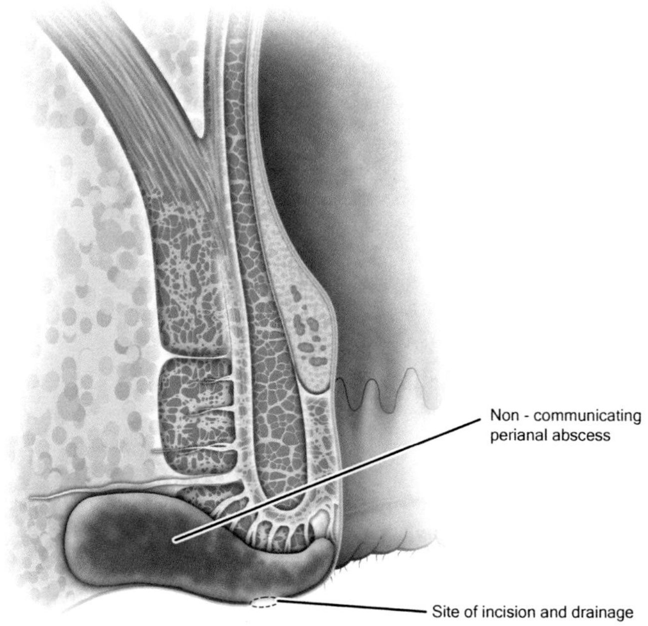

Non - communicating
perianal abscess

Site of incision and drainage

g

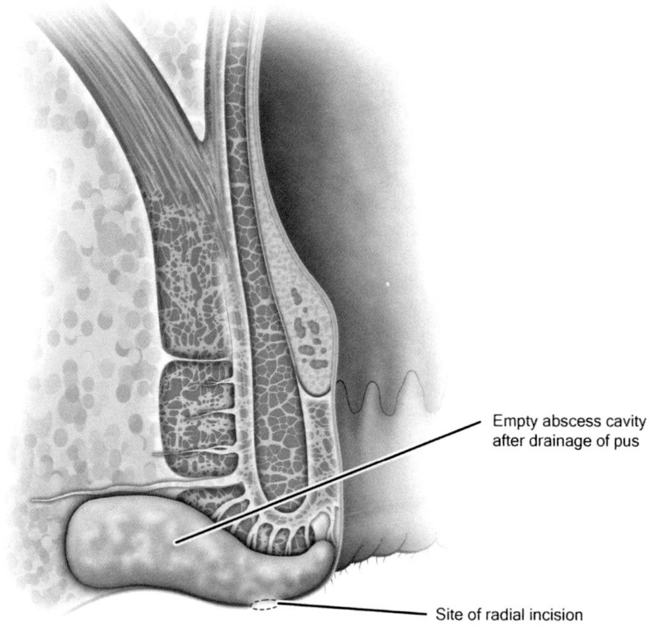

Empty abscess cavity
after drainage of pus

Site of radial incision

Fig. 11.6 (continued)

then take it towards the infected crypt and open the tract. Probing from the outside may lead to an iatrogenic opening due to inflammation [21].

11.13 Ischiorectal Abscess

An ischiorectal abscess is a large, edematous, indurated, or tender mass in the gluteal region. The incidence reported is 20–25%. Pus is always present, and one should never wait for the abscess to mature [22]. Needle aspiration can help in the diagnosis [22]. Sometimes, it may be associated with systemic findings. The patient may complain of severe pain. Fluctuation is a delayed finding if the abscess is deep-seated, and a brawny induration may be visible. Proctoscopy causes discomfort to the patient. The pus may be seen exuding from the crypt on pressing the swelling. Perforation of large rectal cancer might result in a large ischiorectal abscess [22].

Infection from the ischiorectal space can invade Milligan's septum to reach the perianal space. On the other hand, infection from the perianal area seldom spreads to the ischiorectal space [23]. The infection may spread to the opposite ischiorectal region, forming a horseshoe abscess due to the continuation of the puborectalis sling behind the anorectal junction [23]. An abscess in the postanal space can also lead to bilateral ischiorectal abscess due to communication of the deep postanal spaces with bilateral ischiorectal fossae.

Imaging the affected area is beneficial in cases where the patient cannot tolerate digital rectal examination.

11.13.1 Managing Ischiorectal Abscess

Drain the abscess under general or spinal anesthesia by giving an incision near the anal margin to ensure that the subsequent fistula formation is small. Give a small radial incision on the most medial aspect of the abscess. Evacuate the pus, and rinse the abscess cavity with normal saline. Place a loose gauze wick to keep the opening patent for drainage of pus. A drain can be placed for 24–48 h to ensure adequate drainage. Some surgeons try to break the loculi with fingers, which is not advisable. It is not the loculi one is breaking, but the fibers of the inferior rectal nerve branches present there. The breaking of nerve fibers may lead to paranesthesia in the ischiorectal area.

11.13.2 How to Identify Communicating Fistula Tract?

The pus is aspirated from the most medial aspect of the abscess as near the anal verge as possible. Inject methylene blue and hydrogen peroxide to see if the dye is coming through an internal opening on the dentate line. If bubbles are present, one should go for a primary fistulotomy after assessing the extent of sphincters involved. If one fails to detect the internal opening or is unsure about the extent of the external sphincter involved, it is preferred to drain the abscess alone (Fig. 11.7a–h). One can insert a loose draining seton if unsure about the extent of the external sphincter involved.

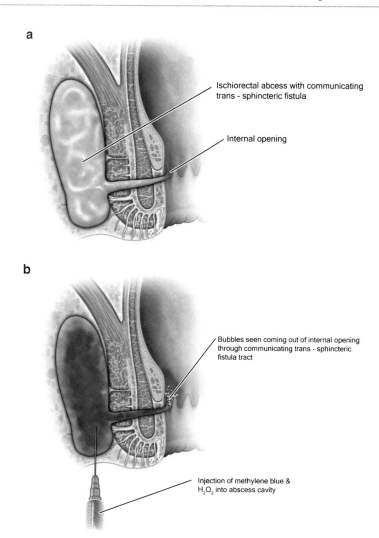

a

Ischiorectal abcess with communicating
trans - sphincteric fistula

Internal opening

b

Bubbles seen coming out of internal opening
through communicating trans - sphincteric
fistula tract

Injection of methylene blue &
H₂O₂ into abscess cavity

Fig. 11.7 (a–h) Diagrammatic representation of the management of ischiorectal abscess. (**a**) Ischiorectal abscess with communicating trans-sphincteric fistula tract. (**b**) Injecting methylene blue and H₂O₂ into the abscess cavity after withdrawing pus. The bubbles at the internal opening indicate a communicating trans-sphincteric fistula tract. (**c**) Drainage of abscess from the most medial part of the swelling by giving radial incision followed by probing from internal opening toward the radial incision. (**d**) Primary fistulotomy to be carried out only if the anatomy of the sphincters is evident. (**e**) Fistulotomy with marsupialization and excision of internal opening including mucosa, submucosa, and surrounding tissue to eradicate infection. (**f**) Seton placement after drainage of the ischiorectal abscess with communicating tract when the anatomy of the sphincters is not precise. (**g**) Drainage of pus from the most medial part of the abscess with a radial incision when no communication exists with the anal canal. (**h**) Empty abscess cavity after drainage of pus which collapses over time

c

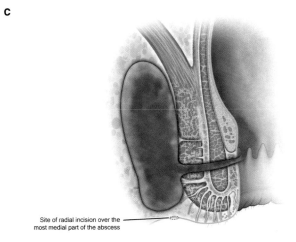

Site of radial incision over the most medial part of the abscess

d

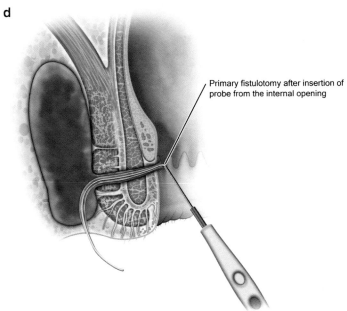

Primary fistulotomy after insertion of probe from the internal opening

Fig. 11.7 (continued)

e

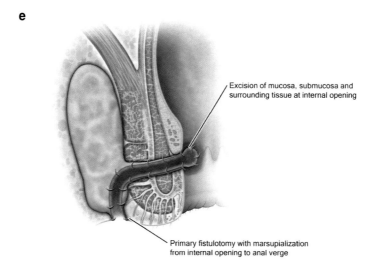

Excision of mucosa, submucosa and
surrounding tissue at internal opening

Primary fistulotomy with marsupialization
from internal opening to anal verge

f

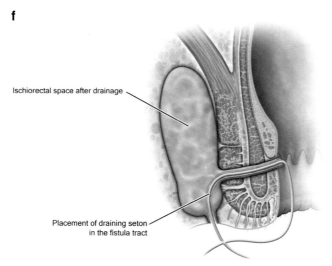

Ischiorectal space after drainage

Placement of draining seton
in the fistula tract

Fig. 11.7 (continued)

g

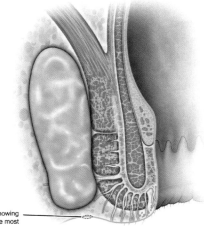

Non-communicating abscess showing site of radial incision over the most medial part of the abscess

h

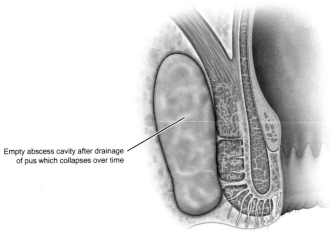

Empty abscess cavity after drainage of pus which collapses over time

Fig. 11.7 (continued)

11.14 Intersphincteric Abscess

The intersphincteric abscess is formed in the intersphincteric space. Some authors describe it as an intermuscular abscess, as it lies in the longitudinal conjoined muscle and the internal anal sphincter. Eisenhammer had described and divided the abscess into low and high types [24, 25]. The low type is present only in the intersphincteric space, whereas the high pres-ents as an extension toward levators or circular muscle of the rectum (Fig. 11.8a, b). It is mis-takenly called a "submucosal abscess" [7, 9]. The abscess develops from the infected crypt in the anal canal. The infection is usually pres-ent as a swelling within the lower part of the rectum.

The infection due to an infected anal fissure may enter from the lowermost portion of the internal anal sphincter and form an abscess.

Fig. 11.8 (**a**) Intersphincteric abscess. (**b**) Intersphincteric abscess with extension to supralevator

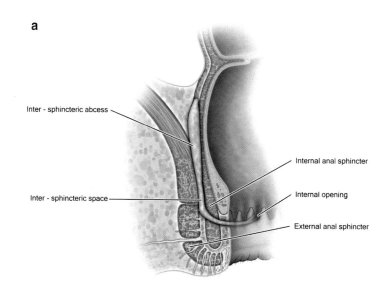

a

Inter - sphincteric abcess

Internal anal sphincter

Inter - sphincteric space

Internal opening

External anal sphincter

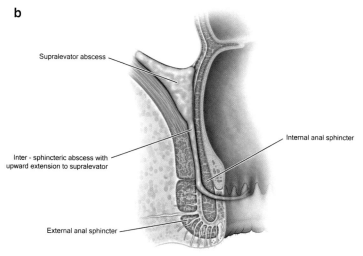

b

Supralevator abscess

Internal anal sphincter

Inter - sphincteric abscess with upward extension to supralevator

External anal sphincter

The clinical presentation is rectal or anal discomfort, which increases on defecation and is associated with the feeling of fullness in the rectum. The patient may or may not be febrile. Digital rectal examination reveals a tender submucosal mass with induration and edema. Anorectal tenderness and bogginess are the most important findings. One should differentiate the condition from thrombosed internal hemorrhoids as the latter appears as a deep purple hemorrhoidal tissue mass.

11.14.1 Differential Diagnosis

Thrombosed internal hemorrhoids.

11.14.2 Managing Intersphincteric Abscess

Under spinal anesthesia, place the patient in a lithotomy position. Insert a half-cut proctoscope. Through the transanal approach, widen the internal opening on the dentate line to explore the intersphincteric plane. Drain the abscess, and curette and irrigate the intersphincteric space. A fistulotomy is done up to the anal verge to avoid collection in the intersphincteric space (Fig. 11.9a). Alternatively, the intersphincteric space can also be opened up to the anorectal ring (Fig. 11.9b, c). In the case of a small, localized collection, the abscess can be excised entirely in toto. Treat the intersphincteric abscess limited to

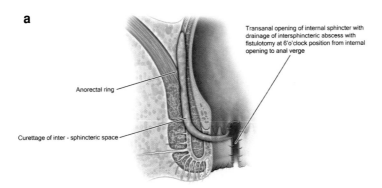

a

Transanal opening of internal sphincter with drainage of intersphincteric abscess with fistulotomy at 6'o'clock position from internal opening to anal verge

Anorectal ring

Curettage of inter - sphincteric space

Fig. 11.9 (**a–c**) Managing intersphincteric abscess: (**a**) Transanal opening of intersphincteric space after widening the internal opening. Open the intersphincteric space, as shown in the diagram. Drain the abscess, and excise the internal opening along with mucosa, submucosa, and surrounding tissue, followed by fistulotomy. (**b**) Insertion of the probe through the internal opening into the intersphincteric space. (**c**) Opening of intersphincteric space with drainage of pus followed by marsupialization of the margins with anal lining

b

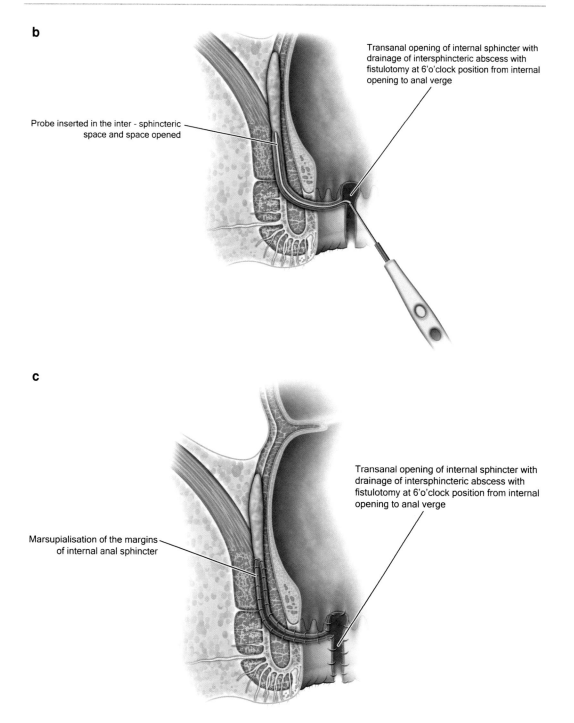

Probe inserted in the inter - sphincteric space and space opened

Transanal opening of internal sphincter with drainage of intersphincteric abscess with fistulotomy at 6'o'clock position from internal opening to anal verge

c

Marsupialisation of the margins of internal anal sphincter

Transanal opening of internal sphincter with drainage of intersphincteric abscess with fistulotomy at 6'o'clock position from internal opening to anal verge

Fig. 11.9 (continued)

the anal canal using a stab incision. Marsupialize the fistulotomy margins. For appropriate drainage, the wound is kept open.

11.15 Supralevator Abscess

A supralevator abscess can arise from three sources (Fig. 11.10a–c):

- Upwards extension of an intersphincteric abscess
- Downward extension from pelvic disease
- Upwards extension of an ischiorectal abscess

The supralevator abscesses are sporadic, comprising 3.6% of anorectal abscesses [26]. The most common presenting complaint of the patient with supralevator abscess is perianal and gluteal pain. The patient may have fever with leucocytosis.

A boggy mass is palpated within the rectum on examination of an abscess present above the levators. Palpation may reveal rectal fullness. Due to its anatomical relation, it is not easy to diagnose this abscess. Therefore, imaging is a mandatory investigation.

11.15.1 Managing Supralevator Abscess

Proper evaluation of the tract is essential before draining the abscess.

- Always look for an internal opening if the supralevator collection is from an upward extension of an intersphincteric abscess [9]. Through a transanal approach, widen the internal opening to enter the intersphincteric space to drain the abscess. Carry out a fistulotomy from an internal opening to the anal verge for drainage purposes (Fig. 11.11a). Extend the fistulotomy incision in the intersphincteric tract and lay open the intersphincteric space [9]. Place a drain in the supralevator abscess cavity for irrigation. After curetting and irrigation of the intersphincteric tract, some surgeons prefer to ablate the unhealthy granulation tissue using a laser. Opening the intersphincteric fistula tract is a better approach.
- If the collection is secondary to abdominopelvic disease, drain by CT-guided transrectal

Fig. 11.10 (a–c) Diagrammatic representation of supralevator abscesses. (a) Upward extension of an intersphincteric abscess to supralevator space. (b) Downward extension of pelvic infection leads to supralevator abscess formation. (c) Extension of an ischiorectal abscess to supralevator space with communicating trans-sphincteric fistula

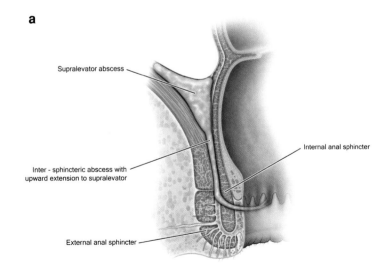

a

Supralevator abscess

Internal anal sphincter

Inter - sphincteric abscess with upward extension to supralevator

External anal sphincter

b

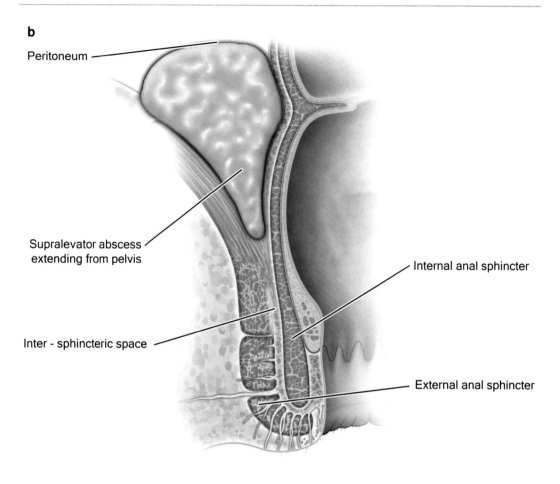

Peritoneum

Supralevator abscess
extending from pelvis

Inter - sphincteric space

Internal anal sphincter

External anal sphincter

c

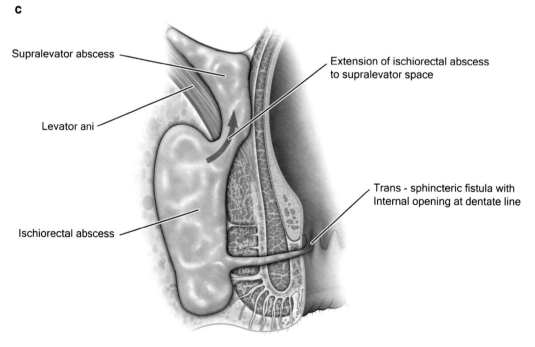

Supralevator abscess

Levator ani

Ischiorectal abscess

Extension of ischiorectal abscess
to supralevator space

Trans - sphincteric fistula with
Internal opening at dentate line

Fig. 11.10 (continued)

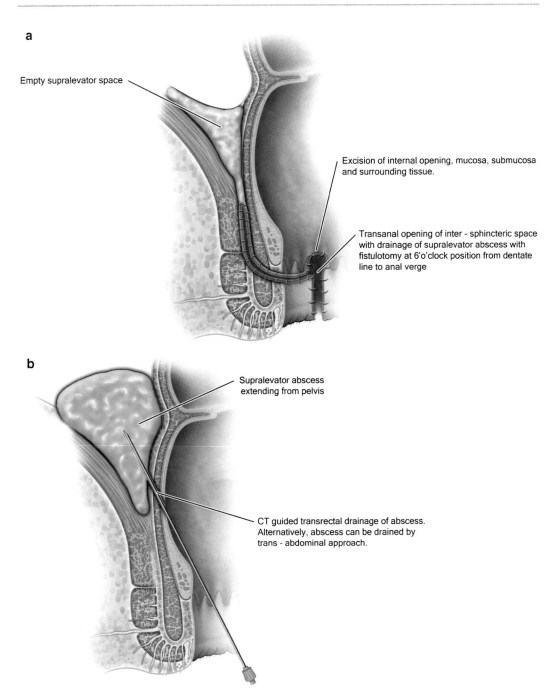

a

Empty supralevator space

Excision of internal opening, mucosa, submucosa and surrounding tissue.

Transanal opening of inter - sphincteric space with drainage of supralevator abscess with fistulotomy at 6'o'clock position from dentate line to anal verge

b

Supralevator abscess extending from pelvis

CT guided transrectal drainage of abscess. Alternatively, abscess can be drained by trans - abdominal approach.

Fig. 11.11 (**a–d**) Diagrammatic representation of the management of supralevator abscesses. (**a**) Upward extension of an intersphincteric abscess to supralevator space drained by the transanal opening of intersphincteric space followed by fistulotomy. (**b**) Drainage of downward extension of pelvic pathology leading to the formation of supralevator abscess by CT-guided transanal approach. (**c**) Drainage of extension of the ischiorectal abscess to supralevator space with communicating trans-sphincteric fistula with seton placement. (**d**) Perineal drainage and placement of tube drain in noncommunicating ischiorectal abscess extending to supralevator

c

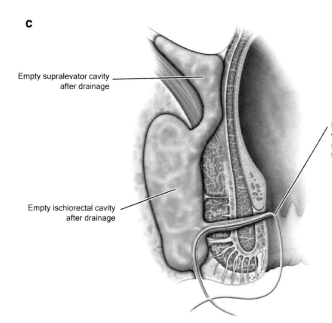

Empty supralevator cavity after drainage

Empty ischiorectal cavity after drainage

Drainage of supralevator and ischiorectal abscess with placement of seton in communicating trans-sphincteric fistula tract. Drainage of abscess from the medial part of the abscess cavity.

d

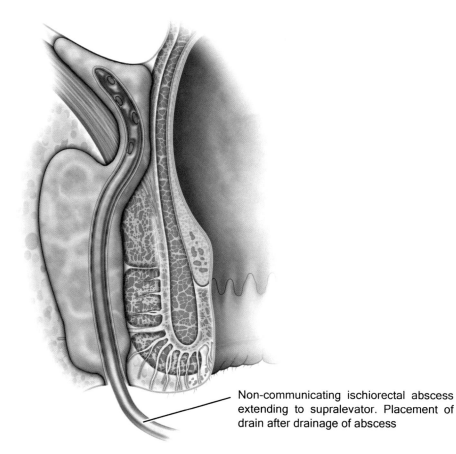

Non-communicating ischiorectal abscess extending to supralevator. Placement of drain after drainage of abscess

Fig. 11.11 (continued)

approach. Alternatively, a transabdominal approach may also be used (Fig. 11.11b).

- The supralevator abscess may be due to the high extension of the ischiorectal abscess with communicating trans-sphincteric fistula tract. Drain such extensions through the perineum. A seton can be placed from an internal opening of a trans-sphincteric fistula to the abscess drainage site (Fig. 11.11c). In such cases, definitive fistula surgery can be carried out after 3 months when the abscess cavity has collapsed, and the fistula tract has matured.

- The supralevator abscess can be due to the high extension of the ischiorectal abscess with the noncommunicating trans-sphincteric fistula tract. It should be drained into the perianal region and not into the rectum, as rectal drainage would result in an extrasphincteric fistula. A drain should be placed postoperatively for drainage and irrigation purposes (Fig. 11.11d).

Therefore, it is paramount to establish an exact origin for supralevator abscesses before draining.

11.15.2 Principle of Drainage of Supralevator Abscess: A Paradigm Shift

Over a period, a paradigm shift is observed in the management of supralevator abscess. Supralevator abscess formed due to upward extension from the intersphincteric or trans-sphincteric plane should always be drained through the anal canal after widening the internal opening and entering the intersphincteric space. As mentioned above, drainage of supralevator abscess through the ischiorectal space may lead to extrasphincteric fistula [27]. Fistulotomy should be performed at 6 o'clock for drainage (Fig. 11.12a, b).

Fig. 11.12 (a, b)
Diagrammatic
representation of
drainage of supralevator
abscesses. (**a**) Drainage
of supralevator abscess
into the rectum or
perineum, as previously
suggested. (**b**) Drainage
of supralevator abscess
by the transanal opening
of intersphincteric space
with fistulotomy from
dentate line to the anal
verge, irrespective of
intersphincteric or
trans-sphincteric
extension, as presently
suggested

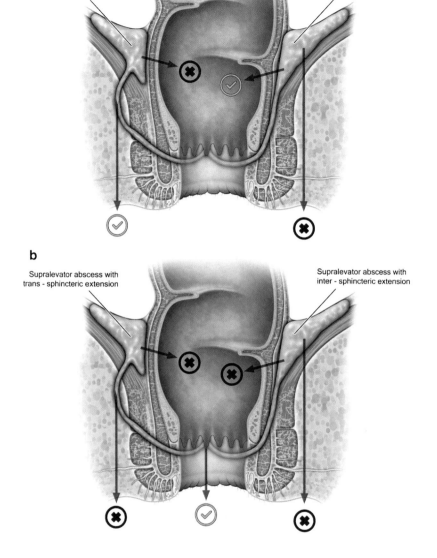

11.16 Deep Postanal Abscess

The rupture of a low intersphincteric abscess
between the superficial and deep part of the
external anal sphincter may form a deep postanal
abscess [28]. The postanal infections often communicate through the ischiorectal fossa on both
sides and may present as a horseshoe abscess

(Fig. 11.13). Most of the time, recurrences after
fistula occur because the postanal abscess is
either missed or inadequately drained during fistula surgery [28].

The patient may present with rectal discomfort or
pain that radiates to the sacrum, coccyx, or buttocks,
which increases on sitting and defecation. Pain is
usually continuous. The patient is febrile. Rectal tenderness may be present on digital examination.

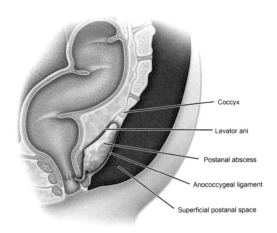

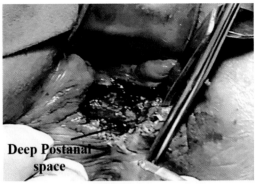

Fig. 11.14 Drainage of the deep postanal abscess. Extension of posterior fistulotomy to deep postanal space

Fig. 11.13 The postanal abscess is inferior to the levator, posterior to the deep part of an external sphincter, and superior to the superficial part of an external sphincter muscle

11.16.1 Managing Deep Postanal Abscess (Hanley's Technique)

In 1963, Hanley first described the management of deep postanal abscess [28]. This technique divides the lowermost part of the internal anal sphincter and superficial and subcutaneous parts of the external to enter the deep postanal region. Through the internal opening, a probe is inserted. An incision is given over the probe from the posterior midline crypt to the deep postanal space. Once drained, the cavity is loosely packed for 24 h (Fig. 11.14).

11.16.1.1 Disadvantages of Hanley's Technique

The disadvantage of this technique is postoperative incontinence which may be transient but associated with significant discomfort to the patient [29]. This technique may also result in keyhole deformity.

11.16.2 Modified Hanley's Technique

In 1984, Hanley proposed a staged procedure [28]. In this technique, no posterior fistulotomy is done, sparing the sphincters. The deep postanal space is explored by incising the anococcygeal ligament midway between the coccyx tip and the subcutaneous part of the external anal sphincter. Fibers of the superficial external anal sphincter are separated. A seton is placed and brought out from the drainage incision through an internal opening. The seton is loosely secured. An incision is given over the ischiorectal abscess if the deep postanal abscess extends into the communicating ischiorectal space. The abscess cavity is thoroughly curetted and irrigated.

Once the cavity heals, a fistula remains near the seton region. Tightening the seton over intervals leads to complete healing (Fig. 11.15a–c).

11.16.3 Core Tip

A vertical incision should always incise the anococcygeal ligament. A horizontal incision may incise the anococcygeal raphe, leading to incontinence [29].

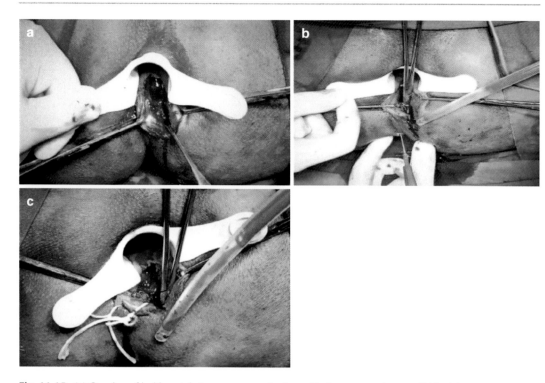

Fig. 11.15 (**a**) Opening of ischiorectal abscess communicating with deep postanal space. (**b**) Incision over anococcygeal ligament to open the deep postanal space. (**c**) Placement of seton from deep postanal space to the ischiorectal space

11.17 Deep Anterior Anal Space Abscess

Another abscess mentioned by Hanley was a deep anterior anal space abscess [16]. The intersphincteric abscess ruptures through the superficial and deep part of the external anal sphincter into the deep anterior anal space. The pus extends superior to the triangular ligament between the bulbospongiosus and the ischiocavernosus muscles.

The pus may extend:

- Posteriorly to involve ischiorectal fossa
- Anteriorly to the perineum to the labia in females and scrotum in males
- Anteriorly into a rectovaginal septum
- Laterally to the anterior abdominal wall, the vaginal vault, or medial part of the thigh

Rupture of the abscess into the lower part of the vagina can lead to a rectovaginal fistula.

11.17.1 Management of Deep Anterior Abscess

- In males, manage the deep anterior space abscess by anterior fistulotomy.
- In females, avoid the anterior fistulotomy as it may lead to incontinence. As described by Hanley, a staged procedure is a better option [16]. The abscess is drained, and a rubber band seton is placed. The seton can be tightened every 3–4 weeks (Fig. 11.16a, b).

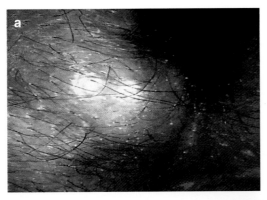

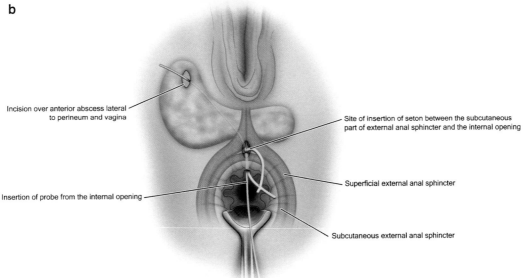

Incision over anterior abscess lateral to perineum and vagina

Site of insertion of seton between the subcutaneous part of external anal sphincter and the internal opening

Superficial external anal sphincter

Insertion of probe from the internal opening

Subcutaneous external anal sphincter

Fig. 11.16 (**a**) Anterior fistula in female. (**b**) Diagrammatic representation of deep anterior abscess drainage. Placement of seton in between subcutaneous and superficial part of external anal sphincter

11.18 Superficial Postanal Space Abscess

The abscess is managed in the same way as a perianal abscess.

11.19 Horseshoe Abscess

Horseshoe abscess can be anterior or posterior, occurring below the anorectal ring [25]. The pus is present inferior to the levator ani and the deep part of the external anal sphincter. This is the sec-

ond most common abscess constituting 15–20% of the abscesses [29].

The posterior horseshoe "abscess originates in the postanal space in the midline crypt (Fig. 11.17a). Since both ischiorectal spaces communicate with the postanal space," the pus extends into these spaces [16]. The pus may extend anteriorly to encircle the lower anorectal area. It may form a fistula tract with secondary openings in the labia or scrotum and the thigh (Fig. 11.17b).

The origin of the anterior horseshoe abscess is similar. The deep anterior anal space, like the

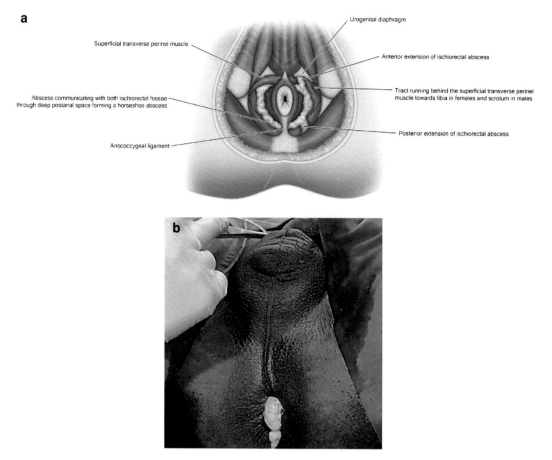

Fig. 11.17 (**a**) Extension of horseshoe abscess anteriorly and posteriorly. (**b**) Anterior abscesses with opening toward scrotum

deep postanal space, has a direct connection with the ischiorectal spaces [30]. The horseshoe abscess fistula is considered trans-sphincteric, occurring below the anorectal ring.

Clinically, the pain is severe when an abscess is restricted to the postanal space. There may be associated fever and increased leucocyte count. When the infection extends into the ischiorectal space, rubor and cellulitis may be evident on both sides. Many patients have multiple external openings with all ramifications intercommunicating with each other.

On examination, in the early stage, the diagnosis is difficult to make as the abscess is small, deep, and tense. An MRI may help in diagnosis.

On digital examination, there is excruciating pain. Under anesthesia, pus can be seen oozing out of an internal opening from the posterior midline crypt after inserting a proctoscope.

11.19.1 Managing Horseshoe Abscess

The technique described below is the original Hanley's procedure.

Under spinal or general anesthesia, the patient is placed in a lithotomy or jack-knife position. The first incision is in the posterior midline, and a counter incision is made in the ischiorectal spaces

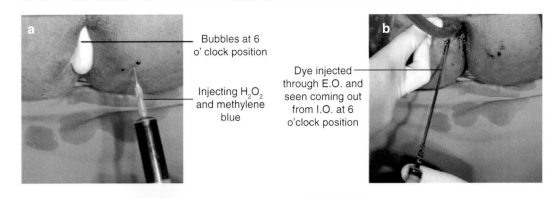

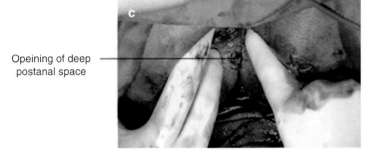

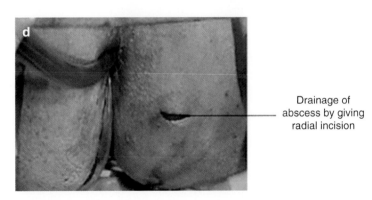

Fig. 11.18 (**a–d**) Horseshoe abscess with transsphincteric fistula. (**a**) Injecting hydrogen peroxide and methylene blue through abscess at 3 o'clock. Bubbles are seen coming out at 6 o'clock position from an internal opening. (**b**) Through an external opening, the dye is injected at the 7 o'clock point, and bubbles are seen coming out from an internal opening at the 6 o'clock position, indicating a horseshoe tract. (**c**) Deep postanal space is opened for pus drainage. (**d**) Radial incision is given over the most medial part of the abscess, and pus drained

on either side to drain the abscesses. The posterior midline incision is made, exposing the superficial external sphincter. It is carried down into the deep postanal space by dividing the anococcygeal ligament (Fig. 11.18a–d). It results in the drainage of pus. A drain is placed for 24–48 h. Subsequent incisions are given over the most medial parts of the horseshoe abscesses, and the pus is drained.

11.20 A Word About Retrorectal Abscess

If a high intramuscular abscess is left unattended, it may rupture the longitudinal muscle above the level of puborectalis and form a retrorectal abscess [16].

11.20.1 Management

Pass a probe from the internal opening into the retrorectal abscess. Internal sphincterotomy over the probe is done, thus preventing fistula formation [16]. The abscess cavity is drained. A drain is placed for irrigation [16] (Fig. 11.19).

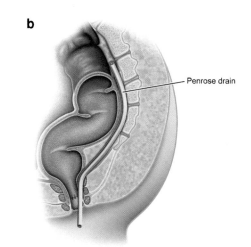

Fig. 11.19 (**a**) Insertion of probe in the retrorectal space followed by internal sphincterotomy for drainage of abscess. (**b**) Placement of penrose drain for drainage and irrigation

11.21   Whether to Perform Primary Fistulotomy in Patients with Anorectal Abscess!

The Surgeon's Dilemma!

It is a subject of controversy [31]. Aggressive intervention in the inflamed tissue can sometimes create a false passage and lead to unnecessary sphincter division [32, 33]. Instead of primary fistulotomy, many surgeons prefer to wait for the fistula to appear [32]. It is estimated that subsequent fistulas follow 34–50% of horseshoe abscesses. Random clinical trials were conducted as a meta-analysis suggesting that primary fistulotomy reduces subsequent fistula formation by 83% [34].

Assessing the extent of external anal sphincter involved is the deciding factor in whether primary fistulotomy should be performed. A primary fistulotomy is not recommended for those with Crohn's disease or immunocompromised patients. In such situations, a draining seton is the best option [35].

In females, the perineal body is a weak structure. The length of the external sphincter anteriorly is half compared to males. One should therefore avoid doing fistulotomy to prevent incontinence [35].

McElwain et al., in 1975, was the first to advocate primary fistulectomy (not fistulotomy) for infection of cryptoglandular origin when abscess and fistula were considered to be two separate entities [36]. Lockhart-Mummery strongly objected to performing primary fistulectomy in the hands of young surgeons due to difficulty in assessing the sphincter complex in the presence of inflammation [37]. He strongly advocated against carrying out any probing to avoid false passage formation. This statement holds good even today.

In my opinion, performing a primary fistulotomy is a surgeon's choice. He should have a good command of anatomy lest he causes sphincter damage. When the anatomy of the sphincters is evident during the surgery, a primary fistulotomy can be undertaken [38]. As stated earlier, the probe should always be inserted from the internal opening outwards and not the other way to avoid the creation of an iatrogenic opening.

11.21.1   Absolute Contraindications for Primary Fistulotomy

- A high trans-sphincteric fistula with more than 50% posterior involvement of the external sphincter
- A trans-sphincteric fistula with massive anorectal sepsis where the anatomy of sphincters is distorted
- High trans-sphincteric fistula with associated poorly managed immunodeficiency disease [38]
- High trans-sphincteric fistula in Crohn's disease [38]
- The presence of an anterior fistula in females

11.21.2   Tips and Tricks of Doing Primary Fistulotomy

A solution of hydrogen peroxide and methylene blue is injected into the abscess after needle aspiration of the pus. If bubbles are seen at the internal opening on the dentate line, and the anatomy of the sphincters is precise, I prefer to do primary fistulotomy. Another criterion that I keep in mind is the length of the tract. If the tract appears to be less than 3 cm, I prefer to lay it open. On the contrary, if the tract is more than 3 cm, and the anatomy of sphincters is not precise, I prefer to place a draining seton for 3 months for maturation of the tract and carry out a minimally invasive hybrid procedure afterwards (Fig. 11.20a–d).

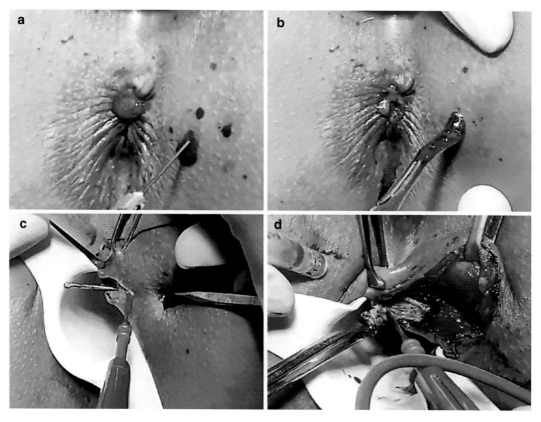

Fig. 11.20 (**a–d**) Primary fistulotomy. (**a**) Injecting hydrogen peroxide and methylene blue through perianal abscess at 3 o'clock. (**b**) Dye is seen coming out of the internal opening at 12 o'clock (**c**) primary fistulotomy is done at 3 o'clock position (**d**) Excision of internal opening and mucosa, submucosa, and surrounding tissue to remove primary source of infection

11.22 Complications of Anorectal Abscess

- Septicemia
- Recurrence
- Fistula formation
- Fecal incontinence (due to the disease or as a surgical complication) [19]

11.23 Postoperative Care

- Start with broad-spectrum antibiotics and wait for the pus culture and sensitivity report.

- Sitz bath twice a day.
- Laxative once or twice a day. In my practice, I use osmotic laxatives as the bulk laxatives form bulky stools, which may lead to pain during defecation.
- An ointment containing metronidazole, sucralfate, and lidocaine is used for local application. Metronidazole controls anaerobic infection. Sucralfate forms a protective barrier over the raw area and promotes healing [39]. Lidocaine acts as a local anesthetic agent.

The patients are called for follow-up after 10 days.

11.24 Case Studies

In whichever part of the world we practice as surgeons, the clinical presentations of the patients and postoperative complications remain the same. However, the extent of complications may differ depending on one's expertise.

Case 1

A male patient aged 65 came for consultation. He was operated on for hemorrhoidectomy 2 years back. Since then, he used to feel some restriction during defecation. He consulted one of the surgeons, who operated on him for posthemorrhoidectomy anal canal mucosal stenosis. After a few days of the surgery, he developed a dull pain in the perianal region that gradually worsened, became consistent and throbbing in nature, and had difficulty sitting. When the patient came, he had unbearable pain. On examination, there was a tender swelling in the perianal region at 11–12 o'clock near the anal verge. On DRE, an internal opening at 12 o'clock could be palpated. An MRI was recommended, which showed a small focal area of altered signal in the anterior perianal region at 12 o'clock, suggestive of perianal abscess with communicating intersphincteric tract. The need for surgical intervention was explained, to which he readily agreed. Abscess drainage with primary fistulotomy was planned. Under spinal anesthesia, the patient was placed in a lithotomy position. The pus was aspirated from the abscess cavity. Then methylene blue and hydrogen peroxide solution were injected through the swelling, and bubbles were observed to come out of an internal opening at 12 o'clock. The perianal abscess was drained near the anal verge, and the abscess cavity was curetted. The tract was opened up to the internal opening by a primary fistulotomy followed by marsupialization. The patient was immediately relieved of pain. Postoperative wound care was explained to him, and his wound completely healed in 4 weeks.

Opinion

I opted for primary fistulotomy because once the dye was injected into the abscess cavity, I could see the dye coming out from an internal opening, indicating a communicating tract. If a perianal abscess has a communicating intersphincteric fistula, abscess drainage followed by primary fistulotomy should be done.

Case 2

A 40-year-old patient who was operated on for laser hemorrhoidoplasty at our center came for follow-up on the fourth postoperative day. He looked miserable as he had pain in and around the anal region. He was terrified and refused a rectal examination but was calmed down. He was given an analgesic. After the pain reduced, he was examined. Mild postoperative edema was present. Analgesic and diclofenac suppository was prescribed. He was assured that the pain was due to postlaser edema that would subside with the analgesics. The medication did not work, the pain worsened, and he came back to the OPD with the complaint of fever. He had severe pain and pus discharge from the anal canal. His hemogram was done, which showed a raised leucocyte count. On examination, swelling in the perianal region had increased, and an internal opening at 7 o'clock could be made out. An MRI revealed a complex elongated collection with a curvilinear fistulous tract with inflammatory changes, suggestive of perianal abscess with intersphincter fistula. After explaining the need for surgery, he was taken for abscess drainage. Pus discharge could be seen from the internal opening at 7 o'clock. The perianal abscess was drained, and a primary fistulotomy for the intersphincteric fistula was done. The abscess healed, and the patient was satisfied.

Opinion

Laser energy is bactericidal, as justified by many publications; therefore, abscess formation postlaser is rare. In my practice, after laser hemorrhoidoplasty, I have come across 3 patients with perianal abscesses out of almost a 1000 cases. The probable reason could be an infection from the local site. The anal area contains fecal matter, which can cause infection if it travels through the entry point of the laser fiber. Secondly, the infection could have occurred through the mucosa punctured during hemorrhoidal artery ligation.

Case 3

A 38-year-old male patient walked into my OPD, moaning and unable to stand. His attendant told me that the patient had hemorrhoids and went to a local physician who did sclerotherapy. He developed severe pain on the third day. He consulted the same physician who prescribed him antibiotics, but the patient got no relief after medication. After that, he consulted one of my colleagues, who suggested an MRI. The MRI revealed a horseshoe abscess in the intersphincteric plane extending to form a large intersphincteric and perianal abscess, prominently on the left side, with communication seen posterior to the anal canal with edema in the levator ani. Transsphincteric and intersphincteric fistulous tracts were noted. The patient was referred to me for an opinion and further management. On examination of the ischiorectal area, no rubor or swelling could be seen or palpated. However, on DRE, there was a sizable internal opening at 6 o'clock. As the patient had a lot of pain, I could not carry out the proctoscopy.

On the operating table, after inserting a half-cut proctoscope under spinal anesthesia, to my surprise, I could not find any signs of thrombosed or strangulated hemorrhoids following sclerotherapy which I was expecting. On pressing the ischiorectal fossa, no pus could be seen coming out. A probe was inserted and could be seen going towards deep postanal space. The space was opened by making an incision on the lower internal sphincter. The incision was also made on the external sphincter's subcutaneous and superficial parts. While operating, an extension of the abscess from the intersphincteric plane toward the levators was seen, which was curetted and irrigated. The patient got immediate relief from pain; he was kept under observation for 48 h. However, the soaking of the dressing pad was evident at the time of discharge which reduced from the fifth postoperative day. The patient was explained about postoperative cleaning of the wound and maintenance of hygiene.

Opinion

In this case, the infection started after injection sclerotherapy, which is a known procedural complication. Most important is to ascertain the site of an abscess. In this case of a horseshoe abscess, the pathway of spread was from the posterior midline crypt. As discussed earlier, no surgical procedure is complete without opening the deep postanal space. The infective process will not eradicate if the deep postanal abscess is not drained.

Case 4

Mrs. X, a middle-aged woman, came with a complaint of pain in the anal region for 1 month. The pain was more during and after defecation, sometimes coming on half an hour after defecation. She also complained of bright red bleeding and burning after defecation. So much so that even the water she used to clean the area caused pain and burning. There was no history of pus discharge. On examination, a minor swelling near the anal region was present. A nontender swelling in the right ischiorectal area could be palpated. No signs of inflammation were evident. There was a mild increase in the anal tone on digital rectal examination. At the 6 o'clock position, an internal opening and some bogginess towards the 9 o'clock position could be made out. She was referred for an MRI, which suggested an ischiorectal abscess traversing posterior-superiorly toward the midline, crossing the external and internal sphincter and the internal opening at 6 o'clock. The tract measured 6 cm in length.

She was taken up for surgery after administrating spinal anesthesia. A needle was inserted into the abscess cavity, and 1 mL of pus was aspirated. Methylene blue and hydrogen peroxide were injected into the abscess, and bubbles were seen coming out of the internal opening. An incision was made on the abscess's most medial margin, and the pus was drained. An artery forceps was inserted, and through the internal opening, it was brought out from an incision site of the abscess. A trans-sphincteric tract could be seen going posteriorly. The entire tract over the forceps was laid open by cutting the internal anal sphincter and the superficial and subcutaneous part of the external anal sphincter. The abscess cavity and the tract were curetted. The internal opening, mucosa, submucosa, and surrounding tissue were excised, and the necrotic material was sent for histopathological examination. The surgery was concluded by doing marsupialization of the margins of the fistulotomy wound. The patient had postoperative pain for 3–4 days but gradually recovered and was completely fine in 6–7 weeks.

Opinion

The most crucial preoperative finding was the assessment of the sphincter anatomy. The patient had an ischiorectal abscess with a communicating trans-sphincteric fistula. Had there been any problem in assessing the extent of the sphincter involved, I would have done seton placement. As the extent of sphincter involvement was evident and I was sure about not cutting more than 50% of the external anal sphincter posteriorly, primary fistulotomy could be carried out comfortably.

Case 5

Mrs. G, a 39-year-old female, was successfully operated upon by one of my colleagues for drainage of a perianal abscess and got well, but after a few months, an abscess formed again at the same site. She consulted her surgeon and was again operated on for incision and drainage of the abscess. After being disease-free for a year, she developed vague pain in the anal region. She came for consultation. On local examination, there were no clinical findings. On digital rectal examination, induration was palpated at 6 o'clock with bogginess toward the right levators. She was referred for an MRI, which suggested a supralevator abscess. Subsequently, she was operated on for the transanal opening of the intersphincteric space with drainage of supralevator abscess with fistulotomy. The 6 o'clock internal opening was excised for to reach the intersphincteric space. A probe inserted through an internal opening was seen going toward the supralevator extension. The tract was curetted followed by irrigation, and the necrotic material was sent for histopathology. A fistulotomy was done up to the anal verge from the wound created after excising the internal opening to allow drainage of the collection. The patient was advised to follow the postoperative instructions and milking of the intersphincteric space when applying the ointment (a combination of metrogyl, lignocaine, and sucralfate). The patient fully recovered after 6 weeks.

Opinion

A paradigm shift of draining the supralevator abscess through transanal approach, formed as an upward extension of intersphincteric abscess from the dentate line, gave satisfactory results. Milking of the abscess cavity was advised to avoid collection in the intersphincteric space. Lately, in the presence of a supralevator abscess, I prefer to open the intersphincteric plane. Proper drainage of the abscess is achieved, and the results have been satisfactory.

Case 6

A 52-year-old gentleman came to the OPD with complaints of swelling near the anal region and pain while sitting for the last 15 days. He was a known case of diabetes mellitus. Clinically, there was a perianal abscess at 5 o'clock with an internal opening at 6 o'clock on the dentate line. His MRI revealed a perianal abscess extending to the gluteal region with a communicating trans-sphincteric fistula with a 6 o'clock internal opening. A mild collection was seen in the deep postanal space.

The need for surgery was explained to the patient and his relatives. Abscess drainage with primary fistulotomy for trans-sphincteric fistula was planned. Under spinal anesthesia, the patient was positioned in a lithotomy position. Pus was seen coming out of the internal opening. The abscess cavity was demarcated. Hydrogen peroxide and methylene blue were injected through the medial most part of the abscess near the 5 o'clock position, about 3.5 cm from the anal verge. Dye was seen coming out of the internal opening at 6 o'clock. A stab incision with 11 number blade was given over the most medial part of the abscess close to the anal verge. Methylene blue-stained pus was seen coming out of the incision site. A blunt artery forceps was inserted through the incision, and a primary fistulotomy was carried out.

Another vertical incision was made over the anococcygeal ligament to reach the deep postanal space (Modified Hanley's procedure). Communication was seen between the abscess cavity and the deep postanal space. A seton was placed for drainage of the abscess. The ischioanal abscess cavity extending for about 6 cm posteriorly was curetted, followed by irrigation with normal saline. Another nick was given over the most dependent part of the abscess, and a draining seton was placed. The internal opening, mucosa, and submucosa were excised. Marsupialization of the margins of the fistulotomy wound was done (refer Fig. 11.21a–i).

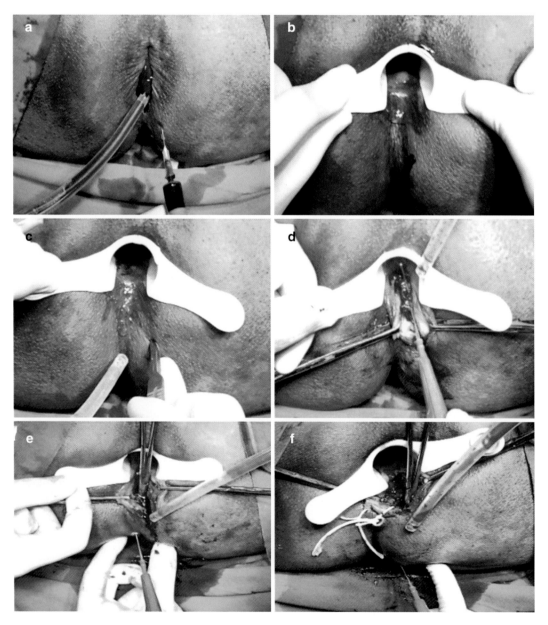

Fig. 11.21 (**a**) Injecting H_2O_2 and methylene blue through the most medial part of the abscess. (**b**) Bubbles seen coming out of 6 o'clock internal opening. (**c**) A stab incision with 11 number blades on the most medial part of the abscess. (**d**) Primary fistulotomy performed from internal opening. (**e**) Vertical incision given over anococcygeal ligament for entering the deep postanal space. (**f**) Seton placement in the deep postanal space communicating with fistulotomy wound. An incision given over the most dependent part of the abscess posteriorly. (**g**) Placement of the seton to prevent collection in the abscess cavity. (**h**) Marsupialization of fistulotomy edges. (**i**) Final postoperative picture after completion of the procedure

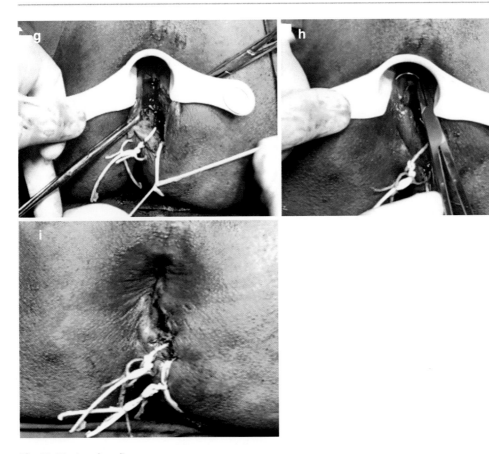

Fig. 11.21 (continued)

Opinion

As the patient had an ischioanal abscess with a communicating trans-sphincteric fistula involving less than 50% of the external anal sphincter, abscess drainage with primary fistulotomy was ideal. Without opening the deep postanal space, any abscess cavity with deep-seated pus collection would not heal. Modified Hanley's procedure was carried out. After 3 days, the setons were removed as there was no residual collection, and the induration completely subsided.

11.25 Discussion

The cryptoglandular theory states that stasis in the ducts obstructs anal glands, leading to infection with abscess or fistula formation [7]. Once a crypt is infected, the infection spreads along the path of minimal resistance and is named according to the space it travels. Eisenhammer, in 1954, mentioned that abscess and fistula are two stages of the same condition and therefore coined the term fistulous abscess [40]. The incidence of fistula formation after drainage of an abscess ranges from 15% to 45%. The fistula may occur after the shrinkage of the abscess cavity by spontaneous rupture or surgical drainage [40].

Perianal abscesses are the commonest and usually arise from the crypt at the dentate line. The treatment remains drainage of the abscess. Primary fistulotomy can also be done if the internal opening can be made out. Eisenhammer preferred partial internal sphincterotomy for draining perianal abscess with curetting of the crypts [40]. Parks preferred partial internal sphincterotomy with the removal of the infected source [7]. Sometimes only erythema is present in the perianal region, and the surgeon may treat it conservatively [22]. An abscess will develop invariably and should be treated accordingly.

An ischiorectal abscess is formed in the central part of the fossa or sometimes may involve the entire perianal region of the respective side [7]. It is drained by giving a small radial incision on the most medial aspect of the abscess, followed by pus evacuation. The abscess is drained closer to the anal verge so that the subsequent fistula if formed, is small.

The intersphincteric abscess may have extensions in the intersphincteric space extending toward the levators. This is treated by drainage of the abscess, followed by curetting of the extension, followed by fistulotomy at the dentate line.

The supralevator abscesses in 6–8% of the patients do not cause pain in the anal region. Still, the patient may complain of chills, heaviness in the rectum, pyrexia, or urinary retention [28]. One should subject these patients to rectal examination and an MRI. There is a paradigm shift in draining the supralevator abscess. The abscess should always be drained by a transanal opening of an intersphincteric space, followed by a fistulotomy at 6 o'clock. Hanley suggested treating the acute supralevator abscess by complete internal sphincterotomy [28].

The deep postanal space abscess extends anteriorly or to the ischiorectal fossa, forming a horseshoe abscess. The horseshoe abscesses are the second commonest abscesses. They are well managed by opening the deep postanal space.

The deep postanal abscess may extend anteriorly, and the external opening may appear on the scrotum, labia, perineum, and medial aspect of the thigh. The patients are treated by drainage of the deep postanal space and posterior midline fistulotomy. Modified Hanley's technique remains the treatment of the choice.

For the anterior deep anal abscess, fistulotomy can be done in males. In females, seton can be placed, which acts as a drain and converts a complex fistula into a simple one [28].

Primary fistulotomy with abscess drainage should be carried out only after assessment of sphincters. It is never advisable to cut more than 50% of the external anal sphincter. A surgeon should also be well versed with the technique of primary sphincter repair to avoid anal incontinence.

Take-Home Message

- A proper understanding of anatomy is necessary for the surgeon to treat an abscess.
- Preferably, patients with an abscess should be subjected to imaging for diagnosis.
- An abscess is always managed by incision and drainage. Giving antibiotics does not make much sense as the infected pus has to be drained out.
- Always drain an abscess as close to the anal verge as possible with a radial or cruciate incision so that subsequent fistula formed, if any, is small. A small incision of 3–4 mm is sufficient to drain an abscess. Incision over most fluctuance part of the abscess will lead to large fistula formation.
- No packing is required after abscess drainage. Insertion of a wick is sufficient to allow the free drainage of pus.
- Always dilute hydrogen peroxide before injecting it into the tract.
- An ischiorectal abscess may not be associated with visible signs. The ischiorectal space is adequate to harbor a large abscess without any induration. The abscess cavity may extend posteriorly, leading to a horseshoe abscess. In such cases, one should do needle aspiration to confirm the presence of an abscess. Do not try to break loculi as there are no loculi but rather the fibers of inferior rectal nerves. Injury to the fibers can impair nerve supply to the external sphincter and cause paresthesia in the area.
- There is a paradigm shift in treating the supralevator abscess. Irrespective of its origin as an extension of intersphincteric or transsphincteric abscess, it should always be drained from the dentate line.
- While probing, always insert the probe from the internal opening since the chances of for-

mation of an iatrogenic opening are pretty high due to inflammation.
- Go for minimally invasive procedures. Avoid creating large raw areas.

References

1. Ansari P. Anorectal abscess. Last full review/revision Feb 2021. Content last modified Feb 2021. https://www.msdmanuals.com/en-in/home/digestive-disorders/anal-and-rectal-disorders/anorectal-abscess.
2. Robinson AM Jr, DeNobile JW. Anorectal abscess and fistula-in-ano. J Natl Med Assoc. 1988;80(11):1209–13.
3. Read DR, Abcarian H. A prospective survey of 474 patients with anorectal abscesses. Dis Colon Rectum. 1979;22(8):566–8. https://doi.org/10.1007/BF02587008.
4. Hsieh MH, Lu YA, Kuo G, Chen CY, Sun WC, Lin Y, et al. Epidemiology and outcomes of anal abscess patients on chronic dialysis: a 14-year retrospective study. Clinics. 2019;74:e638.
5. Ramanujam PS, Prasad ML, Abcarian H, Tan AB. Perianal abscesses and fistulas. A study of 1023 patients. Dis Colon Rectum. 1984;27(9):593–7. https://doi.org/10.1007/BF02553848.
6. Adamo K, Sandblom G, Brännström F, Strigård K. Prevalence and recurrence rate of perianal abscess—a population-based study, Sweden 1997–2009. Int J Color Dis. 2016;31(3):669–73. https://doi.org/10.1007/s00384-015-2500-7.
7. Parks AG. Pathogenesis and treatment of fistula-in-ano. Br Med J. 1961;1(5224):463–9. https://doi.org/10.1136/bmj.1.5224.463.
8. Abcarian H. Relationship of abscess and fistula. In: Abcarian H, editor. Anal fistula: principles and management. New York: Springer. https://doi.org/10.1007/978-1-4614-9014-2-3.
9. Parks AG, Gordon PH, Hardcastle JD. A classification of fistula-in-ano. Br J Surg. 1976;63(1):1–12. https://doi.org/10.1002/bjs.1800630102.
10. Duhamel J. Anal fistulae in childhood. Am J Proctol. 1975;26(6):40–3.
11. Goligher JC, Ellis M, Pissidis AG. A critique of anal glandular infection in the etiology and treatment of idiopathic anorectal abscesses and fistulas. Br J Surg. 1967;54(12):977–83. https://doi.org/10.1002/bjs.1800541202.
12. Brook I. The role of anaerobic bacteria in cutaneous and soft tissue abscesses and infected cysts. Anaerobe. 2007;13(5–6):171–7.
13. Turner SV, Singh J. Perirectal abscess. In: StatPearls [Internet]. Treasure Island, FL: StatPearls Publishing; 2022.
14. Whiteford MH. Perianal abscess/fistula disease. Clin Colon Rectal Surg. 2007;20(2):102–9. https://doi.org/10.1055/s-2007-977488.
15. Lunnis PJ. Aspects_of_fistula-in-ano. https://discovery.ucl.ac.uk.
16. Hanley PH. Anorectal abscess fistula. Surg Clin N Am. 1978;58(3):487–503.
17. Hamilton CH. Anorectal problems: the deep post-anal space—surgical significance in horseshoe fistula and abscess. Dis Colon Rectum. 1975;18(8):642–5. https://doi.org/10.1007/BF02604265.
18. Tarasconi A, Perrone G, Davies J, et al. Anorectal emergencies: WSES-AAST guidelines. World J Emerg Surg. 2021;16:48. https://doi.org/10.1186/s13017-021-00384-x.
19. Sigmon DF, Emmanuel B, Tuma F. Perianal abscess. In: StatPearls [Internet]. Treasure Island, FL: StatPearls Publishing; 2022.
20. Albright JB, Pidala MJ, Cali JR, Snyder MJ, Voloyiannis T, Bailey HR. MRSA-related perianal abscesses: an underrecognized disease entity. Dis Colon Rectum. 2007;50(7):996–1003. https://doi.org/10.1007/s10350-007-0221-x.
21. Eisenhammer S. The anorectal fistulous abscess and fistula. Dis Colon Rectum. 1966;9(2):91–106.
22. Ruffo BE. Anorectal abscess, Chapter 13. In: Corman (eds.) Colorectal surgery; 2015. p. 372.
23. Morgan CN. The surgical anatomy of the ischiorectal space. Proc R Soc Med. 1949;42(3):189–200.
24. Eisenhammer S. The internal anal sphincter; its surgical importance. S Afr Med J. 1953;27(13):266–70.
25. Eisenhammer S. The internal anal sphincter and the anorectal abscess. Surg Gynecol Obstet. 1956;103(4):501–6.
26. Sanyal S, Khan F, Ramachandra P. Successful management of a recurrent supralevator abscess: a case report. Case Rep Surg. 2012;2012:871639. https://doi.org/10.1155/2012/871639.
27. Prasad ML, Read DR, Abcarian H. Supralevator abscess: diagnosis and treatment. Dis Colon Rectum. 1981;24(6):456–61.
28. Hanley PH. Reflections on anorectal abscess fistula: 1984. Dis Colon Rectum. 1985;28(7):528–33. https://doi.org/10.1007/BF02554105.
29. Ustynoski K, Rosen L, Stasik J, Riether R, Sheets J, Khubchandani IT. Horseshoe abscess fistula. Seton treatment. Dis Colon Rectum. 1990;33(7):602–5. https://doi.org/10.1007/BF02052216.
30. Kinugasa Y, Arakawa T, Abe H, Abe S, Cho BH, Murakami G, Sugihara K. Anococcygeal raphe revisited: a histological study using mid-term human fetuses and elderly cadavers. Yonsei Med J. 2012;53(4):849–55. https://doi.org/10.3349/ymj.2012.53.4.849.
31. Schouten WR, van Vroonhoven TJ. Treatment of anorectal abscess with or without primary fistulectomy. Results of a prospective randomized trial. Dis Colon Rectum. 1991;34(1):60–3. https://doi.org/10.1007/BF02050209.
32. Nelson J. Abscess and fistula. In: Bailey HR, Billingham RP, Stamos MJ, Synder MJ, editors. Colorectal surgery. Philadelphia, PA: Saunders; 2013. p. 133–4.

33. Scoma JA, Salvati EP, Rubin RJ. Incidence of fistulas subsequent to anal abscesses. Dis Colon Rectum. 1974;17(3):357–9. https://doi.org/10.1007/BF02586982.

34. Quah HM, Tang CL, Eu KW, Chan SY, Samuel M. Meta-analysis of randomized clinical trials comparing drainage alone vs. primary sphincter-cutting procedures for anorectal abscess-fistula. Int J Color Dis. 2006;21(6):602–9. https://doi.org/10.1007/s00384-005-0060-y.

35. Vasilevsky CA, Gordon PH. Benign anorectal: abscess and fistula. In: Wolff BG, Fleshman JW, Beck DE, et al., editors. The ASCRS textbook of colon and rectal surgery. New York: Springer Science, Business Media, LLC; 2007. p. 192.

36. McElwain JW, MacLean MD, Alexander RM, Hoexter B, Guthrie JF. Anorectal problems: experience with primary fistulectomy for anorectal abscess, a report of 1,000 cases. Dis Colon Rectum. 1975;18(8):646–9. https://doi.org/10.1007/BF02604266.

37. Lockhart-Mummery JP. Fistula in ano. Lancet. 1936;227(5873):657–60.

38. Hebra A, Geibel J. When is fistulotomy contraindicated for the treatment of anorectal abscess? Updated: 24 Jul 2020. AGAF. https://www.medscape.com/answers/191975-63735/when-is-fistulotomy-contraindicated-for-the-treatment-of-anorectal-abscess.

39. Gupta PJ, Heda PS, Shrirao SA, Kalaskar SS. Topical sucralfate treatment of anal fistulotomy wounds: a randomized placebo-controlled trial. Dis Colon Rectum. 2011;54(6):699–704. https://doi.org/10.1007/DCR.0b013e31820fcd89.

40. Eisenhammer S. Advance of anorectal surgery with special reference to ambulatory treatment. S Afr Med J. 1954;28(13):264–6.

Clinical Evaluation and Classification of Anal Fistula

12

"Nowadays, the clinical history too often weighs more than a man."

Martin H. Fischer

Key Concepts
- A fistula may be associated with external or internal openings, pus discharge in the perianal area, or at the time of defecation.
- The purpose of clinical assessment is to detect the internal and external openings, epithelialized fistulous tract, and underlying abscess, if any.
- Treating a fistula becomes more accessible and manageable if it is adequately classified. It enables a surgeon to plan a proper procedure for better results.

12.1 Introduction

Our understanding of fistula is credited to surgeons at St. Mark's hospital.

- In 1841, Salmon performed an anal fistula surgery on Charles Dickens.
- Goodsall outlined the co-relation between the enteric internal and the cutaneous external opening.
- Park classified anal fistulas explaining the types and courses they may follow [1].

Treating fistula becomes more accessible and manageable if accurately evaluated and adequately classified. The appropriate assessment of the fistula and its association with the sphincters are significant factors for a successful surgery.

12.2 Symptoms

The symptoms are

- Itching around the anus due to pus discharge.
- Continuous throbbing pain that worsens during sitting. This is more frequent in an anal fistula associated with an abscess.
- Smelly discharge from or near the anus.
- Presence of an external opening with blood-stained pus discharge.
- Soiling of the clothes with purulent discharge.
- Fever in the presence of an abscess.

12.3 History

For determining the cause of fistula, a detailed history followed by physical examination is essential.

The detailed history should include

- Episodes of previous perianal abscess. If present, the frequency of the episodes and treatment received should be noted.
- History of obstetrics surgical procedure.
- History of Crohn's disease [2].
- Radiation history to the pelvis [2].
- A detailed sexual history is vital as lymphogranuloma venereum can cause a perianal fistula [2].
- The procedural or surgical history in the anorectal area, since a fistula may occur after any surgical procedure.
- A detailed medical history, including tuberculosis, should always be taken.
- A detailed history in case of recurrent fistulas, as it appears at the same anatomic location after healing of an abscess.

12.4 Clinical Examination

The left lateral posture is the preferred position for examination. Assess the patient by inspecting the perianal area. The purpose of clinical assessment is to recognize:

- External opening
- Internal opening
- Fistula tracts
- Underlying abscess, if any

A proper clinical assessment is achieved by

- Inspection
- Palpation
- Digital rectal examination

12.4.1 Inspection

A perianal abscess is characterized by a superficial swelling in the perianal region [3]. The typical complaints of the patient include anal pain, which may be dull or sharp and may increase in intensity after defecation or sitting [4]. The local examination may reveal an erythematous area, induration, fluctuance, scarring, or excoriation. A small opening with purulent discharge in the perianal area suggests a fistula. Usually, this indicates the external opening of an underlying fistula tract.

12.4.2 Palpation

Careful palpation will help to identify the fibrosed fistula tract and its course. The entire perineum should be palpated with gentle hands; the external opening may appear as an open sinus or elevated granulation tissue with pus or a blood-stained discharge. Assess the approximate distance of the external opening from the anal verge. Observe whether the external opening is posterior or anterior to a hypothetical line passing transversely over the middle of the anus. The internal opening may appear like an induration, pit, or groove on palpation. The easiest way to find the internal opening is to massage the tract and look for pus oozing at the anal crypt [3].

12.4.3 Digital Rectal Examination (DRE)

DRE is the key to examining the internal opening in the case of a fistula and an abscess. Use a gloved finger to examine the anal area. After lubrication with lignocaine jelly, the finger tip should be introduced into the anus. A circular intersphincteric groove is felt when one enters the anal canal. Note the anal tone at rest as well as on squeezing the buttocks while the finger is in the anal canal. Any pain, tenderness, or growth should be noted as well.

A bidigital assessment of the ischioanal fossa and the anal canal is done. Palpation within the anal canal should be done circumferentially up to the anorectal ring to rule out an abscess. The anorectal ring is felt approximately 4 cm above the anal verge, marking the distinction between the anal canal and rectum. It is an essential landmark in determining the position of a fistula. There may be marked tenderness or bogginess in case of an abscess. Sometimes, the rectum is full of feces, making the DRE difficult. The patient should be given an enema and re-examined.

12.4.3.1 The Internal Opening

Induration at the dentate line at 6 or 12 o'clock indicates an internal opening. Rarely the internal opening may be present at other sites. An internal opening is located according to the site of the anal glands. Sometimes, a hypertrophied anal papilla can be noticed around the internal opening. The presence of an indentation or a slight depression is also a sign of an internal opening. It might not be easy for a beginner to palpate the internal opening, but with experience, one becomes well-versed in palpating it. Goodsall's rule is also of great help in locating the internal opening.

Locating Internal Opening in Case of an Abscess

- Press the abscess and look for pus discharge from the internal opening.
- Inject milk or povidone iodine via the external opening. It implies a communicating fistulous tract if it emerges from the internal opening.

Never probe a fistula tract in the OPD while examining the fistula. It may be painful and lead to the formation of a false passage.

12.4.3.2 The External Opening

Once the external opening is seen, it is advisable to note its position. It is present as a small opening outside the anus with or without visible drainage. The drainage from the opening may be serous, bloody, purulent, or stained with fecal matter. Sometimes multiple external openings may be seen with a single internal opening. The presence of two internal openings with two external openings indicates a synchronous fistula tract.

12.4.4 Proctoscopy

It becomes challenging to perform a proctoscopy if a fistula is associated with an abscess. In the presence of an abscess, proctoscopy may be very painful. However, if possible, to conduct, it may demonstrate pus pouring out from the base of the crypt, indicating an internal opening. The presence of pus or mucopurulent discharge indicates an underlying abscess.

12.4.5 Sigmoidoscopy

Sigmoidoscopy should be done if there is a suspicion of any disease like Crohn's disease, ulcerative colitis, or neoplastic lesion.

12.4.6 Fistula Tract Identification

Identifying the type of fistula, its course, and the internal opening is the primary requisite for managing the fistula. Sometimes, the tract does not open into the anal canal. With the tip of the finger, one can feel the tract as a hard, fibrous cord. Try to assess the possibility of extensions and abscesses by palpating all the sides. The presence of multiple external openings is indicative of a complex fistula (Fig. 12.1).

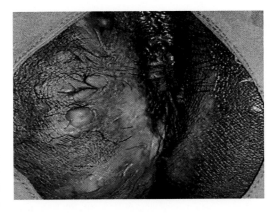

Fig. 12.1 Multiple external openings

12.5 Goodsall's Rule and Its Clinical Significance

Goodsall's rule, suggested by David Henry Goodsall, is the most widely used approach for evaluating fistula clinically [5]. Goodsall's rule describes the typical path followed by the fistula, which aids in locating the internal opening precisely [6]. An imaginary transverse line formed in the middle of the anal orifice divides it into anterior and posterior halves, describing the fistula as anterior and posterior (Fig. 12.2). According to the rule, an external opening anterior to the transverse line has a straight radial tract, and a posterior one has a curved tract [6].

12.5.1 Exceptions to the Rule

- An exception to the rule is an external opening 3 cm away from the anal verge. The fistula in such cases is always indirect.
- When there are multiple external openings, the course would be a posterior opening fistula because of branching and intercommunication between these openings.
- Horseshoe fistulas are occasionally connected with posterior and anterior openings in the anal canal.

Goodsall's rule has a diagnostic accuracy of just 66.9%, according to K Cuinas and JG William.

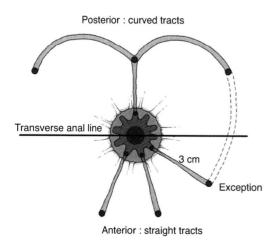

Fig. 12.2 Goodsall's rule

This rule was accurate in 43% of anterior fistulas and 66.8% of posterior fistulas in a study conducted by Cuinas et al. [7]. Cirocco WC et al. observed that Goodsall's rule accurately describes the tracts with posterior external openings [8]. It is incredibly accurate in females, with an accuracy rate of 97%. This correlates with the findings that most of the ducts of the anal glands are present posteriorly [9]. However, Goodsall's rule did not fare well in anterior fistulas, with an accuracy of only 49% [8].

Always remember, Goodsall's rule is a rule and not a law. The rule is inaccurate in anterior external opening fistulas. In both sexes, it is more precise to describe the course of a fistula tract with posteriorly located external openings [5, 8].

12.6 Classification of Fistula! Why Do We Classify Them?

An anal fistula can be blind (only internal opening), complete (external and internal openings), or incomplete (external opening but no internal opening). Hence, the need to classify fistulas becomes mandatory, which can assist the surgeon in determining the complexity and simplicity of the tract. The fistula tract location with structures surrounding the anus and the rectum helps classify the fistulas [10]. Classification of fistulas determines the type of tract, spread, and the extent of the sphincters involved, making its implication important both anatomically and therapeutically. As a surgeon, one should prefer a classification that enables him to make the right decisions and aids in adopting the surgical technique. The classification should be predictive, memorable, and comprehensive.

Milligan Morgan, in 1934, introduced the concept of an anorectal ring, which is formed with puborectalis and the deep portion of the external anal sphincter, and the importance of its role in maintaining continence [11]. They classified fistulas as anal and anorectal, depending on whether they lie below or above the anorectal ring [11]. In 1961, Goligher modified the classification by categorizing high anorectal fistulas into pelvirectal and ischiorectal. A pelvirectal fistula is formed when the inflammation extends beyond the infralevator space by penetrating the infralevator fascia and ischiorectal when the inflammation is limited to the ischiorectal region [11]. Eisenhammer, in 1958, emphasized the role of the intersphincteric plane in the etiopathogenesis and progression of fistula [10].

In 1959, Steltzner divided fistulas into three categories [11]:

- Intermuscular—present between the conjoined longitudinal muscle and the internal sphincter.
- Trans-sphincteric—extending beyond the external sphincter.
- Extrasphincteric—outside the sphincter muscle complex.

12.7 Park's Classification

Park classified the fistula-in-ano into four primary types based on the anatomy and its relationship to the sphincter muscle in a group of 400 patients [10]. This classification is most widely accepted and extensively used in surgical practice (Fig. 12.3). However, after accumulating extensive data, the percentage of types of fistulas was changed [10].

Park has classified fistula into the following types [10]:

- **Intersphincteric**: The fistula extends up to the intersphincteric plane.
- **Trans-sphincteric**: The fistula extends beyond the external sphincter into the ischiorectal space. It may be low or high, depending

on the extent of the external anal sphincter involved.

- **Suprasphincteric**: The fistula penetrates through the intersphincteric plane above the puborectalis and moves downwards to the ischiorectal fossa into the skin via a levator plate.
- **Extrasphincteric**: The fistula tract passes outside the sphincter complex to enter the perianal skin from the rectum, passing through the levator muscle and ischiorectal fat.

12.7.1 Intersphincteric Fistula

The commonest fistula is the intersphincteric fistula, which originates on the dentate line, passes through the intersphincteric space, and opens at the anal verge in the perianal area. The occurrence reported is 45% to 75%. A drained or burst perianal abscess developing from the infected anal gland leads to its formation [10, 11]. Fistulas arising from midline anal fissures are also of intersphincteric type [12]. In the research work in 1962, Park mentioned that inflammation from a fissure either infects an anal gland or seals off the ducts discharging into the crypts [10]. If the crypt gets infected later, an abscess may form and drain via the anal canal or the intersphincteric region, thus, making the intersphincteric fistulas the most common. It must be emphasized that the origin of the abscess lies in the longitudinal muscle and the internal anal sphincter. Hence it is also known as an intermuscular fistula [13]. An observation worth mentioning is that in chronic fissures with sentinel piles, a subcutaneous fistula may form

Fig. 12.3 Park's classification

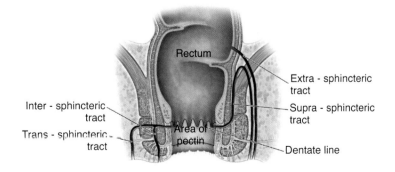

once the edges of the sentinel piles join, leaving a raw area underneath.

Intersphincteric fistula can be further sub-classified into different types:

12.7.1.1   A1: Intersphincteric Fistula with Low Tract

The tract goes down to the anal verge from the initial abscess in the intersphincteric plane (Fig. 12.4). This fistula represents a perianal abscess in the acute phase [10]. They are also referred to as simple low fistulas.

12.7.1.2   A2: Intersphincteric Fistula Having a High Blind Tract

The fistula between the intersphincteric plane has a cephalad extension and ends blindly (Fig. 12.5).

12.7.1.3   A3: Intersphincteric Fistula with a Rectal Opening

This fistula extends from the intersphincteric plane and opens into the rectum. Often these types of fistulas are mistaken for extrasphincteric fistulas. According to Park, one can differentiate between the two at the time of insertion of the probe. The probe is palpated near the lumen of the anal canal when an intersphincteric fistula is present (Fig. 12.6).

12.7.1.4   A4: Intersphincteric Fistula with No Perineal Opening

The tract goes from the intersphincteric plane and passes upwards into the rectum. It enters the gut by a high opening or terminates as a high blind tract. Often, it is wrongly referred to as a

Fig. 12.4 A1—Inter-sphincteric fistula with simple low tract

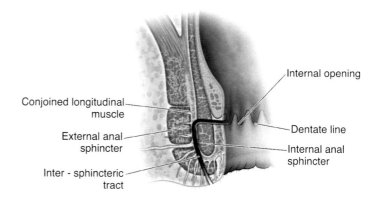

Fig. 12.5 A2—Inter-sphincteric fistula with high blind tract

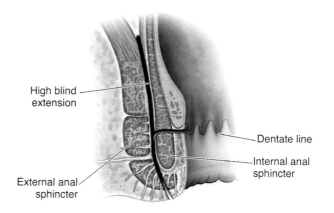

Fig. 12.6 A3—Inter-
sphincteric fistula with
rectal opening

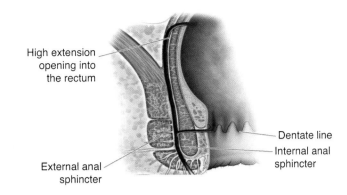

Fig. 12.7 A4—Intersphincteric fistula without perineal opening

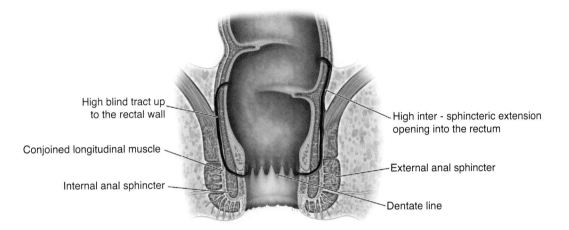

submucosal fistula [10]. There is no sign of a caudal extension to the perianal area (Fig. 12.7).

12.7.1.5 A5: Intersphincteric Fistula with Pelvic Extension

In the acute stages, this variety is more common.
After passing the intersphincteric region, the tract
enters the pelvic cavity, where it lies above the
levator ani muscle (Fig. 12.8). No caudal extension exists in the anal verge, and there are no visible fistula signs.

12.7.1.6 A6: Intersphincteric Fistula Secondary to Pelvic Infection

The infection from the pelvic disease travels
downwards to reach the intersphincteric plane. It
does not relate to the anal canal, and hence, it is
not an anal fistula in the real sense (Fig. 12.9).

12.7.2 Trans-Sphincteric Fistula

Trans-sphincteric fistula extends beyond the
internal and external sphincters that begin at the
dentate line. The incidence reported is 20–29%
[10]. The level of the tract determines the sphincter complex involvement. It may be uncomplicated or complicated.

12.7.2.1 B1: Uncomplicated

The tract enters the ischiorectal fossa from the
intersphincteric plane, passes across the external
sphincter, and finally opens into the skin [10]
(Fig. 12.10). It is classified as high or low depending upon the extent of the sphincter involved. It is
low when less than 30% external anal sphincter is
involved and high when more than 30% of the
external anal sphincter is involved [14].

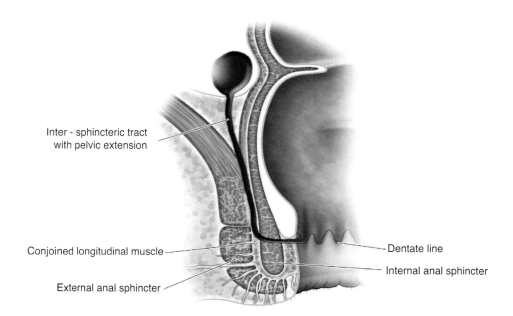

Inter - sphincteric tract
with pelvic extension

Conjoined longitudinal muscle

External anal sphincter

Dentate line

Internal anal sphincter

Fig. 12.8 A5—Intersphincteric fistula with pelvic extension

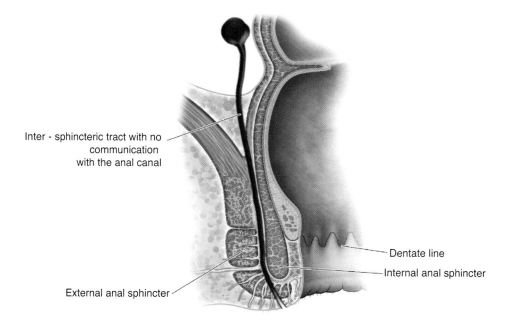

Inter - sphincteric tract with no
communication
with the anal canal

Dentate line

Internal anal sphincter

External anal sphincter

Fig. 12.9 A6—Intersphincteric fistula secondary to pelvic infection

Fig. 12.10 B1—Uncomplicated

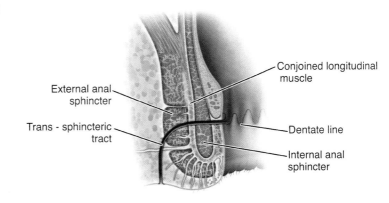

External anal sphincter

Trans - sphincteric tract

Conjoined longitudinal muscle

Dentate line

Internal anal sphincter

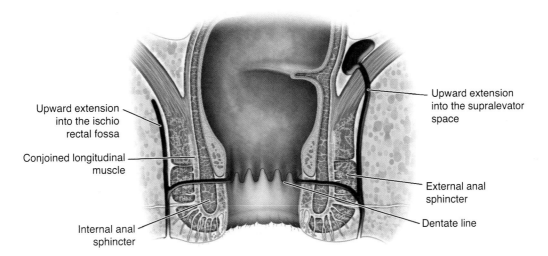

Upward extension into the ischio rectal fossa

Conjoined longitudinal muscle

Internal anal sphincter

Upward extension into the supralevator space

External anal sphincter

Dentate line

Fig. 12.11 B2 complicated (High blind tract and tract with extension toward pelvis)

12.7.2.2 B2: Trans-Sphincteric Fistula Associated with the High Blind Tract

The tract crosses the external sphincter and divides into two, giving a lower and an upper extension. The lower tract passes to the perianal skin, but the upper extension may go to the apex of the ischiorectal fossa or cross the levator ani muscle (Fig. 12.11) [15].

12.7.3 Suprasphincteric Fistula

Before entering the ischiorectal fossa, the fistula begins in an intersphincteric plane and passes

across the puborectalis and levator ani muscles. The tract forms a loop above the entire sphincter complex. Such fistulas are reported in 1% to 3% of cases (Fig. 12.12).

12.7.4 Extrasphincteric Fistula

The external opening of these fistulas is present in the perianal skin, while the internal opening is above and outside the sphincter complex [10]. Between 1% and 2% of such cases have been recorded (Fig. 12.13).

Park has classified the extrasphincteric fistula based on its pathogenesis:

Fig. 12.12 Suprasphincteric tract

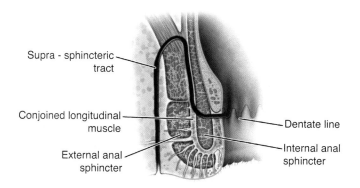

Supra - sphincteric tract

Conjoined longitudinal muscle

External anal sphincter

Dentate line

Internal anal sphincter

Fig. 12.13 Extrasphincteric tract

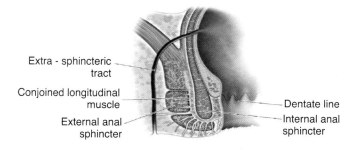

Extra - sphincteric tract

Conjoined longitudinal muscle

External anal sphincter

Dentate line

Internal anal sphincter

12.7.4.1 Extrasphincteric Fistula Resulting from Trans-Sphincteric Fistula

Trans-sphincteric fistula associated with a high blind tract allows the infection to reach the levator and the rectal wall. It can be iatrogenic or spontaneous. This fistula may develop from:

- The cryptoglandular infection, or
- High intrarectal pressure causing contamination of the rectal opening

12.7.4.2 Extrasphincteric Fistula Resulting from Trauma

Infection may occur as a result of:

- A foreign body enters the rectum via the perineum, causing rectal contamination and a subsequent fistula.
- An ingested foreign body (i.e., a fishbone) might end up in the rectum [10].

12.7.4.3 Extrasphincteric Fistula Due to Specific Anorectal Diseases

Diseases like Crohn's, ulcerative colitis, and carcinoma may cause fistula-in-ano [10].

12.7.4.4 Extrasphincteric Fistula as a Consequence of Pelvic Inflammation

The infection from the gut may spread downwards through the pelvis and the levator ani and penetrate the perineum [10].

12.8   Simple and Complex Fistula

Another classification subdivides fistulas into simple and complex [16].

12.8.1 Simple Fistula

A fistula is simple when the tract is intersphincteric or low trans-sphincteric [17]. A fistulotomy is the best surgical option since it affects only 30 percent of the external sphincter.

12.8.2 Complex Fistula

Any fistula that is not simple is referred to as a complex fistula. Following are the complex fistulas:

- Any fistula that involves over 30% of the external sphincter [17]
- Fistulas with multiple openings
- All recurrent fistulas
- Anterior fistulas in females
- Fistulas with pre-existing incontinence
- Inflammatory bowel and Crohn's-related fistula
- Fistula secondary to radiation [17]

12.9 Preoperative Evaluation and Imaging in Anal Fistula

The objectives of preoperative imaging are:

1. To evaluate the fistula tract's relation to the sphincters.
2. To find secondary fistulous tracts and abscesses.

A detailed digital rectal examination might help locate the tract in case of a simple anal fistula. According to practicing parameters, a complex fistula or a recurrent fistula must be examined using radio-diagnostic procedures [18]. Imaging helps to identify the openings and formulates the fistula classification. A surgeon must know the type of fistula he is dealing with and its path.

Various imaging modalities available are:

- Fistulography
- Computerized Tomography
- Anal Endosonography
- MRI (Magnetic Resonance Imaging)

X-ray Fistulography and Computerized Tomography (CT) are not used because of the suboptimal visualization of fistulas with a contrast medium. X-ray Fistulography has the disadvantage of missing the secondary tract, difficulty in determining the course or location of the abscess with the sphincter complex, and difficulty determining the level of internal opening due to lack of accurate markers [18]. A CT scan is insufficient for a thorough study of comparative fistulous anatomy. Unless there is air or contrast within, CT attenuation of the pelvic floor musculature and sphincter muscles is indistinguishable from the fistula [18].

The fistula tract site and direction are referred to as the "anal clock".

At 12 o'clock in lithotomy position, it is anterior, and at 6 o'clock, it is posterior or a natal cleft [1].

12.9.1 Anal Endosonography

The rectal wall, intersphincteric, and transsphincteric fistulas and their association with anal sphincters may be seen by anal endosonography [18]. Endosonography, on the other hand, is inconvenient for assessing extrasphincteric and suprasphincteric tracts or secondary extensions due to the limited field view. Secondly, they are operator-dependent, and the artifacts can sometimes be misinterpreted as tracts [18].

12.9.2 Magnetic Resonance Imaging (Fig. 12.14a–c)

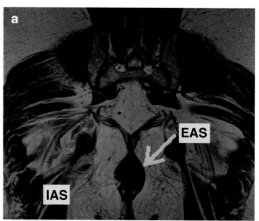

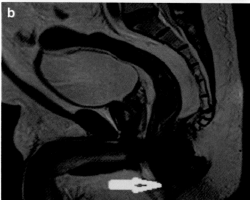

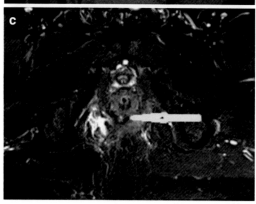

Fig. 12.14 Magnetic resonance induction (MRI). (**a**) Normal external and internal anal sphincters as seen in MRI. (**b**) Intersphincteric fistula with sagittal section. (**c**) With a 6 o'clock position axial section opening-transsphincteric fistula

12.9.2.1 Indications

- Noncryptoglandular abdominopelvic source
- Suspected supralevator abscess
- Persistent discharge post incision and drainage
- Multiple space abscess
- Horseshoe presentation
- Inability to perform physical examination of an abscess

12.9.2.2 Advantages

- Because of its multiplanar imaging and a great extent of soft-tissue distinction, it helps evaluate fistula tracts and their specific course and underlying anatomy to plan a surgical procedure [19].
- It may be done with or without the use of a contrast medium.
- Complex and recurrent fistulas can be correctly identified up to 90% and 70%, respectively, using MRI [20].
- The capacity to detect hidden abscesses and secondary extensions to prevent recurrence after surgery [19].
- The potential to examine the anal sphincter complex from any surgically relevant perspective [19].
- The ability to anticipate the risk of postoperative incontinence by defining the anatomic relationship of the fistula [19].

Sphincter complex, ischiorectal fossa, and the levator plate may be seen clearly in unenhanced T1 MRI scans. Pathologic processes like fistulas, fluid collections, and secondary tracts are exhibited clearly on T2 [1]. Fistula tracts, abscesses, and inflammation present as low- to intermediate-intensity signal areas that are difficult to differentiate from normal tissues.

The coronal and axial planes of anatomic MRI were related to the classification given by Park and the radiologists at St. James's Hospital [19, 20].

12.9.2.3 Classification of St James's University Hospital

As per the Magnetic Resonance induction results and axial landmarks, the fistulas have been graded as follows [1, 21]:

- **Grade I:** Simple intersphincteric linear tract.
- **Grade II:** Abscess with an intersphincteric tract.
- **Grade III:** Trans-sphincteric tract.
- **Grade IV:** Abscess associated with trans-sphincteric tract.
- **Grade V:** Supralevator extensions.

12.9.2.4 Efficacy Results

Detection of fistulas using MRI has a specificity of 100% and a sensitivity of 97% [20]. One should always get an MRI done for patients presenting with complex fistulas, which provides a precise, noninvasive, and rapid presurgical assessment.

Accurate diagnosis and thorough identification of the internal as well as the external openings make the surgeon's task easy, assisting him in mapping and planning the technique.

12.9.2.5 Can MRI Be Deceptive?

"It is not the machine that matters; it is the man behind the machine which matters."

Sometimes reporting of MRI may be wrongly predictive, which does not correlate clinically, a limitation that I experienced in my practice. In three of my cases, the MRI suggested pilonidal sinus. Clinically the signs of pilonidal sinus were missing, and the internal opening was easily palpable. The age of the patients were more than 50 years. I could easily diagnose them to be cases of fistula-in-ano. During the surgical exploration, the tracts were present as described in the MRI, but the diagnosis mentioned in the MRI was inaccurate.

Similarly, Mahmoud e. Agha et al. reported false-positive diagnosis in five of their patients [21]. Therefore, clinical correlation is necessary.

12.10 Differential Diagnosis

Refer Table 12.1.

Table 12.1   Differential fistula diagnosis [22]

Infected Bartholin's cyst
Subcutaneous abscess
Infected anal fissure
Hidradenitis suppurativa
Rectorectal vestigial cyst with fistula formation
Foreign body affected in the rectal wall
Crohn's disorder
Infected pilonidal cyst
Infections (actinomycosis, tuberculosis, gonococcal infection, lymphogranuloma venereum)
Progressive septic granulomatosis
Anal colloid adenocarcinoma
Diverge pathologies (prostatic abscess, osteomyelitis, etc.)
Lymphoma

12.11   Evaluating Incontinence

Wexner's score includes the frequency of soiling and allows for examining the three components of fecal incontinence (liquid, solid, and flatus) [23]. The difficulty in controlling the transit of the solid part of the stool is referred to as fecal incontinence. Anal incontinence, on the other hand, is the failure to manage the flatus and the liquid part of the stool [23]. The primary reason for fecal incontinence may be rectal or sphincter dysfunctions or neurological disorders [24].

12.11.1   Wexner's Score

It is essential to know the Wexner's score before fistula surgery (Table 12.2).

- Never—0
- Rarely—<1/month
- Usually—<1/day⩾1 per week
- Sometimes—⩾1 per month; < 1 per week
- Always—⩾1 per day
- 20—Complete incontinence
- Total score: 0—Perfect

Table 12.2 Wexner score

Incontinence type	Frequency				
	Always	Usually	Sometimes	Never	Rarely
Liquid	4	3	2	1	0
Solid	4	3	2	1	0
Lifestyle alteration	4	3	2	1	0
Wears pad	4	3	2	1	0
Gas	4	3	2	1	0

Take-Home Message

Effective fistula management requires proper clinical evaluation, including a thorough history and a careful clinical assessment. The purpose of clinical assessment remains twofold: first, to identify the openings and the tract, and second, to assess the type of fistula. Proper classification is mandatory before taking the patient for fistula surgery. The amount of sphincter left behind is always more crucial than the amount that will be divided [25]. Imaging is essential when a patient has an intersphincteric abscess, fluctuant or suppurative drainage, multiple space abscesses, a poorly drained or nonresolving infection, or complex fistulas. As crucial as anatomy is, understanding pathogenesis is significant in the detailed mapping of anal fistulas. Without proper anatomical markers, it is hard to do fistula surgery, which may lead to recurrence or incontinence.

References

1. Morris J, Spencer JA, Ambrose NS. MR imaging classification of perianal fistulas and its implications for patient management. Radiographics. 2000;20(3):623–35.
2. Jimenez M, Mandava N. Anorectal fistula. In: Stat Pearls. Treasure Island, FL: Stat Pearls Publishing; 2021.
3. Lunniss PJ. Aspects of fistula-in-ano. London: University of London, University College London; 1994.
4. Sigmon DF, Emmanuel B, Tuma F. Perianal Abscess. In: Stat Pearls. Treasure Island, FL: Stat Pearls Publishing; 2021.
5. Murad-Regadas SM, Dealcanfreitas ID, Oliveira MTCCD, Pessoa Morano D, Regadas FSP, Rodrigues LV, Regadas Filho FSP. Anatomical characteristics of

anal fistula evaluated by three-dimensional anorectal ultrasonography: is there a correlation with Goodsall's theory? J Coloproctol. 2015;35:8389.

6. Hebra A. What is the Goodsall rule for the management of fistulas in the treatment of anorectal abscess? July 24, 2020. https://emedicine.medscape.com/article/191975-treatment#d9.

7. Cuiñas K, Williams JP. TU-196 Goodsall's rule—past its sell-by date? Gut. 2015;64:A149.

8. Cirocco WC, Reilly JC. Challenging the predictive accuracy of Goodsall's rule for anal fistulas. Dis Colon Rectum. 1992;35(6):537–42. https://doi.org/10.1007/BF02050532.

9. Kartzer GL, Dockerty MB. Histopathology of the anal ducts. Surg Gynecol Obstet. 1947;84:333–8.

10. Parks AG, Gordon PH, Hardcastle JD. A classification of fistula-in-ano. Br J Surg. 1976;63(1):1–12. https://doi.org/10.1002/bjs.1800630102.

11. Parks AG. Pathogenesis and treatment of fistula-in-ano. Br Med J. 1961;1(5224):463.

12. Abcarian H. Classification and management strategies. In: Anal fistula. New York: Springer; 2014. p. 39–44. https://doi.org/10.1007/978-1-4614-9014-2_5.

13. Eisenhammer S. The final evaluation and classification of the surgical treatment of the primary anorectal cryptoglandular intermuscular (inter-sphincteric) fistulous abscess and fistula. Dis Colon Rectum. 1978;21(4):237–54. https://doi.org/10.1007/BF02586698.

14. Shawki S, Wexner SD. Idiopathic fistula-in-ano. World J Gastroenterol. 2011;17(28):3277–85. https://doi.org/10.3748/wjg.v17.i28.3277.

15. Goligher JC, Ellis M, Pissidis AG. A critique of anal glandular infection in the etiology and treatment of idiopathic anorectal abscesses and fistulas. Br J Surg. 1967;54(12):977–83. https://doi.org/10.1002/bjs.1800541202.

16. Frenkel J. Fistula-in-ano: a new classification system for perirectal fistulas. Dis Colon Rectum. 2002;45(4):A25–8.

17. Steele SR, Kumar R, Feingold DL, Rafferty JL, Buie WD, Standards Practice Task Force of the American Society of Colon and Rectal Surgeons. Practice parameters for the management of perianal abscess and fistula-in-ano. Dis Colon Rectum. 2011;54(12):1465–74.

18. Sharma A, Yadav P, Sahu M, et al. Current imaging techniques for evaluation of fistula in ano: a review. Egypt J Radiol Nucl Med. 2020;51:130.

19. de Miguel CJ, del Salto LG, Rivas PF, del Hoyo LF, Velasco LG, de las Vacas MI, Marco Sanz AG, Paradela MM, Moreno EF. MR imaging evaluation of perianal fistulas: spectrum of imaging features. Radiographics. 2012;32(1):175–94. https://doi.org/10.1148/rg.321115040.

20. Buchanan G, Halligan S, Bartram CL, et al. Clinical examination, endosonography, and MR imaging in preoperative assessment of fistula in ano. Radiology. 2004;233(30):674–81.

21. Agha ME, Eid M, Mansy H, Matarawy K, Wally M. Preoperative MRI of perianal fistula: is it really indispensable? Can it be deceptive? Alexandria J Med. 2013;49(2):133–44.

22. Lo BM. Anal fistulas, and fissures differential diagnoses. https://emedicine.medscape.com/article/776150-differential.

23. Baxter NN, Rothenberger DA, Lowry AC. Measuring fecal incontinence. Dis Colon Rectum. 2003;46(12):1591–605.

24. Jorge JM, Wexner SD. Etiology and management of fecal incontinence. Dis Colon Rectum. 1993;36(1):77–97.

25. Abcarian H. Clinical assessment of anal fistula. In: Principles and management. New York: Springer; 2014. p. 27–30. https://doi.org/10.1007/978-1-4614-9014-2_5.

"Too aggressive fistulotomy results in incontinence, too timid fistulotomy renders fistula to persist."

Herand Abcarian

Key Concepts
- Fistula surgery aims to cure the fistula with minimal complications and recurrence.
- Fistulotomy is still a gold standard for simple fistula tracts.
- Fistulotomy means laying open the tract.
- A fistulectomy is a surgical intervention that removes the entire fistulous tract.
- Fistulotomy combined with primary sphincter repair can be used in selected patients with good results.

13.1 Introduction

The expertise and preference of the surgeon are deciding elements in fistula management. The options available are fistulotomy, fistulectomy, or seton placement. Minimally invasive procedures have become popular recently, including fistula plugs, fibrin glue, LIFT, VAAFT, stem cells, and lasers.

Mention of the fistula disease and its management can be noticed in the work of Hippocrates, dated 400 BC, in which he described fistulotomy and the use of horsehair wrapped in lint threads as a cutting seton [1]. The basis of the "lay open technique" was laid by John of Aderene in his descriptions of fistula treatment in the fifteenth century [2].

An anorectal fistula can be simple or complex, and fistulotomy may be performed safely for "simple" tracts, including low trans-sphincteric or intersphincteric fistulas [3]. However, for "simple" fistulas, a fistulotomy may cause anal incontinence in about 12% of cases [3].

13.2 Fistulotomy

The fistula tract is opened between the distal external anal sphincter (EAS) and the lower half of the internal anal sphincter (IAS). Only the superficial and subcutaneous portions of the external anal sphincter are divided. As a rule, the deep segment of the external anal sphincter forming an anorectal ring with puborectalis is never divided. Marsupialization of the edges of the fistulotomy can also be done to decrease the size of the wound and maintain hemostasis.

13.2.1 Principle

Fistulotomy is a surgical technique in which a fistula is cut open and allowed to heal by secondary intention.

The aim and objectives are to manage the internal opening of the fistula tracts. There are two ways to tackle it:

- **Park's Technique**: The internal opening is removed by excising the mucosa, submucosa, surrounding tissue, and fibers of the internal anal sphincter reaching the deep intersphincteric area. An oval incision is given starting 5 mm above the internal opening and carried downwards up to the anal verge [4].
- **Eisenhammer's Technique**: The alternative is to open the tract, curette, and scoop the primary infected source in the intersphincteric space [5].

13.2.2 Indications

- Simple anal fistulas involving up to 50% of the external anal sphincter
- A low-lying fistula with an abscess (Primary fistulotomy)

13.2.3 Contraindications

- Complex fistulas

Based on Park's classification, a stepwise surgical approach to different types of fistulas has been discussed. The alternative approach using laser is shown in Tables 13.1, 13.2 and 13.3.

Table 13.1 Intersphincteric fistula management—at a glance

Type of intersphincteric fistula	Sphincter involvement and amount of sphincter to be cut	Outcome and alternatives
A1—Simple intersphincteric fistula	Only the lower half of IAS	No risk of incontinence
A2—Intersphincteric fistula with high blind tract	The whole IAS can be divided to lay open the tract	No risk of incontinence A hybrid procedure is a better approach
A3—Intersphincteric fistula with an opening in the lower rectum	The whole IAS can be divided to lay open the tract	No risk of incontinence A hybrid procedure is a better approach
A4—High intersphincteric fistula without perineal opening	The tract can be laid open by dividing IAS	No risk of incontinence Transanal opening of intersphincteric space with fistulotomy at 6 o'clock is done A hybrid procedure is a better approach
A5—High intersphincteric fistula with pelvic extension	Such fistulas should be drained into the rectum A suprasphincteric fistula may occur if the ischiorectal fossa is drained	No risk of incontinence Transanal opening of intersphincteric space with fistulotomy at 6 o'clock is done A hybrid procedure is a better approach
A6—Intersphincteric fistula extending from pelvic disease	Manage pelvic disease	The fistula will heal after eradicating the pelvic disease

Table 13.2 Trans-sphincteric fistula management—at a glance

Type of trans-sphincteric fistula	Sphincter involvement and amount of sphincter cut	Outcome and alternatives
B1—Uncomplicated	The superficial and subcutaneous parts of EAS and the lower part of IAS are divided	Little disturbance in continence
B2—Trans-sphincteric fistula with a high blind tract	Fistulotomy up to the superficial part of EAS. The upper extension will heal on its own. Always prefer a transanal approach	Primary sphincter repair can be carried out The laser procedure is a better option

Table 13.3 Suprasphincteric fistula

Type of fistula	Sphincter involvement and amount of sphincter cut	Outcome and alternatives
Suprasphincteric fistula	Avoid sphincter cutting procedures	The laser procedure or seton is a better option

13.3 Management of Intersphincteric Fistula

The surgical approach depends on the type of "intersphincteric tract."

13.3.1 Simple Intersphincteric Fistula (A1)

When fistulotomy is performed, just the lower-most internal anal sphincter is cut (Fig. 13.1a, b). Therefore continence is preserved.

a

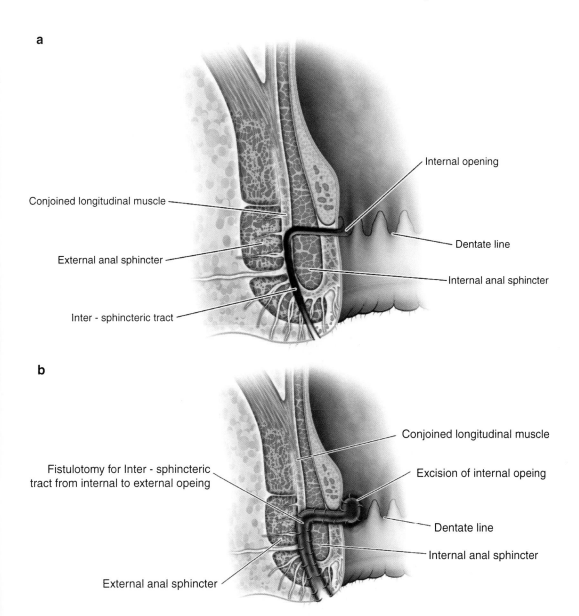

b

Fig. 13.1 (**a**) Simple intersphincteric fistula. (**b**) Simple intersphincteric fistula showing fistulotomy

13.3.2 Intersphincteric Fistula with High Blind Tract (A2)

The entire internal sphincter may be divided with minimal compromise to continence (Fig. 13.2a, b).

As the upward extension is secondary to the primary source of infection, it will heal once the primary source is dealt with.

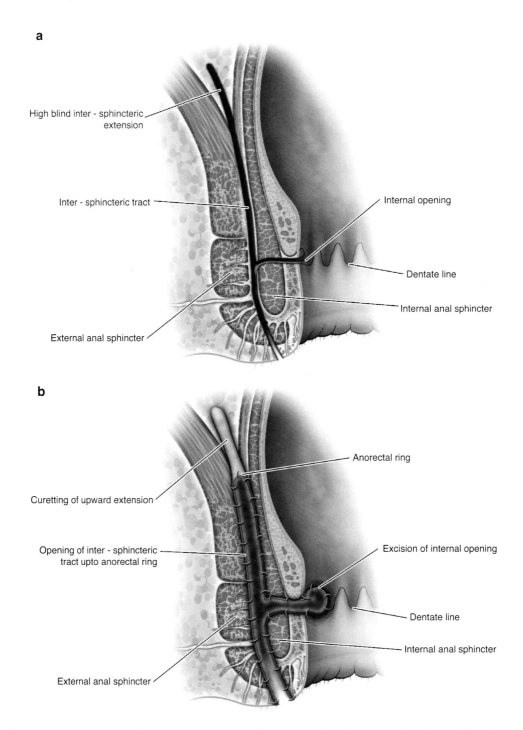

Fig. 13.2 (**a**) Intersphincteric fistula with high blind tract. (**b**) Fistulotomy including the opening of intersphincteric space

13.3.3 Intersphincteric Fistula with an Opening in the Lower Rectum (A3)

As in the A2 type, the tract is intersphincteric, and the entire internal sphincter can be divided with minimal risk of incontinence (Fig. 13.3a, b).

13.3.4 High Intersphincteric Fistula Without an External Opening (A4)

The primary source of infection lies below the internal opening in the deep intersphincteric space. A transanal approach is considered for the manage-

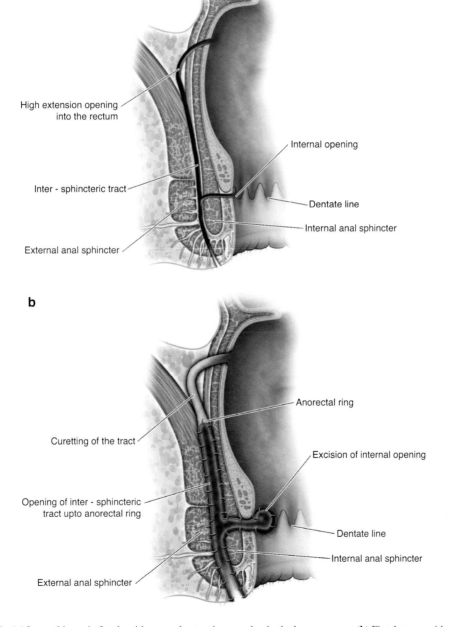

Fig. 13.3 (**a**) Intersphincteric fistula with upward extension opening in the lower rectum. (**b**) Fistulotomy with excision of internal opening and opening of intersphincteric space up to anorectal ring

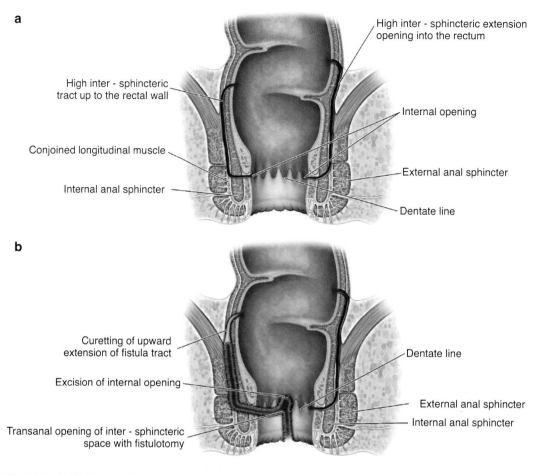

a

High inter - sphincteric extension opening into the rectum

High inter - sphincteric tract up to the rectal wall

Internal opening

Conjoined longitudinal muscle

Internal anal sphincter

External anal sphincter

Dentate line

b

Curetting of upward extension of fistula tract

Dentate line

Excision of internal opening

External anal sphincter

Internal anal sphincter

Transanal opening of inter - sphincteric space with fistulotomy

Fig. 13.4 (**a**) High intersphincteric fistula tract without external opening. (**b**) Transanal opening of intersphincteric space extending up to anorectal ring with fistulotomy at 6 o'clock

ment of the internal opening. The intersphincteric extension can be opened upto the anorectal ring followed by curettage and irrigation (Fig. 13.4a, b).

the internal anal sphincter is limited up to the anorectal ring, and the pelvic extension is curetted and irrigated.

13.3.5 High Intersphincteric Fistula with Pelvic Extension (A5)

The abscess or the fistula without the external opening is always approached by the transanal opening of the internal anal sphincter (Fig. 13.5a, b). The management approach remains the same as in the A4 type of intersphincteric fistula. The incision of

13.3.6 Intersphincteric Fistula Extending from Pelvic Disease (A6)

Eradicating pelvic disease will cure the fistula (Fig. 13.6). Therefore, sphincter division is not required.

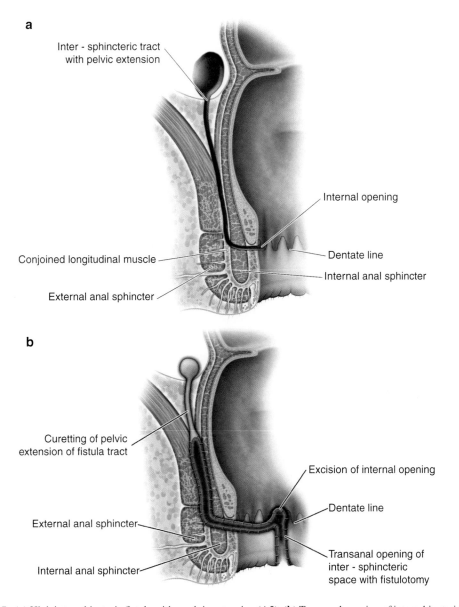

Fig. 13.5 (**a**) High intersphincteric fistula with a pelvic extension (A5). (**b**) Transanal opening of intersphincteric space with fistulotomy

Fig. 13.6 Intersphincteric fistula from pelvic disease

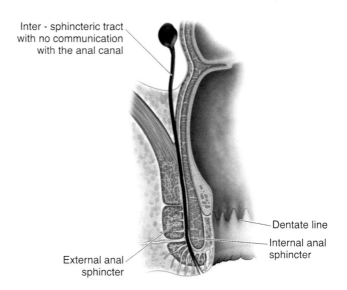

Inter - sphincteric tract with no communication with the anal canal

Dentate line

Internal anal sphincter

External anal sphincter

13.4 Management of Trans-sphincteric Fistula

A trans-sphincteric fistula could be either high or low. Less than 30% of the external anal sphincter is involved in the low trans-sphincteric fistula [6]. In contrast, over 30% of the external anal sphincter is involved in the high trans-sphincteric fistula [6]. However, according to some authors, the differentiation between low and high trans-sphincteric fistula depends upon whether less than or more than 66% of the external sphincter is involved [7, 8]. A low trans-sphincteric fistula crosses the lower one-third of the external anal sphincter, whereas a high trans-sphincteric fistula crosses the upper or middle third of the external anal sphincter [7, 8].

13.4.1 B1 Uncomplicated

- The lowermost internal anal sphincter, superficial, and subcutaneous external sphincter are divided in an uncomplicated low trans-sphincteric fistula. The disturbance to the anal continence is minimal (Fig. 13.7a, b).

13.4.2 B2 Complicated

- Trans-sphincteric fistula with high blind tract or extension to the supralevator space.

  Fistulotomy is performed up to the superficial part of the external anal sphincter. If adequately drained, the upper extension will heal itself. Whenever probing is done, the probe invariably goes straight. Because the trans-sphincteric tract is at a right angle to the main tract, it is challenging to move the probe from the external to the internal opening, as shown (Fig. 13.8a–c). Aggressive probing can lead to the formation of an extrasphincteric fistula. After identification of internal opening, a transanal approach is better (Table 13.2).

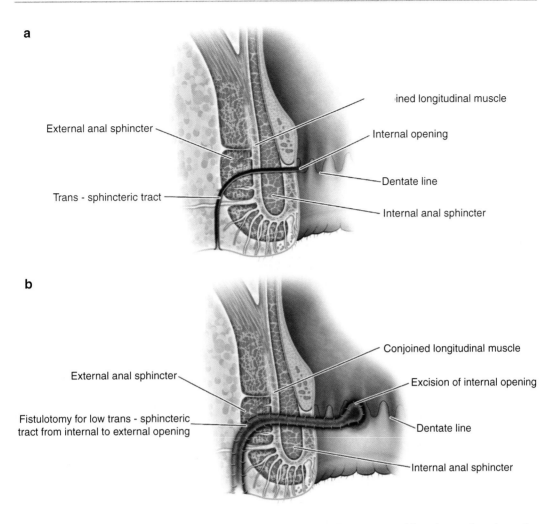

Fig. 13.7 (**a**) Uncomplicated trans-sphincteric fistula. (**b**) Fistulotomy for low trans-sphincteric tract from internal to external opening

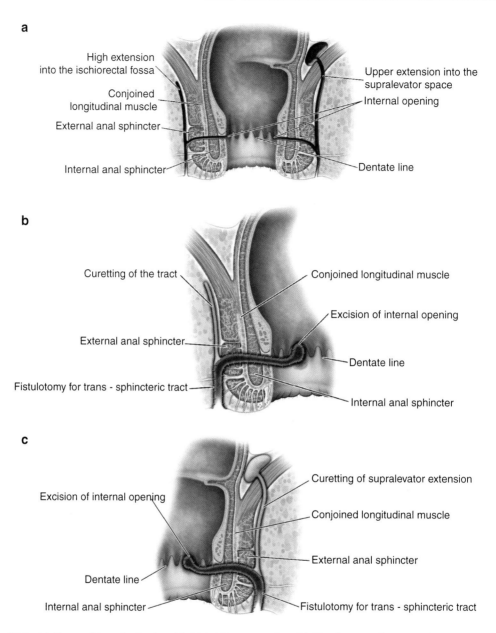

Fig. 13.8 (**a**) Trans-sphincteric fistula with high blind tract and suprasphincteric extension. (**b**) Fistulotomy of trans-sphincteric tract followed by excision of internal opening. (**c**) Fistulotomy of trans-sphincteric tract followed by curetting of supralevator extension

13.5   Management of Suprasphincteric Fistula

This is an uncommon fistula and is challenging to cure.

- The first and most crucial step is to excise the internal opening and surrounding tissue. The intersphincteric part of the tract is opened by dividing the internal anal sphincter up to the anorectal ring. The deep part of the external

anal sphincter should never be cut. The edges of the cut internal sphincter are marsupialized with the anal canal wall. The rest of the tract is curetted. At 6 o'clock, a fistulotomy from the internal opening to the anal verge is performed for drainage (Fig. 13.9a, b).

Park proposed that such fistulas are usually horseshoe and, after a while, form a crescentic fibrous ring, which acts as a sphincter. A staged fistulotomy can be attempted [4] (Table 13.3).

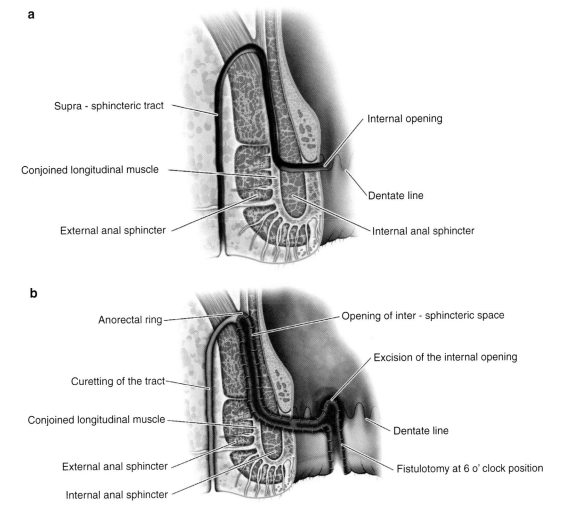

Fig. 13.9   (**a**) Suprasphincteric fistula. (**b**) Fistulotomy at 6 o'clock position with opening of intersphincteric part of the tract

13.6 Management of Extrasphincteric Fistula

1. **Extrasphincteric Tract Secondary to a Trans-sphincteric Fistula**

    One of the openings in this fistula is the primary internal opening of cryptoglandular origin in the anal canal. The second is the trans-sphincteric fistula's rectal opening extending from the extrasphincteric region (Fig. 13.10a). In such fistulas, fistulotomy can be carried out from the internal to the external perineal opening (Fig. 13.10b). The distal tract opening into the rectum may pose a problem in healing due to high rectal pressure leading to contamination. A temporary diversion colostomy may be required to heal the tract completely [4]. These cases, however, are sporadic.

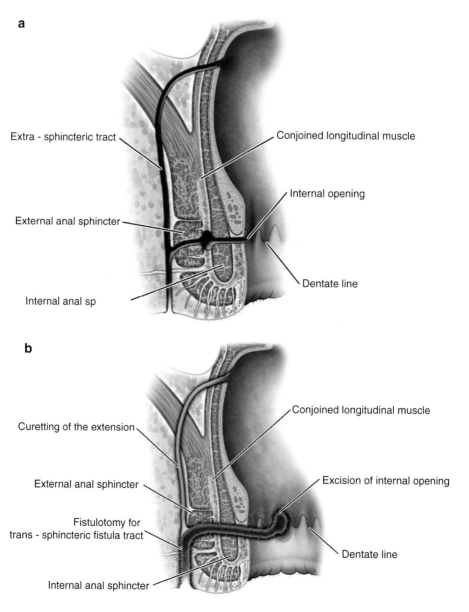

Fig. 13.10 (**a**) Extrasphincteric fistula tract extending from trans-sphincteric tract of cryptoglandular origin. (**b**) Excision of internal opening with fistulotomy done for trans-sphincteric tract. The extrasphincteric extension curetted. Primary sphincter repair can be done incase more than 30% of external sphincter is divided

2. **Extrasphincteric Fistula Due to Trauma**

   The primary cause is foreign body penetration from the perineum (Fig. 13.11). Removing the foreign body is necessary. However, an iatrogenic fistula may also develop by aggressive probing. No sphincter cutting procedure is required. The patient may require a temporary diversion colostomy [4].

3. **Extrasphincteric Fistula Due to Anorectal Diseases**

   The underlying pathologies like Crohn's disease, ulcerative colitis, or malignancy must be treated in this type of fistula [4].

4. **Extrasphincteric Fistula Due to Pelvic Inflammation**

   The primary source of infection in the pelvis should be managed [4] (Table 13.4).

Fig. 13.11 Extrasphincteric fistula tract following trauma

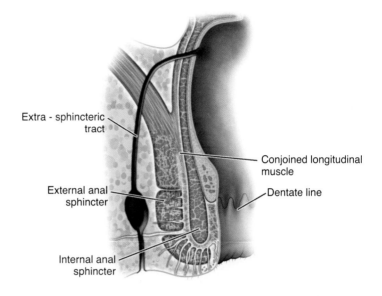

Table 13.4 Extrasphincteric fistula

Type of fistula	Sphincter involvement and amount of sphincter cut	Outcome and alternatives
Extrasphincteric fistula	No sphincter cutting	**The laser procedure is better in iatrogenic extrasphincteric fistulas**

13.7   Simple Fistulotomy Technique

The patient is placed in a lithotomy position under spinal, regional, or general anesthesia. Hydrogen peroxide is injected through the external opening, and bubbles are observed flowing out of the internal opening (Fig. 13.12a). The fistula tract is demarcated by injecting methylene blue (Fig. 13.12b).

A probe is gently inserted into the tract through the external opening and brought out through the internal opening, and the overlying tract is divided (Fig. 13.12c, d). Unipolar cautery or bare laser fiber is used to open the tract over the probe. Once the tract is laid open, the base can be seen stained with methylene blue, an affir-

mative sign of the fistula tract. The tract should be followed to see other branches demarcated by methylene blue. In a low intersphincteric fistula, the subcutaneous part of the external anal sphincter is divided. In a low trans-sphincteric fistula, the subcutaneous and the lower part of the superficial external anal sphincter are always divided. If the superficial part of the external anal sphincter needs to be cut, primary sphincter repair should be done to avoid anal incontinence. The division of the lowermost part of the external anal sphincter can be associated with acceptable postoperative incontinence. The internal opening and the nidus of primary infection in the intersphincteric space are scooped out (Fig. 13.12e, f). The wound base is then curetted and left open to heal by secondary intention. The curetted unhealthy

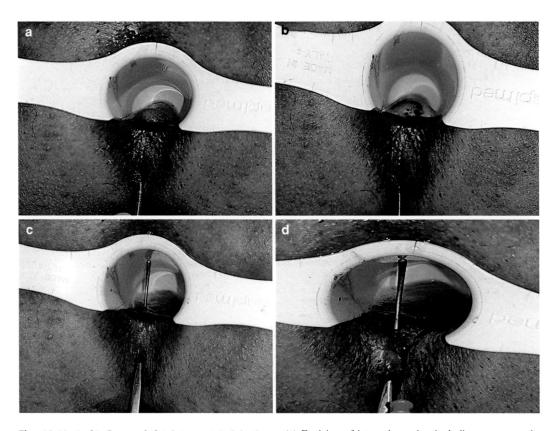

Fig. 13.12 (**a–h**) Steps of fistulotomy. (**a**) Injecting hydrogen peroxide through external opening. Bubbles seen coming out of internal opening at dentate line. (**b**) Demarcation of fistula tract by injecting methylene blue. (**c**) Probe is entered via the external opening and brought out through the internal opening. (**d**) Laying open of fistula tract over the probe using monopolar electrocautery.

(**e**) Excision of internal opening including mucosa, submucosa, and surrounding tissue up to intersphincteric space to eradicate the source of infection. (**f**) Fistulotomy wound showing fibers of internal sphincter. (**g**) Marsupialization of fistulotomy edges using Polyglactin 2-0. (**h**) The final wound as seen at the end of procedure

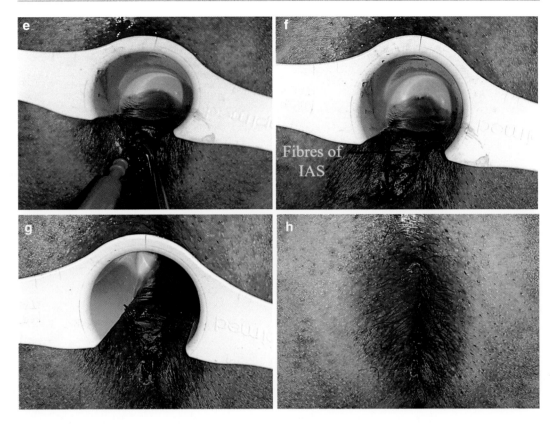

Fig. 13.12 (continued)

granulation tissue is sent for a histopathology examination. Finally, marsupialization of fistulotomy wound edges is done (Fig. 13.12g, h). No packing of the wound is required.

13.7.1 Advantages of Marsupialization

Marsupialization is not a part of the fistulotomy technique but has the following advantages [9]:

- Decreases the size of the wound.
- Maintains hemostasis from the edges of the wound.
- Avoids trapping of the fecal matter underneath the wound margins.

- Prevents the bridging of the margins of the fistula tract.
- Prevents early skin closure. The skin heals faster than mucosa; the underlying raw area can lead to recurrence.

13.7.2 Results

Ho et al. reported faster healing in fistulotomy with marsupialization [10]. Interrupted sutures for marsupialization of margins are taken using 2-0 or 3-0 Polyglactin. Continuous sutures, on the other hand, are recommended by Pescatori et al. because they provide better obliteration of perianal wounds, reducing the risk of bleeding and suppuration after surgery [9].

13.8   Discussion

The most feared complication of fistulotomy is incontinence. The old fallacy is still alive: When the sphincter of the pelvis is disrupted, incontinence is a serious concern [11]. The internal sphincter does not affect the anal continence, and it may be cut without causing any harm [11]. The crux of fistulotomy lies in how much external sphincter is involved. The external sphincter should always be carefully divided as it is of prime importance in maintaining the integrity of continence [11]. The external sphincter is connected both posteriorly and anteriorly to a greater extent. There is no consensus on how much muscle may be divided safely [6]. Posteriorly, up to 50% sphincter can be divided safely, whereas the anterior division should not exceed 30%. The posterior division is not as harmful as the lateral division since the external sphincter fibers are not supported laterally [11].

Fistulotomy has a success rate of 92–97% when patients are carefully selected [6].

13.8.1 Intersphincteric Fistula

Intersphincteric fistula is the commonest, which may or may not be associated with an abscess. The most typical cause of intersphincteric fistula is a cryptoglandular infection in the anal glands. Hill et al. noticed that the anal glands are concentrated mainly posteriorly, less anteriorly, and least laterally [12]. An important aspect of an intersphincteric fistula or perianal abscess is that the glands in the caudal direction have multiple ramifications compared to those extending cephalad [12]. Lymphocytes infiltrate all the anal glands just like lymph nodules [12].

If the intersphincteric fistula is associated with a perianal abscess, primary fistulotomy with abscess drainage can be done in a single sitting. The elimination of the contaminated source in the intersphincteric area below the internal opening remains the crux of a successful operative procedure [5]. The fistula will recur unless the intersphincteric space is cleared of the primary infection. In aged patients with

the lax anal tone, the anal sphincter complex is already weak; therefore, fistulotomy can lead to partial incontinence [4].

13.8.2 Trans-sphincteric Fistulas

The Latin term "trans" means "on the other side" [13]. A trans-sphincteric fistula crosses the external and internal anal sphincters at variable levels, giving rise to low and high variety. The extensions cross the levator ani muscle at right angles to the primary tract [4]. If the probing is done from the external opening, the probe will directly go upwards. Aggressive probing can create an iatrogenic opening, consequently forming an extrasphincteric fistula. At the dentate line, induration may be felt due to the internal opening. Therefore, identifying and eradicating the primary source of infection is essential. Fistulotomy in such cases should be carried out after a thorough assessment of the external anal sphincter. The extensions may be managed by adequate drainage. Fistulotomy in high trans-sphincteric fistula can cause incontinence ranging from 17% to 33% [14]. Even in experienced hands, incision of the deep segment of the external anal sphincter with primary sphincter repair might result in fecal incontinence.

In complicated trans-sphincteric fistulas, sphincter-saving techniques are the treatment of choice to prevent incontinence.

13.8.3 Suprasphincteric Fistula

The tract passes the whole sphincter complex, including the puborectalis and the intersphincteric plane. It may spread in a circumferential manner forming a fibrous ring that may act as a sphincter. A fistulotomy involving the division of the muscles forming the anorectal ring may cause incontinence. According to Park [4], removing all the muscles underneath the ring at once is not recommended since this would result in a broad separation. Staged fistulotomy, if done, will allow the fibrous tissue to develop that will anchor around the partially divided sphincter. Care

Table 13.5 Results and outcomes of fistulotomy

Journal	Year	Success rate (%)
Dis Colon Rectum Multicenter study Neil Hyman et al. [15]	2009	87
Dis Colon Rectum Multi Centre Study Jason F. Hall et al. [16]	2014	94
International Journal of Surgery P. Garg [17]	2018	98
Annals of Medicine and Surgery A prospective randomized controlled trial Olfat I. Al Sebai et al. [18]	2021	93.3
Int J Colorectal Dis Mario Pescatori [19]	2021	96.4

should be taken so that sphincter division in such cases is confined below the puborectalis sling.

If such fistulas are encountered, they can be managed with a hybrid procedure. Since these fistulas are not very common, they should be operated on by experienced surgeons.

13.8.4 Extrasphincteric Fistula

This form of fistula incidence is between 1% and 2%. If the condition is caused by trauma, it is generally treated with a colostomy or by removing the contaminated source from the pelvis. If it is secondary to suprasphincteric or trans-sphincteric fistulas, it is necessary to deal with the primary source of infection.

The results and outcomes of fistulotomy have been mentioned in Table 13.5.

13.9 Points to Ponder

Sometimes I wonder why there is recurrence and so many variations in results after fistulotomy (Table 13.5). There are a few facts based on literature.

- Firstly, Lockhart Mummery, in 1929 [11], described that "*The fundamental principle to follow in operating for fistula is to provide free*

drainage to all parts of the tract. According to him, recurrence will occur due to inadequate drainage of the fistulous tract at the primary operation." It may be seen that initially, the healing process is quick. Still, when the fistula seems to be almost cured, further healing does not occur, indicating a residual infection.

- Secondly, I want to draw readers' attention to Park's original paper on the pathogenesis of anal fistulas, published in 1961 [4]. He stated, "*The crux of the fistula surgery is removing the infecting source, the infected anal gland, and the surrounding inter-sphincteric abscess lying deep to the internal sphincter. The abscess is most easily approached through the anal lumen. Once the internal opening is identified, an oval incision starts 0.5 cm above it. The mucosa, submucosa, the internal sphincter, the inter-sphincteric tissue, and the cryptogenic abscess with surrounding tissue are excised.*"

The procedure recommended by Park is similar to partial internal sphincterotomy [4]. Since this procedure is performed through an intra-anal approach, all the extensions can easily be identified and explored. Park further described that the cause of recurrence is the anal gland epithelium left behind during the procedure.

Eisenhammer, in 1965, proposed that "*The fistula does not persist because of an abscessed anal gland, but because once the chronic infection is established in the deep inter-sphincteric space, connected with the crypt, it will maintain the fistula in an active state connecting the crypt with the external opening. Further, once the infection sets in, the identity of the anal gland is completely lost*" [5].

Instead of excising the infected primary source as recommended by Park to remove necrotic material, Eisenhammer recommended that the best way to cure a tract was to lay it open from its external to the internal opening, followed by curetting [4, 5]. Since both these publications are highly authentic, the surgeon's choice is to excise the internal opening or go for a fistulotomy. If both procedures are thoroughly analyzed, the source of infection in a fistula is found below the internal opening in the deep intersphincteric region. Both procedures aim to avoid recurrence.

- Thirdly, the fistula is opened till the internal opening. Below the internal opening, a deep intersphincteric space lies midway in the anal canal. Although the intersphincteric area is scooped to remove the remnants of the anal glands, the deep intersphincteric space is left unattended. According to some authors, more than the deep postanal area, the deep intersphincteric area is responsible for the spread of the horseshoe abscess [20]. Two spaces should never be confused; the deep postanal space located deep to the anococcygeal ligament and the deep intersphincter located posterior to the internal anal sphincter above the dentate line [21]. These spaces have already been described in detail in Chap. 10.

Sphincter-saving procedures should be undertaken in high-risk patients, such as women with anterior fistula, a history of anorectal surgeries, pre-existing weak sphincter control, and complicated fistulas. Simple fistulas can be best dealt with by fistulotomy. Even complex fistulas, especially recurrent ones, can be managed by fistulotomy, but the same should be combined with primary sphincter repair. Care should be taken to ensure that the extent of sphincter division is confined to below the puborectalis sling. The proximal extension, if any, should be curetted.

13.10 Core Tips

- Before fistulotomy, the extent of the external sphincter involved and the anal tone must be assessed [22]. The external sphincter between the internal opening and the levator ani must be preserved during fistulotomy [22]. The ultimate objective is to preserve at least 2–2.5 cm of the external sphincter [22].
- The primary source of infection in the intersphincteric region is below the internal opening; excising the internal opening with the surrounding tissue through the anal approach decreases the chances of recurrence.
- Exploring the deep intersphincteric space is necessary as the infection can extend due to the ramifications of the anal glands. Even if the glands are destroyed, as proposed by Eisenhammer [5], the infection may still persist from the ramifications of these glands.
- While opening intersphincteric space, the entire internal sphincter can be cut open without risk of incontinence [4].
- Fistulotomy wounds do not require packing. A sitz bath and a local application of an ointment (combination of metrogyl, sucralfate, and lignocaine) are sufficient to manage postoperative wounds.
- A seton placement is a better option when the anatomy of sphincters is undefined.
- Precaution should be taken while operating for an abscess with a primary fistulotomy. If there is a large internal opening resulting from the bursting of an abscess inside, the communicating fistula tract can be approached from the inside out using a probe. However, if the internal opening is insignificant, a blunt artery forceps should be inserted from the abscess incision site toward the internal opening to avoid the formation of an iatrogenic opening. One should remember that there is inflammation in the presence of an abscess, and probing can create an iatrogenic opening.

13.11 Fistulectomy

A fistulectomy is a surgical technique in which a fistulous tract is entirely removed. The tract is laid open and curetted in fistulotomy, but fibrous tissue and glandular epithelium may be left behind. In a controlled trial conducted by Kronborg [23], the fistulectomy patients took longer to heal as more tissue was excised than fistulotomy, whereas the complication rate was the same.

13.11.1 Indications

- Trans-sphincteric and intersphincteric fistulas below the anorectal ring

13.11.2 Technique

Excision of the fistula tract from an external to an internal opening, dividing both the internal and external sphincters and leaving an open wound to recover by secondary intention. The deep area of the external sphincter that forms the anorectal ring is not cut.

13.11.3 Advantages

This procedure gives the surgeon a clear vision of the fistula tract, allowing him to remove it entirely.

13.11.4 Disadvantages

- Longer operative and healing time
- More bleeding
- Larger defects
- No reduction in recurrence rate compared to fistulotomy

Table 13.6 Results of fistulectomy

Procedure	Success rate (%)	Incontinence (%)
Fistulectomy	93–100 [27]	11.5–20

Yansong Xu et al. [24] recorded no significant difference in operating and recovery period between fistulotomy and fistulectomy in a meta-analysis of 565 individuals. Further, no significant difference was observed in the recurrence rate following fistulectomy versus fistulotomy.

Some surgeons have criticized the technique of fistulectomy because of significant tissue loss, leading to delayed healing [25]. Fistulectomy by surgical coring-out has the advantage of accurate determination of the tract and lowers the risk of missing the secondary tracts [26]. Once the tract is cored out, the tunnel can be closed from the inside to prevent fecal matter from entering the tunnel through the anal canal.

In a clinical trial conducted in patients with simple fistulas managed with fistulotomy versus fistulectomy, significant muscular injury caused to the sphincter mechanism was seen mainly in patients who underwent fistulectomy compared to fistulotomy [26]. The results of fistulectomy are shown in Table 13.6.

13.12 Fistulotomy Versus Fistulectomy: A Surgeon's Dilemma!

Fistulotomy is considered a gold standard for treating fistula-in-ano. According to several studies, fistulotomy takes less time to recover than fistulectomy, although the recurrence rate is similar [9]. In most cases, incontinence is minimal, ranging from 11.5% to 20% [28] (Table 13.7).

Table 13.7 Results of fistulotomy versus fistulectomy

Procedure	Postoperative bleeding (%)	Infection (%)	Recurrence (%)
Fistulotomy [29]	0.8	2.2	10.7
Fistulectomy [29]	3.1	3.8	15.3

13.13 Primary Sphincter Repair

An aggressive fistulotomy may lead to postoperative incontinence, whereas inappropriate conservative surgery may cause recurrence. Over 30% division of the external anal sphincter anteriorly or more than 50% posteriorly or laterally can cause incontinence to the flatus and liquid part of fecal matter. Hence these procedures are followed by primary sphincter repair. As mentioned before, one should always refrain from cutting the deep part of the external anal sphincter.

13.13.1 Indications

• To prevent iatrogenic incontinence

13.13.2 Advantages

• Prevents anal incontinence
• Faster healing of the wound
• Creates a less postoperative raw area

13.13.3 Technique

The Allis forceps is applied during fistulotomy at the divided external and internal anal sphincter margins. The internal anal sphincter has white fibers, the conjoined longitudinal muscle has pink fibers, whereas the external anal sphincter has reddish-brown fibers [4].

For reconstruction of the sphincters, the repair always starts from the inside out. The mucosa and the margins of the internal anal sphincter are sutured with 3-0 Polyglactin, taking interrupted sutures starting from the excised internal opening.

Table 13.8 Results of primary sphincter repair

Journal	Recurrence rate	Incontinence
Asian Journal Surgery Farag A. F. A. et al. [30]	9.1%	2.28%
Int J Colorectal Disease Markus Hirschburger [31]	–	6% (flatus incontinence)
J Med Association Thai Jivapaisaarnpong [32]	–	No incontinence
Int J Colorectal Dis Stephen Seyfried [33]	–	23% 15.5% (flatus incontinence) 6.8% (liquid incontinence)
Aging Clin Exp Res Domenico Mascagni [34]	2.3%	

After that, the margins of the external anal sphincter are approximated using 2-0 PDS. Finally, the anoderm is reconstructed, leaving a small opening to allow drainage of any collection.

13.13.4 Postoperative Care

• Antibiotics, analgesics, laxatives, and sitz bath

13.13.5 Core Tips

The margins of the cut sphincters should be approximated and not overlapped. The knot should not be very tight as it can lead to ischemia and stricture formation (Table 13.8).

13.13.6 Discussion

A functional deficiency occurs when more than 30–50% of the external sphincter is divided. Primary sphincter repair preserves the sphincter's function, maintaining continence. The rapid reconstruction of the sphincters following fistulotomy was documented by Parkash and colleagues in 1985 [30].

13.13.7   Core Tips

Before closing the wound, one should ensure that no part of the fistulous tract has been left behind. While doing sphincter repair, there should be no dead space to avoid collection, as it becomes a nidus for infection.

13.14   Case Studies

Case 1

A 38-year-old male patient came to the OPD for consultation. A year ago, he was operated on for fistula-in-ano. His wound did not heal completely. He had a slight discharge which increased over the past 3–4 days. He consulted his surgeon and was given some antibiotics. But there was no relief, and the discharge persisted. On examination, two adjoining external openings could be seen at 1–2 o'clock, approximately 3.5 cm from the anal verge. A single internal opening was felt as an induration at 1 o'clock. The MRI suggested a fistula tract with an intersphincteric extension (Type A2). It was a case of persistent fistula.

Fistulotomy with marsupialization was planned. Methylene blue and hydrogen peroxide were injected from the external openings and could be seen coming out from the internal opening at 1 o'clock. The probe was inserted and could be observed coming out at 1 o'clock. The internal opening was excised along with mucosa, submucosa, and the surrounding tissue. The fibers of internal anal sphincters were divided to enter the deep intersphincteric space, and the nidus of infection was removed. An extension could be seen extending into the intersphincteric space. The extension was curetted, irrigated, and laser ablated. A small fistulotomy was done at 1 o'clock, extending from the excised internal opening wound to the anal verge by cutting the subcutaneous part of the external anal sphincter. The external openings were excised. In the end, the fistulotomy wound was marsupialized. The patient was discharged the next day. He did well after 1½ years of regular follow-up.

Opinion

The patient did not have complete cessation of pus discharge following the previous surgery, and hence, it was a case of persistent fistula. As the length of the tract was approximately 3.5 cm, fistulotomy was an appropriate decision. Park's technique was performed as the primary source of infection was in the intersphincteric region, and all the extensions were secondary. If the internal opening is tackled precisely, the secondary tracts heal subsequently.

Case 2

Mr. D, a 25-year-young man, came to the OPD complaining of pus discharge from the anal region. He narrated that he had pain in the perianal region and difficulty in sitting. The pain was continuous and throbbing and made him miserable. He was unable to perform his duties. He went to a surgeon who diagnosed it as a perianal abscess. The abscess was drained. He got immediate relief from pain and remained well for a few months, but then developed pus discharge which constantly irritated him. On examination, there was an external opening at the 6 o'clock position, 3 cm from the anal verge. An internal opening was palpated at the 6 o'clock position on the dentate line. His endosonography perineum revealed a fistula in the posterior region leading to a well-defined tract measuring 6 mm in diameter. The tract coursed superiorly for 2.4 cm to open into the anterior wall of the anal canal at a depth of 1.5 cm from the anal verge.

The patient was operated on for fistulotomy with marsupialization.

Opinion

It was a simple case of perianal abscess with an intercommunicating intersphincteric fistula tract. Initially, the patient was operated on for drainage of a perianal abscess. A second surgery could have been avoided if a primary fistulotomy had been attempted simultaneously.

Case 3

Mrs. F, a woman in her late forties, gave a history of pus discharge from an opening in the perianal region, along with itching and mild pain on and off for 6 months. She consulted many physicians and tried different treatments but got no relief. On examination, there was an external opening at 6 o'clock, 2.5 cm from an anal verge, and an internal opening at 6 o'clock on the dentate line. MRI showed an intersphincteric fistula with an intersphincteric collection.

Fistulotomy with marsupialization was planned. Methylene blue was injected into the external opening and was seen coming out through the internal opening. A probe was inserted and passed from the dentate line's internal opening. The internal opening was excised along with mucosa, submucosa, and the surrounding tissue. The fibers of internal anal sphincters were divided to enter the deep intersphincteric space, and the nidus of infection was removed. A methylene blue-stained tract was seen going superiorly. A probe was inserted and seen going superiorly into the deep intersphincteric space for about 1.5 cm. The deep intersphincteric space was curetted, irrigated, and laser-ablated. Fistulotomy was done up to the anal verge. The margins of the fistulotomy wound were marsupialized.

Opinion

As a result of staining with methylene blue, the extension in the deep intersphincteric space was easily identified. Laser ablation of the extension is an appropriate way of managing such tracts. The alternative is to lay it open.

Take-Home Message

- Fistulotomy and Fistulectomy are sphincter cutting procedures, and their use has been undisputed over the years. Sometimes fancy procedures can be technically demanding and not required. Fistulotomy is the best procedure when the tract is short and straightforward. In complex fistulas, excellent results can be achieved with hybrid procedures.

- In the fistulotomy procedure, there are two options: to follow Park's procedure or follow Eisenhammer's. Both techniques are equally good. Both aim to remove the primary source of infection in the intersphincteric space. My personal preference is Park's technique. The extensions can be best managed by laser ablation after curetting. A laser is an optional tool but a good one.

- When one is excising the internal opening, always palpate for induration. The excision is done till the intersphincteric space is reached. If the external opening crosses the ischiorectal fossa, the external and internal openings are separated by a bridge between the intervening ischiorectal fat and the skin [9]. One can always go for coring as a fistulotomy wound will create a large raw area.

- As already mentioned about the importance of marsupialization, the literature by Park also advocates the same. According to Park, if the mucosal edges are allowed to bridge over the wound, it will cause the fistula to form again. This is because the anal-gland epithelium lining the fistula is made to form a part of the wall of the anal canal. If this gland epithelium remains intact, it will line the new tract again, leading to recurrence [4].

- Once the primary source of infection is tackled, the secondary tracts are taken care of by the hybrid procedures.

- Anatomically high anal fistulas are a challenge to treat. Sphincter reconstruction is an excellent technique that prevents anal incontinence. Literature research, including observational studies and randomized clinical trials in PubMed, Cochrane, and Google Scholar on surgically managing the simple anal fistulas, conclude that sphincter-cutting procedures provide outstanding cure rates in selected patients.

References

1. Malik AI, Nelson RL. Surgical management of anal fistulae: a systematic review. Colorectal Dis. 2008;10(5):420–30. https://doi.org/10.1111/j.1463-1318.2008.01483.x. PMID: 18479308

2. Arderne J. Treatises of fistula in ano: hemorrhoids, and clysters. Routledge; 2019.

3. Dudukgian H, Abcarian H. Why do we have so much trouble treating anal fistula? World J Gastroenterol. 2011;17(28):3292–6. https://doi.org/10.3748/wjg.v17.i28.3292. PMID: 21876616; PMCID: PMC3160532

4. Parks AG. Pathogenesis and treatment of fistula-in-ano. Br Med J. 1961;1(5224):463–9. https://doi.org/10.1136/bmj.1.5224.463. PMID: 13732880; PMCID: PMC1953161

5. Eisenhammer S. The final evaluation and classification of the surgical treatment of the primary anorectal cryptoglandular intermuscular (inter-sphincteric) fistulous abscess and fistula. Dis Colon Rectum. 1978;21(4):237–54. https://doi.org/10.1007/BF02586698. PMID: 657933

6. Steele SR, Kumar R, Feingold DL, Rafferty JL, Buie WD, Standards Practice Task Force of the American Society of Colon and Rectal Surgeon. Practice parameters for the management of perianal abscess and fistula-in-ano. Dis Colon Rectum. 2011;54(12):1465–74.

7. Garcés-Albir M, García-Botello SA, Esclapez-Valero P, Sanahuja-Santafé A, Raga-Vázquez J, Espi-Macías A, Ortega-Serrano J. Quantifying the extent of fistulotomy. How much sphincter can we safely divide? A three-dimensional endosonographic study. Int J Colorectal Dis. 2012;27(8):1109–16.

8. Van Onkelen RS, Gosselink MP, van Rosmalen J, Thijsse S, Schouten WR. Different characteristics of high and low trans-sphincteric fistulae. Colorectal Dis. 2014;16(6):471–5. https://doi.org/10.1111/codi.12578. PMID: 24471695

9. Pescatori M, Ayabaca SM, Cafaro D, Iannello A, Magrini S. Marsupialization of fistulotomy and fistulectomy wounds improves healing and decreases bleeding: a randomized controlled trial. Colorectal Dis. 2006;8(1):11–4. https://doi.org/10.1111/j.1463-1318.2005.00835.x. PMID: 16519632

10. Ho YH, Tan M, Leong AF, Seow-Choen F. Marsupialization of fistulotomy wounds improves healing: a randomized controlled trial. Br J Surg. 1998;85(1):105–7. https://doi.org/10.1046/j.1365-2168.1998.00529.x. PMID: 9462396

11. Lockhart-Mummery JP. Discussion on fistula-in-ano. Proc R Soc Med. 1929;22:1331–41.

12. Hill MR, Sheryock EH, ReBell FG. Role of anal glands in the pathogenesis of the anorectal disease. JAMA. 1943;121:742.

13. Jimenez M, Mandava N. Anorectal fistula. In: StatPearls [Internet]. Treasure Island, FL: StatPearls Publishing; 2022. PMID: 32809492.

14. Abcarian H. Classification and management strategies. In: Abcarian H, editor. Anal fistula. New York: Springer; 2014. p. 39–44.

15. Hyman N, O'Brien S, Osler T. Outcomes after fistulotomy: results of a prospective, multicenter regional study. Dis Colon Rectum. 2009;52(12):2022–7. https://doi.org/10.1007/DCR.0b013e3181b72378. PMID: 19934925

16. Hall JF, Bordeianou L, Hyman N, Read T, Bartus C, Schoetz D, Marcello PW. Outcomes after operations for anal fistula: results of a prospective, multicenter, regional study. Dis Colon Rectum. 2014;57(11):1304–8.

17. Garg P. Is fistulotomy still the gold standard in the present era, and is it highly underutilized? An audit of 675 operated cases. Int J Surg. 2018;56:26–30. https://doi.org/10.1016/j.ijsu.2018.06.009. Epub 2018 Jun 8. PMID: 29886281

18. Al Sebai OI, Ammar MS, Mohamed SH, El Balshy MA. Comparative study between inter sphincteric ligation of perianal fistula versus conventional fistulotomy with or without seton in the treatment of perianal fistula: a prospective randomized controlled trial. Ann Med Surg. 2021;61:180–4.

19. Pescatori M. Surgery for anal fistulae: state of the art. Int J Colorectal Dis. 2021;36(10):2071–9.

20. Kurihara H, Kanai T, Ishikawa T, Ozawa K, Kanatake Y, Kanai S, Hashiguchi Y. A new concept for the surgical anatomy of posterior deep complex fistulas: the posterior deep space and the septum of the ischiorectal fossa. Dis Colon Rectum. 2006;49(10 Suppl):S37–44. https://doi.org/10.1007/s10350-006-0736-6. PMID: 17106814

21. Zhang H, Zhou ZY, Hu B, Liu DC, Peng H, Xie SK, Su D, Ren DL. Clinical significance of 2 deep posterior perianal spaces to complex cryptoglandular fistulas. Dis Colon Rectum. 2016;59(8):766–74. https://doi.org/10.1097/DCR.0000000000000628. PMID: 27384095

22. Burney RE. Long-term results of surgical treatment of anal fistula in a case series of 483 patients. Int J Surg Open. 2021;33:100350.

23. Kronborg O. To lay open or excise a fistula-in ano: a randomized trial. Br J Surg. 1985;72(12):970.

24. Xu Y, Liang S, Tang W. Meta-analysis of randomized clinical trials comparing fistulectomy versus fistulotomy for low anal fistula. Springerplus. 2016;5(1):1722. https://doi.org/10.1186/s40064-016-3406-8. PMID: 27777858; PMCID: PMC5052239

25. Lunniss PJ, Phillips RKS. Anal fistula, fistulectomy. In: Colorectal surgery. 5th ed. 2014. https://www.sciencedirect.com/topics/medicine-anddentistry/fistulectomy.

26. Belmonte Montes C, Ruiz Galindo GH, Montes Villalobos JL, Decanini Terán C. Fistulotomía vs fistulectomía. Valoración ultrasonográfica de lesión al mecanismo de esfínter anal [Fistulotomy vs fistulectomy. Ultrasonographic evaluation of lesion of

the anal sphincter function]. Rev Gastroenterol Mex. 1999;64(4):167–70. Spanish. PMID: 10851578

27. Tozer P, Sala S, Cianci V, Kalmar K, Atkin GK, Rahbour G, Ranchod P, Hart A, Phillips RK. Fistulotomy in the tertiary setting can achieve high rates of fistula cure with an acceptable risk of deterioration incontinence. J Gastrointestinal Surg. 2013;17(11):1960–5. https://doi.org/10.1007/s11605-013-2198-1. Epub 2013 Sep 4. PMID: 24002754

28. Sheikh P, Baakza A. Management of fistula-in-ano-the current evidence. Indian J Surg. 2014;76(6):482–6. https://doi.org/10.1007/s12262-014-1150-2. Epub 2014 Aug 15. PMID: 25614724; PMCID: PMC4297991

29. Irfan Ali S, Irfan S, Muhammad Shoaib H, Muhammad Misbah R, Noman K, Saad A. Fistulotomy vs. fistulectomy in treating simple low anal fistula of male patients. Pak Armed Forces Med J. 2015;65(6):798–802.

30. Farag AFA, Elbarmelgi MY, Mostafa M, Mashhour AN. One stage fistulectomy for high anal fistula with the reconstruction of anal sphincter without fecal diversion. Asian J Surg. 2019;42(8):792–6.

31. Hirschburger M, Schwandner T, Hecker A, Kierer W, Weinel R, Padberg W. Fistulectomy with primary sphincter reconstruction in treating high trans-sphincteric anal fistulas. Int J Colorectal Dis. 2014;29(2):247–52. https://doi.org/10.1007/s00384-013-1788-4. Epub 2013 Dec 15. PMID: 24337835

32. Jivapaisarnpong P. Core out fistulectomy, anal sphincter reconstruction, and primary repair of internal opening in treating complex anal fistula. J Med Assoc Thai. 2009;92(5):638–42. PMID: 19459524

33. Seyfried S, Bussen D, Joos A, Galata C, Weiss C, Herold A. Fistulectomy with primary sphincter reconstruction. Int J Colorectal Dis. 2018;33(7):911–8. https://doi.org/10.1007/s00384-018-3042-6. Epub 2018 Apr 12. PMID: 29651553

34. Mascagni D, Pironi D, Pontone S, Tonda M, Eberspacher C, Panarese A, Miscusi G, Grimaldi G, Catania A, Santoro A, Filippini A, Sorrenti S. Total fistulectomy, sphincteroplasty and closure of the residual cavity for trans-sphincteric perianal fistula in the elderly patient. Aging Clin Exp Res. 2017;29(Suppl 1):101–8. https://doi.org/10.1007/s40520-016-0652-0. Epub 2016 Nov 9. PMID: 27830517

"More sphincters are injured by aggressive surgeons rather than aggressive disease."

John Alexander Williams

Key Concepts

- Minimally invasive fistula treatment aims to obliterate the internal opening and fistula tracts with no sphincter division.
- The mucosal advancement flap aims to cover the internal opening, interrupt the course of the fistula, and encourage healing.
- Fibrin glue and fistula plugs offer reasonable healing but are associated with complications like infection and extrusion.
- A seton is a surgical thread placed in the fistula tract and left for several weeks. This allows the fistula to drain without the need for cutting the sphincter.
- LIFT is a procedure of fistula tract ligation in an intersphincteric space with separation and curettage of the distal tract.
- VAAFT is a technique that is carried out under direct endoluminal vision.
- Stem cell transplantation increases the number of cells. It restores normal cell healing by matrix remodeling and secretion of growth-factor.
- SLOFT aims to obliterate the internal opening by ligating it and disconnecting the distal tract near the internal opening.

14.1 Introduction

The sphincter-saving techniques are minimally invasive procedures for treating a fistula without cutting the sphincters. They increase the possibility of proper healing and avoid surgery-related complications like incontinence, which may result after sphincter cutting procedures.

14.2 Principle

The principle of minimally invasive techniques in fistula treatment is to obliterate the epithelialized tracts and any internal fistulous opening without dividing the sphincter. The various minimally invasive techniques are discussed below.

14.3 Endorectal Advancement Flap

First described by Noble in 1902, the mucosal advancement flaps were used in rectovaginal fistulas. The technique aims to mobilize partial-thickness flaps comprising muscle fibers, rectal submucosa, and mucosa [1]. Elting, in 1912, was the first to apply this principle of anorectal advancement flap for fistula surgery with a desire to preserve the normal function of the sphincters. He stated that the underlying essential principle for curing the anal fistula is comprised of:

1. Severance of communication between the fistulous tract and bowel
2. Removing the affected part of the bowel and the fistulous opening [2]

In his study in 1948, Laird reported using the anterior rectal mucosal flap principle for successfully dealing with complex anal fistula [3]. Over the years, numerous changes were made to this method described originally by Elting.

14.3.1 Principle

The core principle is that the healing of the anal fistula involves separating the communication between the bowel and tracts with the removal of the affected part, including its internal opening [2]. Mucosal advancement flap aims at covering the internal fistulous opening, thus interrupting the course of the fistula and encouraging healing.

14.3.2 Indications

- Complex anal fistulas
- Rectovaginal fistulas

14.3.3 Contraindication

- Presence of an abscess

14.3.4 Some Aspects of the Surgical Technique

14.3.4.1 Type of Flap

A vertical incision on the flap's lateral sides is the fundamental distinction between the types of flaps [4]. Some authors utilized a rhomboid flap, while Elting and Aguilar et al. employed an elliptical flap (Fig. 14.1). Theoretically, elliptical flaps enable an improved blood supply to the flap's tip because of the lack of corners; this claim is not supported by previous studies [4]. However, studies reported no difference in recovery time between individuals who used rhomboid and elliptical flaps in trials [4].

14.3.4.2 Shape of Flap

Authors have described numerous shapes over the past 20 years [4] (Fig. 14.2):

- Narrow round flaps
- Wide-angular flaps
- Wide round flaps

14.3.4.3 Flap Thickness

Over time, many techniques have been proposed, which are:

Fig. 14.1 Insertion of fistula plug in the tract

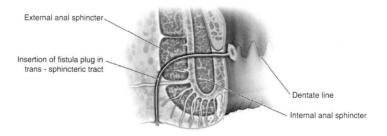

External anal sphincter

Insertion of fistula plug in
trans - sphincteric tract

Dentate line

Internal anal sphincter

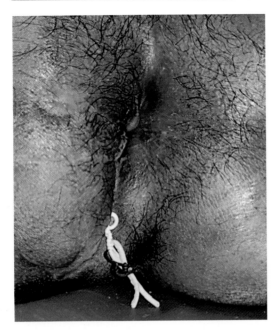

Fig. 14.2 Placement of seton

- Mucosal flap: Includes mucosa and submucosa.
- Partial-thickness flap: The flap plane is submucosal, consisting of mucosa, submucosa, and muscle fibers.
- Full-thickness flap: The flap plane is intersphincteric, including full muscle thickness of the internal sphincter.

According to studies, creating advanced flaps that surround the full thickness or circular fibers of rectal walls leads to improved recovery rates with minor incontinence [4].

14.3.5 Technique

After positioning the patient, the external opening is enlarged, followed by excision of the fistulous tract as far as possible without including the external sphincter. The internal opening is exposed. The overlying tissue is excised. The internal opening is occluded with 2–3 stitches. This helps in the plication of muscles. Dissection of the submucosal area creates a big buttonhole shape flap with no sharp edges. The mucosal flap hence raised, is used to cover the plicated muscle. Normal saline is injected at the end of the procedure through an external orifice to verify the occlusion of the internal opening [5]. Before applying the flap, some surgeons prefer to do a partial fistulectomy or coring out of the tract from an external opening till the sphincter is accessed [6].

14.3.6 Core Tip

To maintain an adequate blood supply, the width of the flap should gradually rise until the width of the base is double that of the apex [6].

14.3.7 Advantage

The procedure can preserve the external sphincter while securely closing the interior opening [7].

14.3.8 Results

The endorectal advancement flap is technically challenging. Even though the sphincter mechanism is not divided, up to 31% of patients experience moderate incontinence, and up to 12% of patients experience significant incontinence [8]. The overall results are mentioned in Table 14.1.

Some surgeons prefer to insert a seton and leave it for nearly 3 months before using a mucosal advancement flap as seton helps form a fibrotic wall near the fistula, allowing easy dissection [9].

Table 14.1 Endorectal advancement flaps

Journal	Year	Success rate (%)
International Journal Colorectal Dis Clinical Trial Uribe N. et al. [7]	2007	92.9
International Journal of Colorectal Disease Michele Podetta [9]	2018	78.1
BMC Surgery Claudia Sefarith [10]	2021	56

14.4   Fibrin Glue

A general term for denoting all the sealants based on fibrin is "Fibrin Glue." The application of fibrin glue dates back to 1940 when Tidrick applied the glue to immobilize skin grafts. Young and Medawar used fibrinogen and bovine thrombin for nerve anastomosis [11]. However, both studies were not successful [11].

Fibrinogen and its components are used to make the biological Fibrin glue [12]. The glue can be applied in surgical procedures to achieve a water-tight seal and hemostasis [12]. Occlusion of the fistula tract with sealant helps prevent tract contamination with mucus, stool, pus, and blood and helps in promoting wound healing and tissue growth.

14.4.1 Principle

Fibrin glue stimulates the terminal stages of a clotting cascade to occur naturally. It provides fluid-and air-tightness through fibrinogen polymerization within a fistula tract and provides a medium where fibroblasts can infiltrate. Together with other components, these fibroblasts contribute to re-epithelization and neovascularization [13].

14.4.2 Mechanism of Action

The action is twofold: First, in immediate effect, the fibrin sealant halts the ongoing contamination due to pus, blood, mucus, and stool. Second, proteins in a sealant activate scaffold wound healing and tissue growth [13].

14.4.3 Indications

Simple fistula.

14.4.4 Technique

Patients are laid in a jack-knife posture. Both external and internal openings are identified. The tract length is assessed, curetted, the unhealthy granulation tissue is removed, and the tract is cleaned using normal saline. Fibrin glue is allowed to reach room temperature and as per the procedure mentioned by the manufacturer, the glue is prepared. The glue is then instilled in the tract from an external opening using a feeding tube. A solid bubble is seen at the internal opening, confirming that the tract is filled with glue. This is followed by the gradual withdrawal of the feeding tube and syringe, thus filling the tract with glue. The external opening is not dressed.

14.4.5 Results

The overall success rate of fibrin glue in treating fistulas is low, ranging from 63% to 69% [12–15]. This may be attributed to the standardization of the products, fistula characteristics like the length of the tract, and complex or recurrent fistulas. Sometimes, the procedure may require two to three attempts (Table 14.2).

Table 14.2 Fibrin glue

Journal	Year	Success rate (%)
Coloproctology Wael Khafagy et al. [14]	2001	80
Diseases of Colon and Rectum Sentovich, Stephen M. [15]	2003	69
J Korean Surg Soc Gokturk et al. [12]	2011	63.04
Colorectal Disease Mathias Vidon [16]	2020	63

14.4.6 Advantages

The advantages include minimum discomfort to the patient, no or low risk of damaging the sphincter complex, and ease of application.

14.4.7 Complications with Fibrin Glue

Generally, the infection develops at the external opening site after fistula glue application [17]. It is important to remember not to suture the external opening after injecting the fibrin glue [17]. Some complications like bronchospasm, hypotension, flushing, etc., have been reported [17].

14.5 Fistula Plugs

Fistula-in-ano has been treated with a variety of biological agents. Cook Medical Surgisis invented the first fistula plug in the United States [18]. The plug is comprised of a lyophilized swine small bowel submucosal matrix containing 90% collagen and which is resistant to infection [18].

The fistula plugs are made of acellular organic components of varied forms and sizes [18]. They act as a framework for fibroblasts and native tissues to grow and close the fistula tract [18].

14.5.1 Principle

The porcine collagen anal fistula plug induces tissue remodeling, resulting in complete closure of the fistula tract.

14.5.2 Indications

- Trans-sphincteric fistula
- Anovaginal and Rectovaginal fistula
- Intersphincteric fistula
- Extrasphincteric fistula

Earlier, a fistula plug was recommended for trans-sphincteric fistulas with no associated infection due to the risk of dislodgement. Later it was realized that the dislodgement of the plug was due to the technique of plug placement [19].

14.5.3 Contraindications

- A small intersphincteric fistula that can easily be drained by fistulotomy
- Infected fistulas
- Allergy to porcine products
- Acute abscess cavity
- Failure to detect an internal opening

14.5.4 Technique

Identify the internal opening and clean the tract with a fistula brush or a curette. Irrigate the tract with normal saline. Pass the probe from an internal opening and take it out through the external opening. Tie a thread to the eye of the probe and pass it through the tract. Take the plug from the sterile pack and hydrate with sterile saline for 1–3 min. Tie it with one end of a thread to an internal opening. Pull this plug inside the tract with tail-first till resistance is felt. Once this plug buries in the internal opening, trim the plug up to the mucosa level, and with the suture, fix it using 2-0 Polyglactin, taking a figure of eight stitch (Fig. 14.1). The outer end of the plug is then trimmed, leaving the external opening to drain [18].

14.5.5 Core Tips for Fistula Plug Usage

- Submerge the anal fistula plug in sterile saline for 2 min [18].
- If the internal opening is epithelialized, debride the tract, and minimize the mobilization of the mucosal margins before suturing [18].

- Trim the plug to the internal opening level and suture it with 2-0 Polyglactin [18].
- From an internal opening through the external opening, the narrow end of the plug is pulled with a suture till it snugs [18].
- The biological fistula plug's composition should allow for vascular ingrowth and good tissue formation while also being resistant to extrusion and infection [18].

14.5.6 Complications

- Extrusion—is attributed to inadequate supporting tissue associated with the fistula [20]
- Infection
- Erosion
- Fistula recurrence
- Seroma
- Abscess
- Allergic reactions [18]

14.5.7 Results

Refer Table 14.3.

Table 14.3 Fistula plugs

Journal	Year	Success rate (%)
Colon and the Rectum Diseases C. Neal Ellis [19]	2010	81
Dis Colon Rectum Christoforidis, Dimitrios et al. [20]	2009	32
Electron Physician Reza Bagherzadeh Saba [21]	2016	83.3
Colorectal Disease Ursula Aho Falt et al. [22]	2020	31

14.6 Seton

A seton is a surgical thread inserted into the fistula tract and left for several weeks to keep it patent [23]. This facilitates the fistula to drain without requiring the sphincter to be severed. Sushruta and Hippocrates were the first to advocate for seton, with the former advocating the Kshar sutra [24] and the latter recommending the insertion of a slender thread composed of raw lint directly into the fistula [25]. The word seton comes from "seta," which means bristle [25].

14.6.1 Principle

The seton works on the principle of

- Draining the pus and sepsis control before starting definitive treatment
- Stimulating fibrosis
- The cutting seton results in slow transection of an external sphincter muscle due to pressure necrosis with the cut ends being minimally separated [25]

14.6.2 What All to Include While Placing Seton?

After skin incision, the following are included:

- The deep external sphincter
- Subcutaneous portion of the external sphincter muscle
- Internal sphincter muscle
- Subcutaneous tissue

14.6.3 Types of Seton

Two types of setons can be used to heal a fistula

- **Draining Seton**: This type of seton is mainly used for drainage purposes. The seton is left to drain the intersphincteric space, boosting fibrosis in the deep sphincter muscle.

- **Cutting Seton**: This type of seton gradually cuts the sphincter muscle, followed by fibrosis.

These can be tied in two ways, loose or tight.

14.6.4 Loose Setons

Usage of loose setons reduces incontinence risk. These can be used for drainage and definitive treatment of trans-sphincteric fistula. They help the primary tract to mature and promote the secondary tract to heal [26]. Loose seton placed after abscess drainage encourages a fibrotic reaction that might close the fistula tract [27]. Many surgeons support that the placement of loose seton is a must for treating a complex fistula [28].

14.6.5 Tight Setons

These setons are used to cure the fistula by slowly cutting through the fistula tract. Cutting seton works on the principle that in fistula tracts, the nonabsorbable materials result in reactive and inflammation fibrosis [27]. Sequential tightening of a seton leads to the sphincter being cut slowly with staged fistulotomy, allowing adequate fibrosis to ensure the sphincter integrity [27]. Many cutting setons employ chemicals that remove debris and promote healthy granulation tissue, resulting in the healing of fistulas [26].

To summarize, the seton is used to cut a sphincter in a phased way or mature the tract for other surgical procedures [29].

14.6.6 Materials Used for Setons

- Ayurvedic-medicated sutures (Kshar sutra)
- Thread rubber band
- Braided sutures
- Penrose drains
- Cable tie setons [26]
- Nonabsorbable silk or nylon sutures [26]

14.6.7 Indications

- Drainage of an abscess, thus preventing further sepsis
- Trans-sphincteric fistula
- In a complex fistula to promote healing of the secondary tracts
- Two-staged fistulotomy where the seton is used to heal the divided sphincter [30]

14.6.8 Complications

- Abscess
- Induration
- Redness
- Severe burning pain
- Slippage of thread [30]
- Frequent changes lead to pain

14.6.9 Technique

Place the patient in a lithotomy posture and curette the tract. A probe is inserted with an eye from an external opening and taken out through the internal opening. The seton is inserted through the eye, and the probe is pulled out with the seton. The knot of the seton is tied (Fig. 14.2). The seton is changed at regular intervals, usually every 2 weeks, and gradually tightened.

14.6.10 Seton and Staged Fistulotomy

The staged fistulotomy is one of the procedures conducted by many surgeons to treat high fistulas. This technique involves carrying out fistulotomy in two stages:

- In the first step, the tract is probed, the skin and fat are separated, but the muscles are left

intact. A seton is tied to facilitate drainage of the fistula tract, constricting any accompanying cavities. Over time, the tissue within the seton thins and scars, causing the seton to loosen, gradually filling the tract. Once this process is over, it is time for the second stage of fistulotomy.

- The second stage involves the division of the remaining tissue within the seton. The wound is cleaned and left open to heal secondarily. The seton is tightened gradually.

Gracia Aguilar et al. concluded that cutting seton and two-staged fistulotomy were equally effective in eradicating fistulas [31].

14.6.11 Snug Seton Technique

"Snug" means "very tight or close-fitting." Hammond et al. described this technique using 1 mm of silastic seton, snugly tied around the sphincter muscles and dividing the sphincter with minimal tension. None of his patients had recurrence; however, 25% had minor incontinence [32].

14.6.12 Double Seton Technique

Walfisch et al. described a modified technique of seton placement, the double seton technique. Two approaches were described in this technique:

1. Tightening of one seton every other day.
2. Tying the second seton for several weeks till it erodes and falls out of the anal tissue. Two threads of silk were passed from the tract to achieve this. The first was left untied for 1 month, and the second was tied. After 1 month, the first seton was tied, and the second was removed. All the patients in the study attained healing by 8 weeks without incontinence [33].

14.6.13 Kshar Sutra

Kshara means to cut, and Sutra means thread, which means cutting with thread.

This is the oldest seton coated with Kshar prepared from herbs and is extensively used in Ayurveda to treat anal fistulas. It is a chemical seton working by "excision, scraping, draining, penetrating, debriding, sclerosing, and healing simultaneously without surgical excision." The standard technique is to insert the Kshar sutra through an external opening of the anal fistula with a metal probe [34].

A comparative study between Kshar Sutra and fistulotomy by G. Dutta et al. showed severe postoperative pain in the fistulotomy group. At the same time, wound discharge was more prevalent in the Kshar sutra group. Both groups had similar wound scarring, bleeding, and infection rates [35].

14.6.14 Results

Refer Table 14.4.

Table 14.4 Seton

Journal	Year	Results (Success rate) (%)
J Nat Sci Biol Med Gauranga Datta [35]	2015	97.2
J of colorectal surgery P. Srivastva and M. P. Sahu [36]	2010	97.3
Annl Saudi Med Salah M. Raslan [37]	2016	90.2
Annl Transl Med Lihua Zheing [38]	2020	100

14.6.15 Core Tips

- Tying the Lockhart-Mummery probe to a seton without a hole or an eye at the tip can be difficult because the seton slides off the probe repeatedly until it goes into the fistula tract. Many surgeons face this issue. A simple method of avoiding this slippage has been described by R. Canter Cid et al. [39]. A short piece of Abbocath is cut, and a 2-0 silk suture is passed through it [39]. The Abbocath's one end is firmly connected to the probe tip. The probe is then removed from the tract, enabling the ligature to slip through without difficulty. This method is comparable to the Seow Cheon railroad method of inserting a seton [39].
- There should be constant tension on the seton to ensure proper cutting of the sphincters.

14.7 Ligation of Intersphincteric Fistula Tract (LIFT)

LIFT is an approach that Dr. Arun Rojanasakul designed in 2007 as a sphincter-sparing procedure [40].

14.7.1 Principle

Fistula tract ligation in an intersphincteric space close to an internal opening with separation of the distal tract.

14.7.2 Indication

- Trans-sphincteric fistulas

14.7.3 Technique

The external and the internal openings are identified by injecting water or a metallic probe from either opening. The intersphincteric groove is palpated, and a curvilinear incision is made parallel to the anal canal to enter the intersphincteric space. Dissection is carried out close to the external sphincter to prevent injury to the internal sphincter or breach of the anal mucosa.

The fistula tract is identified, divided, and isolated. Suture ligations on the distal and proximal end of the tract are done using 3-0 polyglactin. An additional suture is applied to reinforce tract closure. The fistula tract next to the suture site is divided. Saline is injected through the external opening after excision of the intersphincteric tract to ensure that the right tract is removed. The internal and external sphincters are approximated again. The surrounding skin is then sutured loosely. The infected granulation tissue is removed by curetting of the distal tract and sent for a histopathology examination.

14.7.4 Results

The initial LIFT results were more than 90%, and no disturbance was noted in the continence rate. Nevertheless, as more evidence accumulated, the success rate declined to 76% [41] (Table 14.5).

14.7.5 Advantages of LIFT

As it is a sphincter-saving procedure, there is no chance of incontinence. Even when the procedure is unsuccessful, the risk of incontinence is nil [43].

Table 14.5 LIFT

Journal	Year	Results (%)
Tech Coloproctol Rojanasakul [40]	2007	94.4
Journal of Coloproctology Fakhrosadat Anaraki [42]	2016	63.8
Elsevier A meta-analysis Sameh Hany Emile [41]	2020	76.5

14.7.6 Pitfalls of LIFT

Performing the LIFT procedure in an anterior fistula in females has always been difficult as the perineal body lies anteriorly, and an external anal sphincter is deficient in females. There is a fear of misidentifying the plane and dissecting between the external sphincter and the vagina [44].

14.7.7 Complications After LIFT

After the procedure, complications were noted in nearly 14% of patients [41]. The most important complication after LIFT is dehiscence and infection [41].

14.8   Video-Assisted Anal Fistula Treatment (VAAFT)

P. Meinero first designed VAAFT in 2006 [43].

14.8.1 Principle

The VAAFT approach is based on three principles:

- Identification of internal opening
- Destruction of a tract from inside
- Preserving the function of the anal sphincter

The VAAFT technique helps detect and close the internal opening and destroy the distal tract for proper healing. With the VAAFT procedure, an internal opening is detected in almost 82.6% of the cases. The main feature of VAAFT is that the procedure is carried out under direct endoluminal vision [43]. Fistuloscopy also aids in identifying possible chronic abscesses or secondary tracts [44].

The technique has two phases

- **Diagnostic Phase**: Locates the internal opening, abscess cavities, and secondary tracts [43]. The fistuloscope light seen inside helps locate the internal opening [45].

- **Operative Phase**: Destroys the epithelized fistula tract and unhealthy granulation tissue from inside using a unipolar electrode followed by internal opening closure [43].

14.8.2 Indications

- All tracts in which internal opening is challenging to locate

14.8.3 Contraindications

- Tracts with a curved path and multiple extensions. These cannot be adequately explored due to the rigid structure of the scope.
- Tracts with a small diameter. The tract diameter should be wide enough to allow passage of the fistuloscope.

14.8.4 Equipment

The equipment is attached with a camera for surgical videoendoscopy [43]. The equipment consists of

- A monopolar electrode
- A rigid fistuloscope
- Endoscopic forceps
- Brush

A fistuloscope is equipped with a rigid telescope angled on 8° with 18 cm of operative length and 3.3 × 4.7 mm diameter. It has an irrigation, working and an optical channel. The irrigation channel relates to taps; an irrigation solution is attached to one. Both the channels have a handle for facilitating maneuvering. The scope is connected to the videoendoscopy equipment. The entire technique can be video recorded.

14.8.5 Technique

14.8.5.1 Operative Phase
The fistuloscope is inserted through the external opening, and the obturator is removed. The whitish material adherent to the fistula tract is removed with a brush and forceps, followed by cauterization. Continuous irrigation with glycine eliminates the necrotic material into the rectum through the internal opening. Finally, the internal opening is closed with a stapler, an advancement flap, or a suture. As per the position of the internal opening, a semicircular or linear stapler can be used [45]. A mucosal or cutaneous flap is raised to close the internal opening if thick and fibrotic tissue is found near the internal opening.

14.8.6 Advantages

- VAAFT technique provides visualization of the course of the tract and helps identify the fistula branches and internal opening.
- Small surgical wound.
- Destruction of fistula tract under direct vision.

14.8.7 Results

Refer Table 14.6.

Table 14.6 VAAFT procedure

Journal	Year	Results
Tech Coloproctol P. Meinero and L. Mori [45]	2011	73.5% (primary healing) 87.1% (after 1-year follow-up)
Gastroenterology Research and practice Michal Romanizskyn [46]	2017	54.51%
Tech Coloproctol L. Regusci [47]	2020	84.4%

14.8.8 Pitfalls of VAAFT

- Although the fistuloscope provides direct vision, since the tracts are usually curved, it becomes challenging to explore the entire fistula tract with a rigid instrument [46, 48].
- The diameter of the fistuloscope makes it challenging to explore narrow tracts with stiff fibrous walls [46].
- Excessive cauterization may result in collateral injury to tissues outside the fistula [46].

14.9   Stem Cells

Some authors believe that the recurrence of the fistula is due to a defect in the wound healing process [49]. Stem cell transplantation increases cell numbers and restores normal cell healing through matrix remodeling and growth-factor secretion [49].

14.9.1 Principle

Stem cells heal the fistula by local suppression of inflammation and immunoregulation [49].

14.9.2 Indications

- Anal fistula with Crohn's disease

14.9.3 Technique

A metal curette is used to perform vigorous curettage on the track, followed by irrigation with normal saline. The internal opening is closed by direct suturing or with a mucosal flap.

Two vials containing stem cells are injected near the internal opening by the transanal approach. In the perianal approach, stem cells are injected, from an external opening forming tiny deposits of cell suspension within the fistula tract. The stem cell suspension is injected as per the guidelines given by the manufacturer after the preparation and re-suspension of stem cells.

The fistula is massaged gently after the injection, and a sterile bandage is applied to the anal region. After the procedure, there are no restrictions relating to mobility, and the patient is discharged the same day [50].

14.9.4 Results

Some authors recommend using stem cells with fibrin glue. Results vary from 50–71% [29] (Table 14.7).

Table 14.7 Stem cells

Journal	Year	Success rate (%)
Tech Coloproctol S. Choi et al. [51]	2019	62.8
Stem Cell Research and Therapy Chungen Zhou [52]	2020	63.6
Stem Cell Research and Therapy Yantian Cao [53]	2021	71

14.9.5 Core Tip

14.9.5.1 Choosing Stem Cells

Mesenchymal stem cells are used for treating fistula-in-ano. These cells are present in fat and bone marrow. For the stem cell to fulfill the criteria, they must have

- Adherence to the plastic
- Specific surface antigen expression
- Differentiation potential [49]

Syringe liposuction is used for sucking out the fat from a patient's outer or inner thigh or lower abdomen under anesthesia. Cells derived from the fat are known as adipose-derived stem cells. The fistula tract must be detected more than 2 weeks before the adipose stem cell procedure.

The intralesional cells are derived from bone marrow and expanded ex-vivo for use in fistula-in-ano [49].

14.10 Submucosal Ligation of Fistula Tract (SLOFT)

Dr. D. U. Pathak from India first described this procedure in 2014 [54], aiming to obliterate the internal opening and separate the distal tract.

14.10.1 Principle

The procedure is performed to obliterate the internal opening and separate the distal tract by ligating and disconnecting it near the internal opening. The ligation is superficial and at the internal opening, thus leaving behind no stump.

14.10.2 Indications

- Mature straight fistula tract. The internal opening can be reached in stages in curved or horseshoe tracts.

14.10.3 Contraindications

- High internal opening
- Non-negotiable internal opening
- Unable to find an internal opening
- Friable anorectum secondary to inflammatory bowel disease

The procedure may be challenging in an obese patient with a deep natal cleft and scarred anorectum in recurrent fistulas.

14.10.4 Technique

A malleable metal probe is inserted from the external opening and taken out from the internal opening. A figure of eight suture is taken using a 5/8 circle of 27 mm 2-0 Polyglactin, circumambulating the fistula tract at the internal opening. The probe is gently withdrawn before tying the knot. While withdrawing the probe from the internal opening, a sudden jerk while tightening the knot indicates that the suture is placed behind a tract. Normal saline is injected through the external opening to check that the internal opening is duly closed. The probe is inserted again in the fistula tract, and its tip is palpated nearly 2–3 mm proximal to the internal opening, towards the anal verge. The distal tract is separated at the probe's tip using monopolar cautery or bare laser fiber, isolating the distal tract containing the cryptoglandular infection. The normal saline is injected again through the external opening. It can be seen coming out from the tract at the point of division, indicating the separation of the distal tract. One should ensure that the tract is completely separated as a partial separation may lead to recurrence. Finally, the distal tract is curetted, and the external opening is enlarged for drainage.

14.10.5 Results

Refer Table 14.8.

Table 14.8 SLOFT

Journal	Year	Success rate (%)
Ambulatory Surgery D. U. Pathak [54]	2003	90
IJSS Journal of Surgery Mahendra Singh [55]	2018	90
Colorectal Dis N. K. Raja Ram [56]	2020	80.9
International Journal of Recent Scientific Research Kamal Gupta et al. [57]	2019	93.5

Fig. 14.3 Submucosal ligation of fistula tract (SLOFT)

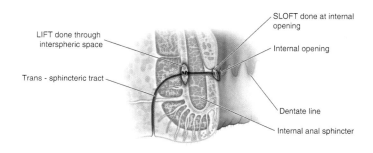

14.10.6 Comparison with LIFT

SLOFT is a simplified version of LIFT:

- In SLOFT, the tract is easier to dissect with the indwelling probe than in LIFT.
- The dissection is close to the internal opening, leaving no stump compared to LIFT (Fig. 14.3).
- In SLOFT, ligation is superficial and easy, whereas in LIFT it is 3–4 cm deep to the skin.
- In case of recurrence in LIFT, the collection is deep in intersphincteric space, which must be dealt with under anesthesia. In contrast, in SLOFT, the recurrence is a small submucosal abscess that bursts by itself or can be drained under local anesthesia.

14.11 Discussion

Minimal invasive techniques have gained popularity over time as they are sphincter-saving, less painful, and offer speedy recovery. Every procedure aims at reducing the recurrence rate. Mucosal advancement flaps are challenging technically, and their recurrence rate varies from 2% to 54%, which may be attributed to structural mobilization or the tendency of a flap to retract or dehiscence [45]. Minimal incontinence has been reported in some patients. Fibrin glue has a success rate of 16% [45].

Similarly, the fistula plugs' recurrence rate ranges from 31% to 80% [22, 23]. Both types of setons, i.e., cutting and loose seton, are used widely, and the selection of the seton is based on the surgeon's choice. The principle behind using a seton is similar to a wire cutting through ice. The ice remains adherent after the division by the wire [58]. A drainage seton can be utilized to control sepsis in the long term or as a preliminary step before a procedure [58].

LIFT and VAAFT are two minimally invasive methods for securing the tract at the internal opening. The LIFT procedure involves ligation of a tract in the intersphincteric space, suture closure of a defect on the external sphincter, and curettage of the tract [45]. LIFT's drawback is that it is technically difficult for high fistulas and fistula tracts with extensions that ascend in the intersphincteric plane and cross the external anal sphincter at a higher level [45]. The exposed intersphincteric space can sometimes disrupt the blood supply to an internal sphincter, which further breaches the anal mucosa, resulting in failure [45]. In the VAAFT technique, one closes the internal opening and destroys the fistula tract.

SLOFT is a simplified LIFT version that allows the tract to be separated near an internal opening. In case of recurrence in LIFT, the collection is deep in intersphincteric space, which is left unattended. The same holds good for SLOFT, as the infection below the internal opening is again not addressed.

Park developed a technique for managing high anal fistulas by excising the internal opening and removing a segment of the internal anal sphincter without cutting the external anal sphincter. Hybrid techniques follow the same principle and aim at sparing the sphincters.

Take-Home Message

- Though these sphincter-saving techniques have recently gained popularity, the success rate varies. Endorectal advancement flaps are highly applied procedures with no incontinence risk because they avoid full-thickness anal sphincter division. Fibrin glue and fistula plugs offer a reasonable healing rate but are associated with complications like infection and extrusion. Setons can either cut or drain and be placed in the fistula tract or abscess cavity to remove residual sepsis. All these procedures have their advantages and disadvantages.
- LIFT is a commonly practiced sphincter-saving technique. It aims to transect and ligate a fistula via an intersphincter space and has mixed results. VAAFT technique creates minor wounds and provides a direct vision of the internal opening. SLOFT needs further studies and trials to gain popularity.
- Lasers have emerged as a practical futuristic approach for anal fistula treatment, which I shall be discussing in the next chapter.

References

1. Bubbers EJ, Cologne KG. Management of complex anal fistulas. Clin Colon Rectal Surg. 2016;29(1):43–9. https://doi.org/10.1055/s-0035-1570392. PMID: 26929751; PMCID: PMC4755767
2. Elting AWX. X. The treatment of fistula in ano: with especial reference to the Whitehead operation. Ann. Surg. 1912;56(5):744–52. https://doi.org/10.1097/00000658-191211000-00010. PMID: 17862924; PMCID: PMC1407359
3. Hilsabeck JR. Transanal advancement of the anterior rectal wall for vaginal fistulas involving the lower rectum. Dis Colon Rectum. 1980;23(4):236–41. https://doi.org/10.1007/BF02587089. PMID: 7389518
4. Zimmerman DD, Wasowicz DK, Gottgens KW. Transanal advancement flap repair: the current gold standard for cryptoglandular transsphincteric perianal fistulas. Turkish J Colorect Dis. 2019;29(3):104–10.
5. Kim DS. Advancement flap for the treatment of a complex anal fistula. Ann Coloproctol. 2014;30(4):161–2.
6. Jensen CC. Endorectal advancement flap. In: Abcarian H, editor. Anal fistula. New York: Springer; 2014. p. 97–108.
7. Uribe N, Millán M, Minguez M, Ballester C, Asencio F, Sanchiz V, Esclapez P, del Castillo JR. Clinical and manometric results of endorectal advancement flaps for complex anal fistula. Int J Colorectal Dis. 2007;22(3):259–64. https://doi.org/10.1007/s00384-006-0172-z. Epub 2006 Aug 2. PMID: 16896993
8. Song KH. New techniques for treating an anal fistula. J Korean Soc Coloproctol. 2012;28(1):7–12. https://doi.org/10.3393/jksc.2012.28.1.7. Epub 2012 Feb 29. PMID: 22413076; PMCID: PMC3296947
9. Podetta M, Scarpa CR, Zufferey G, Skala K, Ris F, Roche B, Buchs NC. Mucosal advancement flap for recurrent complex anal fistula: a repeatable procedure. Int J Colorectal Dis. 2019;34(1):197–200. https://doi.org/10.1007/s00384-018-3155-y. Epub 2018 Sep 5. Erratum in: Int J Colorectal Dis. 2018 Dec 20; PMID: 30187157
10. Seifarth C, Lehmann KS, Holmer C, Pozios I. Healing of rectal advancement flaps for anal fistulas in patients with and without Crohn's disease: a retrospective cohort analysis. BMC Surg. 2021;21(1):283. https://doi.org/10.1186/s12893-021-01282-4. PMID: 34088303; PMCID: PMC8178918
11. Ardakani MR, Hormozi AK, Ardakani JR, Davarpanahjazi AH, Moghadam AS. Introduction of potent single-donor fibrin glue for vascular anastomosis: an animal study. J Res Med Sci. 2012;17(5):461–5. PMID: 23626612; PMCID: PMC3634273
12. Maralcan G, Başkonuş I, Gökalp A, Borazan E, Balk A. Long-term results in the treatment of fistula-in-ano with fibrin glue: a prospective study. J Korean Surg Soc. 2011;81(3):169–75. https://doi.org/10.4174/jkss.2011.81.3.169. Epub 2011 Sep 26. PMID: 22066118; PMCID: PMC3204547
13. Cintron JR. Fibrin sealant. In: Abcarian H, editor. Anal fistula. New York: Springer; 2014. p. 69–81.
14. Khafagy W, Zedan S, Setiet A, et al. Autologous fibrin glue in treatment of fistula in ano. Coloproctology. 2001;23:17–21.
15. Sentovich SM. Fibrin glue for anal fistulas: long-term results. Dis Colon Rectum. 2003;46(4):498–502. https://doi.org/10.1007/s10350-004-6589-y. PMID: 12682544

16. Vidon M, Munoz-Bongrand N, Lambert J, Maggiori L, Zeitoun JD, Corte H, Panis Y, Seksik P, Treton X, Abramowitz L, Allez M, Gornet JM. Long-term efficacy of fibrin glue injection for perianal fistulas in patients with Crohn's disease. Colorectal Dis. 2021;23(4):894–900. https://doi.org/10.1111/codi.15477. Epub 2020 Dec 29. PMID: 33278859

17. Cirocchi R, Farinella E, La Mura F, Cattorini L, Rossetti B, Milanite D, Ricci P, Covarelli P, Coccetta M, Noya G, Sciannameo F. Fibrin glue in the treatment of anal fistula: a systematic review. Ann Surg Innov Res. 2009;3:12. https://doi.org/10.1186/1750-1164-3-12. PMID: 19912660; PMCID: PMC2784785

18. Eisenstein S, Ky AJ. Biologic fistula plugs. In: Abcarian H, editor. Anal fistula: principles and management. New York: Springer; 2014. https://doi.org/10.1007/978-1-4614-9014-2_12.

19. Ellis CN, Rostas JW, Greiner FG. Long-term outcomes with the use of bioprosthetic plugs to manage complex anal fistulas. Dis Colon Rectum. 2010;53(5):798–802. https://doi.org/10.1007/DCR.0b013e3181d43b7d. PMID: 20389214

20. Christoforidis D, Pieh MC, Madoff RD, Mellgren AF. A comparative study is the treatment of transsphincteric anal fistulas by endorectal advancement flap or collagen fistula plug. Dis Colon Rectum. 2009;52(1):18–22. https://doi.org/10.1007/DCR.0b013e31819756ac. PMID: 19273951

21. Saba RB, Tizmaghz A, Ajeka S, Karami M. Treating anal fistula with the anal fistula plug: case series report of 12 patients. Electron Physician. 2016;8(4):2304–7. https://doi.org/10.19082/2303. PMID: 27280009; PMCID: PMC4886575

22. Aho Fält U, Zawadzki A, Starck M, Bohe M, Johnson LB. Long-term outcome of the Surgisis® (Biodesign®) anal fistula plug for complex cryptoglandular and Crohn's fistulas. Colorectal Dis. 2021;23(1):178–85. https://doi.org/10.1111/codi.15429. Epub 2020 Dec 26. PMID: 33155391; PMCID: PMC7898619

23. Treatment anal fistula. https://www.nhs.uk/conditions/anal-fistula/treatment/.

24. Panigrahi HK, Rani MR, Padhi MM. Clinical evaluation of Kshara sutra therapy in the management of Bhagandara (fistula-in-ano)-a prospective study. Ancient Sci Life. 2009;28(3):29.

25. Subhas G, Singh Bhullar J, Al-Omari A, Unawane A, Mittal VK, Pearlman R. Setons in the treatment of anal fistula: a review of variations in materials and techniques. Dig Surg. 2012;29(4):292–300. https://doi.org/10.1159/000342398. Epub 2012 Aug 31. PMID: 22948115

26. Velchuru VR. Seton (loose, cutting, chemical). In: Abcarian H, editor. Anal fistula. New York: Springer; 2014. p. 45–52.

27. Kelly ME, Heneghan HM, McDermott FD, Nason GJ, Freeman C, Martin ST, Winter DC. The role of loose seton in the management of anal fistula: a multicenter study of 200 patients. Tech Coloproctol. 2014;18(10):915–9.

28. Sileri P, Cadeddu F, D'Ugo S, Franceschilli L, Del Vecchio Blanco G, De Luca E, Calabrese E, Capperucci SM, Fiaschetti V, Milito G, Gaspari AL. Surgery for fistula-in-ano in a specialist colorectal unit: a critical appraisal. BMC Gastroenterol. 2011;11:120. https://doi.org/10.1186/1471-230X-11-120. PMID: 22070555; PMCID: PMC3235969

29. Sheikh P, Baakza A. Management of fistula-in-ano-the current evidence. Indian J Surg. 2014;76(6):482–6. https://doi.org/10.1007/s12262-014-1150-2. Epub 2014 Aug 15. PMID: 25614724; PMCID: PMC4297991

30. Nottingham JM, Rentea RM. Anal fistulotomy (seton placement); 2020.

31. García-Aguilar J, Belmonte C, Wong DW, Goldberg SM, Madoff RD. Cutting seton versus two-stage seton fistulotomy in the surgical management of high anal fistula. Br J Surg. 1998;85(2):243–5. https://doi.org/10.1046/j.1365-2168.1998.02877.x. PMID: 9501826

32. Hammond TM, Knowles CH, Porrett T, Lunniss PJ. The Snug Seton: short- and medium-term results of slow fistulotomy for idiopathic anal fistulae. Colorectal Dis. 2006;8(4):328–37. https://doi.org/10.1111/j.1463-1318.2005.00926.x. PMID: 16630239

33. Walfisch S, Menachem Y, Koretz M. Double seton—a new modified approach to high transsphincteric anal fistula. Dis Colon Rectum. 1997;40(6):731–2. https://doi.org/10.1007/BF02140905. PMID: 9194470

34. Kumar A, Kumar M, Jha AK, Kumar B, Kumari R. The easiest way to insert Ksharsutra with the help of an infant feeding tube instead of a metallic probe. Indian J Surg. 2017;79(4):371–3. https://doi.org/10.1007/s12262-017-1668-1. Epub 2017 Jun 21. PMID: 28827918; PMCID: PMC5549058

35. Dutta G, Bain J, Ray AK, Dey S, Das N, Das B. Comparing Ksharasutra (Ayurvedic Seton) and open fistulotomy in the management of fistula-in-ano. J Nat Sci Biol Med. 2015;6(2):406–10. https://doi.org/10.4103/0976-9668.160022. PMID: 26283840; PMCID: PMC4518420

36. Srivastava PD, Sahu MP. Efficacy of Kshar Sutra (medicated seton) therapy in managing fistula-in-ano. World J Colorectal Surg. 2010;2(1):6.

37. Raslan SM, Aladwani M, Alsanea N. Evaluation of the cutting seton as a treatment method for perianal fistula. Ann Saudi Med. 2016;36(3):210–5. https://doi.org/10.5144/0256-4947.2016.210. PMID: 27236393; PMCID: PMC6074548

38. Zheng L, Shi Y, Zhi C, Yu Q, Li X, Wu S, Zhang W, Liu Y, Huang Z. Loose combined cutting seton for patients with high intersphincteric fistula: a retrospective study. Ann Transl Med. 2020;8(19):1236. https://doi.org/10.21037/atm-20-6123. PMID: 33178768; PMCID: PMC7607110

39. Cantero Cid R, Salinas Gómez J, García Olmo D. How to place a seton and prevent it slipping: mission impossible? Tech Coloproctol. 2014;18(6):603.

https://doi.org/10.1007/s10151-013-1118-4. Epub 2014 Feb 14. PMID: 24526396

40. Rojanasakul A. LIFT procedure: a simplified technique for fistula-in-ano. Tech Coloproctol. 2009;13(3):237–40.

41. Emile SH, Khan SM, Adejumo A, Koroye O. Ligation of intersphincteric fistula tract (LIFT) in treatment of anal fistula: an updated systematic review, meta-analysis, and meta-regression of the predictors of failure. Surgery. 2020;167(2):484–92. https://doi.org/10.1016/j.surg.2019.09.012. Epub 2019 Oct 21. PMID: 31648932

42. Anaraki F, Bagherzade G, Behboo R, Etemad O. Long-term results of ligation of intersphincteric fistula tract (LIFT) for management of anal fistula. J Coloproctol. 2016;36(4):227–30.

43. Meinero P, Mori L, Gasloli G. Video-assisted anal fistula treatment: a new concept of treating anal fistulas. Dis Colon Rectum. 2014;57(3):354–9. https://doi.org/10.1097/DCR.0000000000000082. PMID: 24509459

44. Schwandner O. Video-assisted anal fistula treatment (VAAFT) combined with advancement flap repair in Crohn's disease. Tech Coloproctol. 2013;17(2):221–5. https://doi.org/10.1007/s10151-012-0921-7. Epub 2012 Nov 23. PMID: 23179892

45. Meinero P, Mori L. Video-assisted anal fistula treatment (VAAFT): a novel sphincter-saving procedure for treating complex anal fistulas. Tech Coloproctol. 2011;15(4):417–22. https://doi.org/10.1007/s10151-011-0769-2. Epub 2011 Oct 15. Erratum in: Tech Coloproctol. 2012;16(1):111. PMID: 22002535; PMCID: PMC3226694

46. Romaniszyn M, Walega P. Video-assisted anal fistula treatment: pros and cons of this minimally invasive method for treatment of perianal fistulas. Gastroenterol Res Pract. 2017;2017:9518310. https://doi.org/10.1155/2017/9518310. Epub 2017 Jun 7. PMID: 28680443; PMCID: PMC5478827

47. Regusci L, Fasolini F, Meinero P, Caccia G, Ruggeri G, Serati M, Braga A. Video-assisted anal fistula treatment (VAAFT) for complex anorectal fistula: efficacy and risk factors for failure at 3-year follow-up. Tech Coloproctol. 2020;24(7):741–6. https://doi.org/10.1007/s10151-020-02213-w. Epub 2020 Apr 21. PMID: 32318991

48. Parks AG, Gordon PH, Hardcastle JD. A classification of fistula-in-ano. Br J Surg. 1976;63(1):1–12. https://doi.org/10.1002/bjs.1800630102. PMID: 1267867

49. Garcia-Olmo D, Guadalajara-Labajo H. Stem cell application in fistula disease. In: Abcarian H, editor. Anal fistula. New York: Springer; 2014. p. 129–38.

50. Park MY, Yoon YS, Kim HE, Lee JL, Park IJ, Lim SB, Yu CS, Kim JC. Surgical options for perianal fistula in patients with Crohn's disease: a comparison of seton placement, fistulotomy, and stem cell therapy. Asian J Surg. 2021;44(11):1383–8. https://doi.org/10.1016/j.asjsur.2021.03.013. Epub 2021 May 6. PMID: 33966965

51. Choi S, Jeon BG, Chae G, Lee SJ. A meta-analysis of the clinical efficacy of stem cell therapy for complex perianal fistulas. Tech Coloproctol. 2019;23(5):411–27. https://doi.org/10.1007/s10151-019-01994-z. Epub 2019 May 2. PMID: 31049792

52. Zhou C, Li M, Zhang Y, Ni M, Wang Y, Xu D, Shi Y, Zhang B, Chen Y, Huang Y, Zhang S, Shi H, Jiang B. Autologous adipose-derived stem cells for the treatment of Crohn's fistula-in-ano: an open-label, controlled trial. Stem Cell Res Ther. 2020;11(1):124. https://doi.org/10.1186/s13287-020-01636-4. PMID: 32183875; PMCID: PMC7079384

53. Cao Y, Su Q, Zhang B, Shen F, Li S. Efficacy of stem cells therapy for Crohn's fistula: a meta-analysis and systematic review. Stem Cell Res Ther. 2021;12(1):32. https://doi.org/10.1186/s13287-020-02095-7. PMID: 33413661; PMCID: PMC7792029

54. Pathak DU, Agrawal V, Taneja VK. Submucosal ligation of fistula tract (SLOFT) for anorectal fistula: an effective and easy technique. Ambulatory Surg. 2014;20(3):42–3.

55. Singh M, Godse S. Simple new approach for anorectal fistula: submucosal ligation of fistula tract. IJSS J Surg. 2018;4(2):47–8.

56. Raja Ram NK, Chan KK, Md Nor SF, Sagap I. A prospective evaluation of the outcome of submucosal ligation of the fistula tract. Colorectal Dis. 2020;22(12):2199–203. https://doi.org/10.1111/codi.15305. Epub 2020 Oct 6. PMID: 32780561

57. Gupta K, Mital K, Gupta R, Bakshi T. Distal laser proximal fistulotomy-a new sphincter-saving technique. A comparative study with other sphincter-saving procedures. Int J Recent Sci Res. 2020;11(03):37892–4.

58. Corman ML, Bergamaschi RC, Nicholls RJ, Fazio VW. Corman–cirurgia colorretal. Thieme Revinter Publicações LTDA; 2017.

"Continuous improvement is better than delayed perfection."

Mark Twain

Key Concepts
- Fistula Laser Closure (FiLaC) is a sphincter-saving technique that "ablates" the fistula tract with a radial laser fiber and destroys the unhealthy granulation tissue.
- The laser tip does not damage the sphincters.
- At the time of the invention of the procedure for FiLaC, the internal opening was closed with an anorectal advancement flap or by a simple suture.

15.1 Introduction

Treating anal fistulas while conserving the anal sphincters remains a challenge. Simple fistulotomy can be used to treat low trans-sphincteric or low intersphincteric fistulas. The sphincter-saving approach is better for high trans-sphincteric and complex fistulas, which involve a significant sphincter complex. During surgical intervention in this type of fistula, damage to sphincters may lead to fecal incontinence. Fistula Laser Closure is a sphincter-saving technique that "ablates" a fistula tract with a radial laser fiber and destroys unhealthy granulation and the fistula walls, leading to shrinkage and sealing of the tract [1]. Biolitec coined the term FiLaC. However, most surgeons prefer to use the nomenclature "LAFT," which means laser ablation of the fistula tract [1].

Wilhelm from Germany first described FiLaC in 2011 for fistula treatment [2]. As the penetration of laser energy occurs only for a few millimeters, it helps in reducing the collateral damage to the sphincter muscle fibers [3]. Therefore, it is preferred as a sphincter-saving procedure [2, 3]. In the FiLaC method, the internal opening was closed using an anorectal flap or a simple stitch [2]. Later, Giamundo hypothesized obliteration of the internal opening and rest of the fistula tract using the shrinking effect of laser [4].

15.2 Principle

The principle of laser fistula surgery is to ablate the entire fistula tract with a diode laser source, followed by the internal opening closure [5]. The fiber used is a 360-degree corona radial fiber.

15.3 Indications

FiLaC procedure can be performed in the following types of fistulas:

- Intersphincteric
- Trans-sphincteric
- Suprasphincteric

- Anterior fistulas in females
- Complex or high fistulas
- In patients with weak sphincters, to prevent incontinence

15.4 Contraindications

- Fistulas associated with abscesses

15.5 Technique

Hydrogen peroxide is injected in the tract's external opening. Bubbles can be seen coming out of the internal opening (Fig. 15.1a). The tract is curetted, and the necrotic material is sent for histopathology examination (Fig. 15.1b). A 6F infant feeding tube is inserted from the external opening into the internal opening. A 360-degree

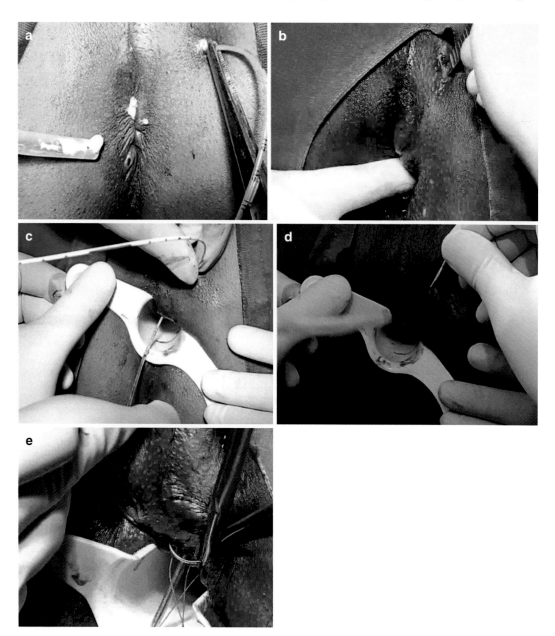

Fig. 15.1 (**a**) Injecting hydrogen peroxide in external opening of a tract to identify its internal opening. (**b**) Curetting of a fistula tract. (**c**) Insertion of laser fiber by railroad method. (**d**) Laser ablation of the fistula tract from internal to external opening. (**e**) Internal opening closure by circumambulation technique using Polyglactin 2-0

corona radial laser fiber is taken through the tube to avoid injury to the tip of the fiber. Alternatively, the infant feeding tube may be inserted into the internal opening and taken out from the external opening (railroad method Fig. 15.1c).

The laser fiber delivers energy radially. The energy is released continuously, and a dosage of 10 W/mm/s is administered. The shrinkage effect occurs due to the vaporization of the water content from the cytoplasm of cells lining the fistula tract. Simultaneously, the unhealthy granulation tissue present in the tract is "ablated" (Fig. 15.1d).

The tract is again curetted, followed by irrigation with normal saline to remove the debris. Using Polyglactin 2-0, the internal opening is then closed. A circumambulation stitch taken with a probe inside the tract is a good way of closing, as it ensures complete closure of the internal opening (Fig. 15.1e). Before tying the knot, the probe is pulled out. The stitches are taken perpendicular or parallel to the dentate line. Internal anal sphincter fibers are also included for proper transfixation (Fig. 15.2a, b). Otherwise, the stitches may give away during defecation due to increased anal canal pressure. A purse-string suture may also be taken to close the internal opening (Fig. 15.2c). Some authors believe that internal opening closure with primary sutures has no advantage in fistula healing [6]. Moreover, they observed that it did not matter which way the internal opening was closed, as the recurrence rates were similar.

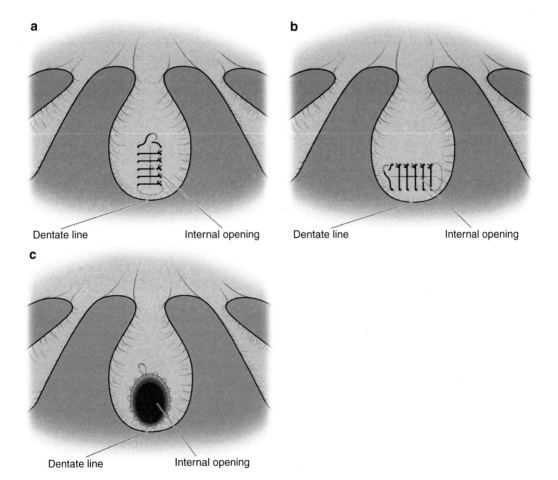

Fig. 15.2 (**a**) Closure of internal opening perpendicular to dentate line. (**b**) Closure of internal opening parallel to dentate line. (**c**) Closure of internal opening by purse-string suture

15.6 Pitfalls

1. As this is a blind procedure, the tracts are not visualized. Moreover, the branching tracts cannot be adequately assessed [1].
2. Increasing the power of the laser energy could result in damage to the sphincter complex [1].
3. One has to rely on the bactericidal effect of the laser beam to destroy the infection in the intersphincteric plane.

15.7 Results

The procedure's success rate ranges from 71.4% to 88.89% (Table 15.1). In Crohn's disease, the success rate is 55% to 69.2% (Table 15.2).

Table 15.1 Results of FiLaC

Year	Name of the journal	No. of patients	Success rate
2013	Colorectal Disease P. Giamundo [4]	35	71.4%
2014	Dis Colon Rectum Oztruk [3]	37	82%
2016	Tech Coloproctol A Wilhelm [2]	117	88%
2017	Turkish Journal of Colorectal Disease Turgut Donmez [5]	27	88.89%
2018	Tech Coloproctol Lauretta A [7]	30	33.33% (initial results)
2019	Tech Coloproctol I Marref [8]	69	60% (high trans-sphincteric fistula)
2019	International Journal of Recent Scientific Research Kamal Gupta et al. [9]	42	84%

Table 15.2 Results of FiLaC in Crohn's disease

Journal	Success rate
Coloproctology A Wilhelm [10]	69.2%
Techniques in Coloproctology Amine Aalam et al. [11]	55%

15.8 Discussion

Fistulotomy remains the gold standard treatment for simple fistulas. However, fistulotomy in complex fistulas may be associated with recurrence and incontinence. Fistula laser closure is a minimally invasive approach for sphincter-saving. According to Wilhelm [2], there are certain advantages of the fistula laser closure technique. The primary benefit is that the radial energy application helps destroy the remnants of granulation tissue and fistula epithelium, which is considered a cause of recurrence after fistula surgery. Another advantage is that the laser energy shrinks the fistula tract, similar to what occurs in blood vessels in laser varicose veins treatment by endovenous ablation. Thirdly, the laser tip does not damage the sphincters [2].

The initial Wilhelm's series comprised only 11 patients with a success rate of 81.8% [2]. In his subsequent study of 5-year follow-up, the success rate was 88% [10]. The anorectal flap was used for closing the tract's internal opening. As mentioned in the previous chapters, the success rate of the anorectal flap is 56% to 92%. Wilhelm has proposed using the VAAFT scope to tackle the side branches, making it more like a hybrid procedure than a standalone [2]. Giamundo advocated that an internal opening could be closed entirely by the shrinkage effect of laser energy, and no anorectal flaps were required [4]. Kursat R. Serin and colleagues, for the first time, used internal opening closure using a purse-string with Polyglactin 2-0 after debridement of the internal opening. No significant improvement was observed in the results [6].

In other sphincter-saving procedures like fistula plugs or fibrin glue, it is presumed that the glue or plug will take care of the internal opening. In a procedure like LIFT, the emphasis is on separating the tract near the internal opening rather than dealing with it [12]. All these concepts are absolutely against the basic pathogenesis of fistula formation, as it is evident that the source of infection lies below the internal opening. Similar are the views of Altomare [13].

It is worth mentioning that the laser beam may have a bactericidal effect [14]. The laser beam emits energy at 80 °C to 100 °C, and the bactericidal effect, especially in organisms like E. coli [15], occurs at 65 °C. Moreover, as mentioned earlier, the laser energy causes protein denaturation leading to the sealing of the blood vessels. This prevents the transmission of infection through blood.

The penetration depth of the laser is 2–3 mm using radial fiber with 1470 nm wavelength, causing minimal sphincter collateral damage [10]. A laser fiber capable of 360° radial emissions is preferred because it causes negligible thermal diffusion. Consequently, it diminishes the peri-fistula collateral thermal damage [4]. The energy delivered by laser destroys the fistula tract epithelial wall and the endoluminal granulation tissue [5], allowing the tissue to repair by fibroblasts and macrophages [13]. The laser tip does not damage the sphincters [3, 5, 6]. Simple diathermy does not achieve the same results as it does not create the tissue shrinkage effect [5]. Moreover, trauma to the sphincters may be high due to the hyperthermic effect of diathermy [5].

The amount of energy delivered through the laser is directly proportional to the length of the tract. It has been opined that a longer tract crossing both the internal and the external sphincters increases the chances of tract closure, in contrast to the small tracts, which cross the minimal adipose tissue as in intersphincteric tracts [8, 16]. According to the literature review, FiLaC has been ineffective in suprasphincteric fistulas with a healing rate of 18% because of poor drainage from the intersphincteric space [8, 17]. Marref et al. found a better success rate of 60% in large trans-sphincteric fistulas [8].

Lauretta et al. conducted their research on the fistula length, the "Achilles' heel" of the laser treatment [7]. According to their study, the shrinkage effect of thermal energy is better if the length of the fistula tract is short. A study conducted by Lauretta et al. reported a primary healing rate of 58.3% for the tracts less than 30 mm, while tracts longer than 30 mm had a healing rate of 16.6% [7]. The tracts with 4–5 mm diameter have better results than larger ones [7, 18]. The tracts with larger diameters may be associated with skip areas as the laser energy delivered may not be sufficient [18].

Another question that needs to be addressed is the energy dosage required to close the fistula tract. There are no standard guidelines regarding dosage, but the broad recommendations are a release of energy of 10 W/mm/s in continuous mode. De Bonnechore et al. have opined that fistula tracts requiring less than 400 joules heal better than those requiring more than 400 Joules [16]. Releasing excess energy to a shorter tract (a few millimeters) might result in tissues being over-burnt.

Similarly, too little energy may not be sufficient for shrinkage of the tract [16]. Ozturk had approximately used 90 J/cm [3], Wilhelm 39 J/cm [2], and P. Giamundo used 120 J/cm [4] for shrinkage of the tracts. I use 100 J/cm in my practice. The use of setons before the laser procedure for anal fistula is also recommended [4]. The setons lead to the maturation of tracts and make the insertion of fibers easy.

The distal part of the fistula tract, which extends from the outer margin of the external anal sphincter to the ischiorectal fossa, has a low potential to shrink because of less fibrotic tissue [19]. Coring of the tact, including the external opening, is recommended.

Another point that needs to be highlighted is that sometimes while withdrawing the fiber, the tissue sticks to the fiber and offers resistance to pulling. The fiber should be taken out, cleaned with a wet gauge, and reinserted in such a case. Otherwise, the proper release of energy will be hampered due to carbonization.

Regarding the selection of the wavelength of 980 versus 1470 nm, a wavelength of 1470 nm is more effective in creating shrinkage, protein denaturation, and better water absorption [10]. In patients treated with 980 nm wavelength, severe anal pain has been reported, attributed to the higher laser energy required with a shorter wavelength [5, 10].

The main reasons for the failure of any surgical procedure for fistula-in-ano are: untreated or missed internal opening, missed side tracts, inadequate drainage of intersphincteric space, and persistent primary tract with remnants of granulation tissue or fistula epithelium [2]. In cases of persistent fistula, it is advisable to repeat the procedure.

15.9 Core Tips

The required dosage should not be given in a pulse mode. As recommended by some authors, do not keep on withdrawing fiber every 5 mm [10]. It will lead to skipping areas of unhealthy granulation tissue leading to a high recurrence rate (Fig. 15.3).

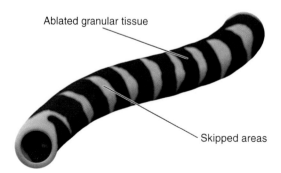

Fig. 15.3 Skip areas. The dark areas show burnt granulation tissue and the gray areas show unburnt skip areas

Take-Home Message

- Many colleagues advocate that laser energy helps in the complete closure of the tract by shrinkage. However, I have yet to see the closure of fistula tracts by laser. I agree about the shrinkage effect, as it is based on the principle of thermal energy. Further, I support the observation of many colleagues who say that no matter how we close the internal opening, the sutures invariably give away.

- In my practice, I did not get satisfactory results with FiLaC [9]. The procedure was entirely abandoned at our center.

- In a study conducted at our center from "March 2017 to October 2019" on 114 patients with different laser techniques, 42 patients underwent the FiLaC procedure, out of which seven (7) showed recurrence, indicating 84% success rate [9]. Literature review gathered from research publications and my experience with lasers fascinated me to combine the different sphincter-saving techniques. I thought of modifying the laser techniques and hybridizing them with other surgical procedures, which decreased the recurrence rate substantially. All the hybrid procedures will be discussed subsequently in the next chapter.

15.10 Your Queries! My Answers!

1. **Is internal orifice closure a must in FiLaC procedure?**

    According to some authors, one of the critical views of fistula management is should the internal opening be closed or not [13]. FiLaC consists of blind ablation of the tracts without addressing its internal opening, with a 71% success rate [18]. Nowadays, the proponents of the LIFT procedure advocate that the interruption of the fistula tract close to the internal opening is sufficient to achieve a 70% or higher rate of healing, even in complex anorectal fistulas [12, 13, 20]. In my opinion, complete removal of the primary infection is the only way to prevent a recurrence.

After going through the literature, I have seen different authors approach the internal opening differently. Some feel that closure of the internal opening occurs on its own due to laser energy's shrinkage effect, and hence no closure is required [4]. Most recurrences occur early, resulting from the reopening of the tracts and the presence of epithelial remnants of the undetected secondary extensions. Others do advocate the closure with Polyglactin 2-0. As I previously mentioned, I am not convinced about the FiLaC procedure. To date, I have not seen any fistulous opening closure by laser. So, it is an individual's call.

References

1. Stijns J, van Loon YT, Clermonts SHEM, Göttgens KW, Wasowicz DK, Zimmerman DDE. Implementation of laser ablation of fistula tract (LAFT) for perianal fistulas: do the results warrant continued application of this technique? Tech Coloproctol. 2019;23(12):1127–32. https://doi.org/10.1007/s10151-019-02112-9.
2. Wilhelm A. A new technique for sphincter-preserving anal fistula repair using a novel radial emitting laser probe. Tech Coloproctol. 2011;15(4):445–9. https://doi.org/10.1007/s10151-011-0726-0.
3. Oztürk E, Gülcü B. Laser ablation of fistula tract: a sphincter-preserving method for treating fistula-in-ano. Dis Colon Rectum. 2014;57(3):360–4. https://doi.org/10.1097/DCR.0000000000000067.
4. Giamundo P, Geraci M, Tibaldi L, Valente M. Closure of fistula-in-ano with a laser—FiLaC™: an effective novel sphincter-saving procedure for complex disease. Color Dis. 2014;16(2):110–5. https://doi.org/10.1111/codi.12440.
5. Donmez T, Hatipoglu E. Closure of fistula tract with FiLaC™ laser as a sphincter-preserving method in anal fistula treatment/Anal Fistul Tedavisinde Sfinkter Koruyucu Yontem Olarak FiLaC™ Lazer Yontemiyle Fistula Traktinin Kapatilmasi. Turk J Colorectal Dis. 2017;27(4):142–8.
6. Serin KR, Hacim NA, Karabay O, Terzi MC. Retrospective analysis of primary suturing of the internal orifice of perianal fistula during FiLaC procedure. Surg Laparosc Endosc Percutan Tech. 2020;30(3):266–9. https://doi.org/10.1097/SLE.0000000000000774.
7. Lauretta A, Falco N, Stocco E, Bellomo R, Infantino A. Anal fistula laser closure: the length of the fistula is the Achilles' heel. Tech Coloproctol. 2018;22(12):933–9. https://doi.org/10.1007/s10151-018-1885-z.
8. Marref I, Spindler L, Aubert M, Lemarchand N, Fathallah N, Pommaret E, Soudan D, Pillant-le Moult H, Safa Far E, Fellous K, Crochet E, Mory B, Benfredj P, de Parades V. The optimal indication for FiLaC® is high trans-sphincteric fistula-in-ano: a prospective cohort of 69 consecutive patients. Tech Coloproctol. 2019;23(9):893–7. https://doi.org/10.1007/s10151-019-02077-9.
9. Gupta K, Mital K, Gupta R, Bakshi T. Distal laser proximal fistulotomy—a new sphincter-saving technique. A comparative study with other sphincter-saving procedures. Int J Recent Sci Res. 2020;11(3):37892–4.
10. Wilhelm A, Fiebig A, Krawczak M. Five years of experience with the FiLaC™ laser for fistula-in-ano management: long-term follow-up from a single institution. Tech Coloproctol. 2017;21(4):269–76. https://doi.org/10.1007/s10151-017-1599-7.
11. Alam A, Lin F, Fathallah N, Pommaret E, Aubert M, Lemarchand N, Abbes L, Spindler L, Portal A, de Parades V. FiLaC® and Crohn's disease perianal fistulas: a pilot study of 20 consecutive patients. Tech Coloproctol. 2020;24(1):75–8. https://doi.org/10.1007/s10151-019-02134-3.
12. Zirak-Schmidt S, Perdawood SK. Management of anal fistula by ligation of the inter-sphincteric fistula tract—a systematic review. Dan Med J. 2014;61(12):A4977.
13. Altomare DF. Anal fistula closure with FiLaC: new hope or the same old story? Tech Coloproctol. 2015;19:441–2. https://doi.org/10.1007/s10151-015-1347-9.
14. Gutknecht N, Franzen R, Schippers M, Lampert F. Bactericidal effect of a 980-nm diode laser in bovine teeth root canal wall dentin. J Clin Laser Med Surg. 2004;22(1):9–13.
15. Elagin V, Smirnov A, Yusupov V, Kirillov A, Ignatova N, Streltsova O, et al. The bactericidal effect of continuous wave laser with strongly absorbing coating at the fiber tip. J Innov Opt Health Sci. 2018;11(5):1850029.
16. De Bonnechose G, Lefevre JH, Auber M, Lemarchand N, Fathallah N, Pommaret E, Soudan D, Spindler L, de Parades V. Laser ablation of fistula tract (LAFT) and complex fistula-in-ano: the ideal indication is becoming clearer. Tech Coloproctol. 2020;24(7):695–701. https://doi.org/10.1007/s10151-020-02203-y.
17. Garg P. Understanding and treating supralevator fistula-in-ano: MRI analysis of 51 cases and a review of literature. Dis Colon Rectum. 2018;61(5):612–21. https://doi.org/10.1097/DCR.0000000000001051.
18. Giamundo P, Esercizio L, Geraci M, Tibaldi L, Valente M. Fistula-tract laser closure (FiLaC™): long-term results and new operative strategies. Tech Coloproctol. 2015;19(8):449–53. https://doi.org/10.1007/s10151-015-1282-9.
19. Giamundo P. Laser treatment for anal fistulas: what are the pitfalls? Tech Coloproctol. 2020;24(7):663–5.
20. Schulze B, Ho YH. Management of complex anorectal fistulas with seton drainage plus partial fistulotomy and subsequent ligation of inter-sphincteric fistula tract (LIFT). Tech Coloproctol. 2015;19(2):89–95. https://doi.org/10.1007/s10151-014-1245-6.

Hybrid Procedures-Future of Fistula Surgery!

16

"Technique is just a means of arriving at a statement."

Jackson Pollock

Key Concepts
- Fistulotomy is a gold standard treatment for simple fistulas.
- A hybrid procedure is a synergistic combination of two or more surgical techniques to yield a better outcome.
- Hybrid procedures can precisely tackle the internal opening and obliterate the fistula tract with minimal or no sphincter cutting.
- Hybrid techniques are the most preferred amongst all sphincter-saving procedures as they create minimal raw areas, especially in long tracts.
- Complex fistulas can be well managed with hybrid procedures.

16.1 Introduction

A hybrid procedure is a synergistic combination of two or more surgical techniques to yield a better outcome. They are not just procedures but concepts of thinking out of the box to treat complex fistulas. Hybrid procedures are an opportunity to combine the various surgical techniques, which are genuinely novel, with less morbidity, faster recovery, and least recurrence.

Various hybrid procedures that a surgeon may find helpful have been discussed in detail to elucidate this vital topic further.

16.2 Why Hybrid Procedures! Aims and Objectives!

- To tackle internal opening more precisely
- To obliterate the fistula tract with minimal or no sphincter cutting
- To create less raw areas, especially in long tracts
- To prevent incontinence in complex fistulas
- Early return to work
- Low recurrence rate

16.3 Indications

All complex fistulas.

16.4 Contraindications

Fistula tracts less than 3 cm. Fistulotomy remains the procedure of choice.

16.5 Hybrid Procedures

The different procedures are:

- Distal laser and proximal SLOFT (DLPS)
- Distal laser and proximal SLOFT with distal tract coring (DCPS)
- Distal laser with proximal LIFT
- VAAFT with LIFT with laser ablation of the distal tract (VA-LIFT)
- Distal coring with proximal fistulotomy with laser ablation (DCPF)

16.6 Distal Laser Proximal SLOFT (DLPS)

This procedure combines submucosal ligation of the proximal fistula tract and laser ablation of the separated distal tract.

16.6.1 Principle

- Closing the internal opening with separation of the distal tract [1].

16.6.2 Indications

- Simple and complex fistulas

16.6.3 Advantages

- Reproducible
- Easy to perform

16.6.4 Technique

Half an hour before the surgery, the patient is given intravenous antibiotics. The patient under the effect of spinal anesthesia is placed in the lithotomy position. A half-cut proctoscope is inserted into the anal canal (Fig. 16.1a–e). Hydrogen peroxide is injected through the external opening, and bubbles are seen coming out from the internal opening (Fig. 16.1a). Laser ablation of the tract up to the internal opening is done using 360° radial fiber inserted through the external opening (Fig. 16.1b). The laser equipment used is of 1470 nm wavelength. The energy is given in continuous mode at 10 W/s/mm. The unhealthy granulation tissue and the tract are destroyed. The tract is curetted and irrigated using normal saline to remove the ablated tissue.

A malleable metal probe is inserted from the external opening and taken out from the internal opening (Fig. 16.1c). A figure of eight suture is taken using a 5/8 circle 27 mm 2-0 Polyglactin, circumambulating the fistula tract at the internal opening (Fig. 16.1d). The probe is gently withdrawn before tying the knot. While withdrawing the probe from the internal opening, a sudden jerk while tightening the knot indicates that the suture is placed behind a tract. Normal saline is injected through the external opening to check that the internal opening is duly closed. The probe is inserted again in the fistula tract, and its tip is palpated nearly 2–3 mm proximal to the internal opening, toward the anal verge. The distal tract is separated at the probe's tip using monopolar cautery or bare laser fiber, isolating the distal tract containing the cryptoglandular infection (Fig. 16.1e). The normal saline is injected again through the external opening. It can be seen coming out from the tract at the point of division, indicating the separation of the distal tract. One should ensure that the tract is completely separated as a partial separation may lead to recurrence. Finally, the external opening is enlarged for draining the remaining ablated tissue.

In the original SLOFT procedure, the distal tract was identified after inserting a probe, and then the mucosa over the probe was incised. The tract was dissected, and a circumferential stitch was taken near the internal opening using an aneurysm needle, followed by the separation of the tract. Finally, the incised mucosa was approximated by suturing with a 2-0 Polyglactin suture.

I modified the technique, hence the name "modified SLOFT." In the modified technique, the mucosa over the tract is not incised to reach behind the tract, unlike the original procedure [1]. Moreover, in the original SLOFT procedure, the distal tract was only curetted and not laser-ablated. However, the basic principle of both techniques remains the same.

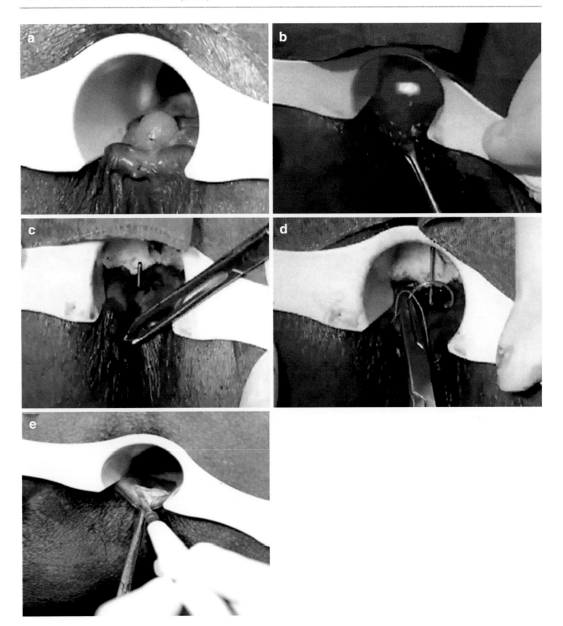

Fig. 16.1 (a–e) Steps of distal laser proximal SLOFT (DLPS). (a) Hydrogen peroxide injected through external opening and bubbles are observed coming out of internal opening. (b) Laser ablation of the fistula tract after curetting and irrigation. (c) Insertion of probe from external opening. (d) Circumambulation stitch taken using Polyglactin 2-0. (e) Separation of distal tract using monopolar cautery

16.6.5 Results

Refer Table 16.1.

Table 16.1 Distal laser proximal SLOFT (DLPS)

Procedure	Success rate (%)
FiLaC [2]	84
DLPS [2]	93.6 [2]

16.6.6 Discussion

Although submucosal ligation with laser ablation of the fistula tract is a minimally invasive
and promising hybrid procedure, there are a
few limitations. The internal opening is closed,
as in FiLaC, which may give way during defecation due to stretching and increased anal
canal pressure. Since the internal opening is
ablated and not removed as in fistulotomy, the
residual infection in the deep intersphincteric
space can lead to recurrence. Since the separation of the distal tract creates a small wound,
some colleagues feel that a new internal opening is created in this procedure, which is not the
case. The wound created at the separated distal
tract should not be confused with the primary
internal opening.

16.7 Distal Coring Using FiXcision with Proximal SLOFT (DCPS)

Excision of the internal opening followed by surgical coring of the fistula tract was described first
in 1961 by Park [3]. FiXcision is a technique of
coring out the fistula tract by making a controlled
circumferential cut around the entire tract [4].
The FiXcision instrument can minimize the circumference of coring without causing injury to
the surrounding sphincter muscles [4].

16.7.1 Principle

FiXcision: Coring out of the distal fistula tract
without creating large raw areas.

The principle of submucosal ligation of the
fistula tract and laser has already been discussed.

16.7.2 Indications

Any fistula tract up to 5 mm in diameter and 5 cm
in length.

16.7.3 Contraindications

- Previous radiation on the pelvic area or his-
  tory of malignancy
- Presence of immunodeficiency disorder
- Crohn's disease
- Fistula tract with an abscess

16.7.4 FiXcision Instrument

The FiXcision instrument consists of

- A malleable probe: This locates the fistula tract
  and allows the guide to be inserted later [4].
- A guide: Controls the circular blade and compresses the tissue around the fistula tract [4].
- Base Plate: Provides resistance at the internal
  opening to ensure complete transection of the
  fistula tract [4].
- Circular blade allows for precise and uniform
  circular fistula tract cutting [4].

16.7.5 Technique

The initial steps are the same as in proximal submucosal ligation and distal laser of the fistula
tract. Once DLPS is completed, methylene blue
is injected to demarcate the tract. The malleable
probe is fixed over the guide, inserted from the
external opening, and taken out through the incision where the distal tract has been separated
after SLOFT (Fig. 16.2a). The probe is separated,
and a base plate is fixed over the guide
(Fig. 16.2b). A small cut in circular motion is
made by pushing the cutting sleeve over a guiding rod, enabling the fistula tract to be cored out
(Fig. 16.2c–e).

After coring, a circumambulation stitch is
taken using 2-0 Polyglactin at the site of the
cored-out tract to prevent the liquid part of motion
from entering the tunnel created after coring. The
stitch is taken by going behind the guiding shaft
as in SLOFT to ensure complete closure of the

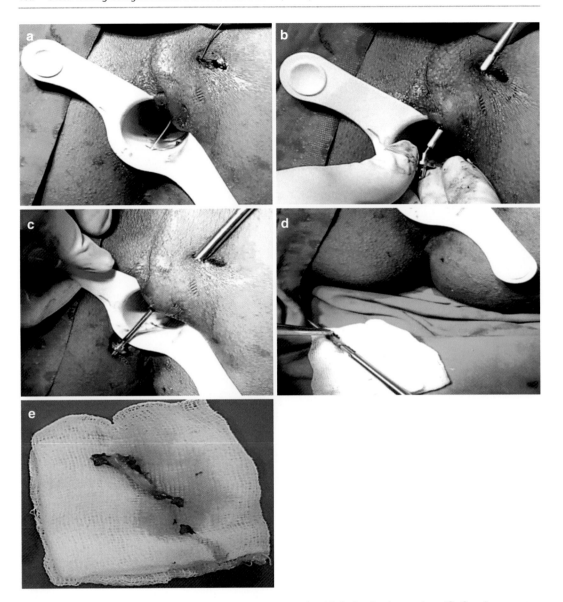

Fig. 16.2 (a–e) Steps of distal coring proximal SLOFT. (a) Insertion of malleable probe from external opening to the separation of the distal tract after SLOFT. (b) Fixation of base plate over the guide. (c) Coring out of tract using cutting blade in circular motion. (d) Cored-out tract as seen over the guide. (e) Completely cored-out tract. Methylene blue-stained inner part and clean outer surface indicates complete coring

tunnel through the anal wound. This prevents infection and leads to faster wound healing.

16.7.6 Pitfalls

FiXcision has limitations because tracts more than 5 mm in diameter and more than 5 cm in length cannot be cored out [5].

16.7.7 Discussion

FiXcision is a wonderful tool for surgeons to completely core out the fistula tract without creating large raw areas. Many surgeons want to know why laser ablation is done before coring the tract. My personal view is that since laser energy helps shrink the tract, it becomes easier to core out the whole tract in toto, especially in those fistulas where the diameter of the fistula tract is slightly more than 5 mm.

It is postulated that the fistula tract in the ischiorectal fat close to the external opening is soft and less fibrotic, leading to less shrinkage with laser energy [6]. Although I am skeptical about this hypothesis, coring out the tract appears to be a good option.

16.8   Distal Laser with Proximal LIFT (DLPL)

This procedure combines "Ligation of the Intersphincteric Fistula Tract" (LIFT) with laser ablation of the distal tract.

16.8.1 Principle

LIFT works by ligating the fistula tract near the internal opening and separating the distal tract [7]. Because the cryptoglandular infection exists in the distal tract, laser ablation of the distal tract is performed.

16.8.2 Technique

The internal opening is disconnected from the fistula tract at the intersphincteric plane. For the distal tract, laser ablation is done after curetting unhealthy granulation tissue (Fig. 16.3a–e).

16.8.3 Results

The success rate of LIFT, as reported, varies from 47% to 90% [8–10]. The advantages of this technique are difficult to define [8–10]. Since I did not get satisfactory results, the procedure was discontinued at our center.

16.8.4 Discussion

Since it is the proximal part where the recurrence occurs, the laser ablation of the distal tract seems to have a limited role. It will lead to faster healing of the distal tract but cannot prevent a recurrence. A few surgeons recently advocated a hybrid procedure that combines the LIFT technique with fistulotomy for the distal tract. Since the recurrence is always from the proximal part, I see no advantage of the distal fistulotomy as it will not improve the success rate. Carrying out such an extensive surgical procedure, especially in longer tracts, defeats the purpose of a minimally invasive procedure.

In SLOFT and LIFT, the internal opening is not removed, below which lies the disease. In LIFT, a small part of the proximal tract near the internal opening is left behind, which may later become infected, resulting in recurrence. This condition is similar to stumpitis when a large stump is left behind after an appendicectomy. Moreover, recurrence may also occur after the LIFT procedure as the extensions of the fistula tract, if any, have not been tackled.

I always ablate the internal opening using laser energy, even in the LIFT procedure. It is difficult for me to comment whether it is the bactericidal effect of the laser beam or the subsequent procedure that is effective.

Few surgeons opine that even if the curetting of the distal tract is done with no laser ablation, the results will be similar. Well, I could not find any literature to support this. In my opinion, the healing time is much faster when curetting is followed by laser ablation of the distal tract.

All said and done, I know a few colleagues are getting good results with LIFT and SLOFT. I think one should opt for a procedure one is good at.

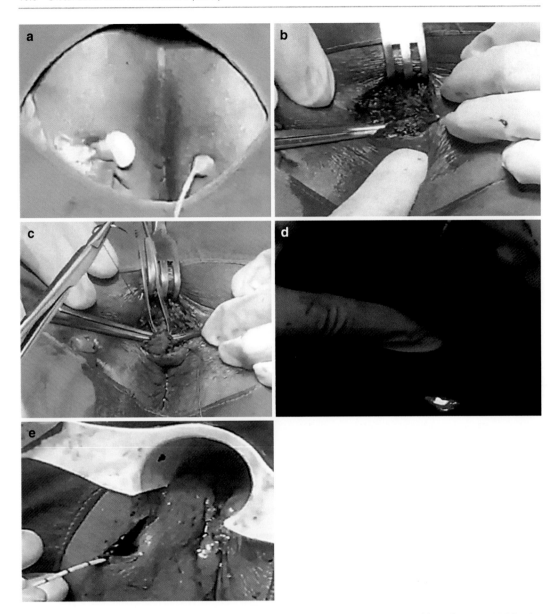

Fig. 16.3 (**a–e**) Steps of distal laser proximal LIFT. Patient in Jack-knife position. (**a**) Horseshoe fistula—Hydrogen peroxide injected from external opening at 7 o'clock and seen coming out of internal opening at 6 o'clock and external opening at 5 o'clock. (**b**) Dissection of fistula tract through intersphincteric space. (**c**) Ligation of tract close to internal opening with Polyglactin 2-0 followed by separation of distal tract (LIFT procedure). (**d**) Laser ablation of the distal tract at 7 o'clock. (**e**) Laser ablation of distal tract at 5 o'clock

16.9   VAAFT with LIFT with Laser Ablation of the Distal Tract (VA-LIFT)

"Video-Assisted Anal Fistula Treatment" is a minimally invasive procedure that treats fistulas under vision using a rigid small-caliber fistuloscope [11]. Studies show that the technique of internal opening closure, which might be a stapler, suture, or an advanced flap, affects the outcome of VAAFT [12]. Some authors have observed that ligation of the fistula tract near the internal opening under direct view may yield better results than the LIFT procedure alone, as the extensions can be visualized with the VAAFT scope [13].

16.9.1   Principle

Combining LIFT with VAAFT is based on the principle that fistuloscopy improves LIFT results [13]. The accessory branches, frequently over-looked in the LIFT procedure, can be visualized and addressed.

16.9.2   Indications

- Trans-sphincteric fistula

16.9.3   Technique

Patients are placed in a Jack-knife position if the fistula tract is posterior, whereas the lithotomy position is preferred in the anterior tracts. Through the external opening, a fistuloscope is inserted to locate the internal opening. Bright light is seen at the internal opening. Demarcation of accessory tracts can be done by injecting diluted methylene blue. The tract is curetted, and the necrotic material is removed with a grasper and a brush. The procedure is followed by ablation of the tract and the extensions with monopolar cautery or laser using 360° radial fiber. After that, the LIFT procedure is carried out under vision (Fig. 16.4a–e).

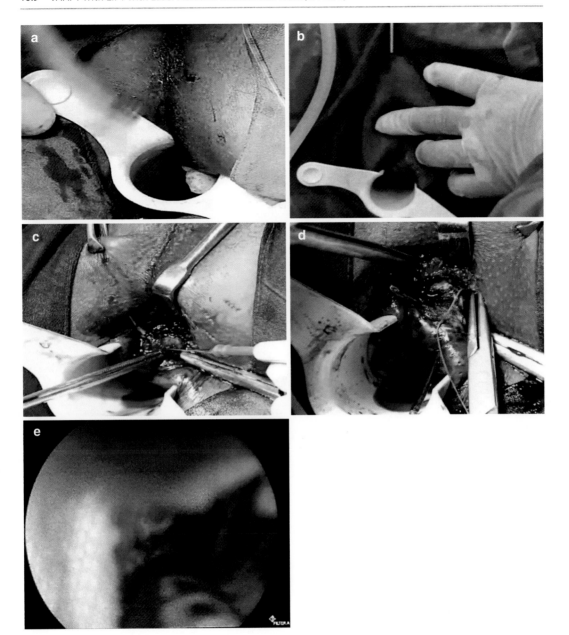

Fig. 16.4 (**a**–**e**) Steps of VAAFT with LIFT with laser ablation. (**a**) Hydrogen peroxide injected through an external opening. Bubbles are seen coming out of the internal opening at 12 o'clock. (**b**) VAAFT scope inserted through the external opening. Bright light visible at the internal opening. (**c**) Fistula tract identified in the intersphincteric space. (**d**) Ligation and separation of fistula tract. (**e**) Ablation of distal fistula tract after brushing and removal of necrotic material

16.9.4   Results

See Table 16.2.

Table 16.2   VAAFT with LIFT with laser ablation of the distal tract (VA-LIFT)

Procedure	Success rate (%)
VAAFT [13]	54.41
VA-LIFT [13]	68.75
LIFT [13]	66.67

16.9.5 Discussion

Overall results of VAAFT are not very encouraging. VAAFT by itself has a limited role. It has more of a diagnostic than therapeutic significance. In a curved tract, it is not easy to negotiate the fistuloscope. The advantage of using laser energy over the monopolar cautery to ablate the distal tract is that the laser does not cause lateral damage to the surrounding tissue.

Moreover, since the ablation of the distal tract is done under vision, the chances of leaving skip areas are negligible. The outcome of this technique is mainly dependent upon the success of the LIFT procedure. This hybrid technique is helpful when it becomes challenging to identify the internal opening.

16.10 Distal Coring with Proximal Fistulotomy and Laser Ablation (DCPF)

This procedure combines proximal fistulotomy with coring of the distal tract using FiXcision after laser ablation of the distal fistula tract (Fig. 16.5a–e).

16.10.1 Principle

- The principle of fistulotomy is to lay open the fistula tract with the healing of the fistulotomy wound by secondary intention [14].
- The principle of coring is to core out the infected distal part of the tract extending from the fistulotomy wound to the external opening [3, 6].
- Laser energy leads to the ablation of unhealthy granulation tissue and coagulation of blood vessels by protein denaturation, limiting the further spread of infection [15]. As mentioned earlier, the laser energy also leads to vaporization of the water from the cytoplasm of the epithelial cells lining the tract, leading to shrinkage. Therefore, the diameter of the tract is reduced, making it easier to core out without creating large raw areas [16].

16.10.2 Indications

- Complex fistulas

16.10.3 Technique

Hydrogen peroxide is injected through an external opening to identify the internal opening. Through the transanal approach, an oval-shaped incision is given 5 mm above the internal opening and extended towards the white line of Hilton. The mucosa, submucosa, surrounding tissue, and the internal opening are excised up to the deep intersphincteric space (Park's technique). A probe is inserted through the external opening and brought out through the excised internal opening wound. The fistulotomy is done over the probe extending up to the subcutaneous part of the external anal sphincter. This is followed by marsupialization of the margins. The distal tract is laser-ablated and cored out using FiXcision (Fig. 16.5a–e).

In the case of multiple external openings, all the communicating external tracts can be curetted and laser-ablated without creating extensive raw areas. Since only the subcutaneous part of the external sphincter and the lower part of the internal sphincter are divided in fistulotomy, there are no chances of incontinence.

16.10.4 Discussion

16.10.4.1 The Difference Between Park's Procedure and Our Approach

Distal coring proximal fistulotomy is the most reliable procedure with a high success rate. The credit for the success goes to proximal fistulotomy. This is the only procedure where the internal opening, mucosa, submucosa, and surrounding tissue are entirely excised. All branches or extensions from the internal opening are disconnected from the primary source. The deep intersphincteric space is explored to eliminate the central focus of infection.

So, what is the difference between a standard fistulotomy for long tracts versus distal coring with proximal fistulotomy? Well, the

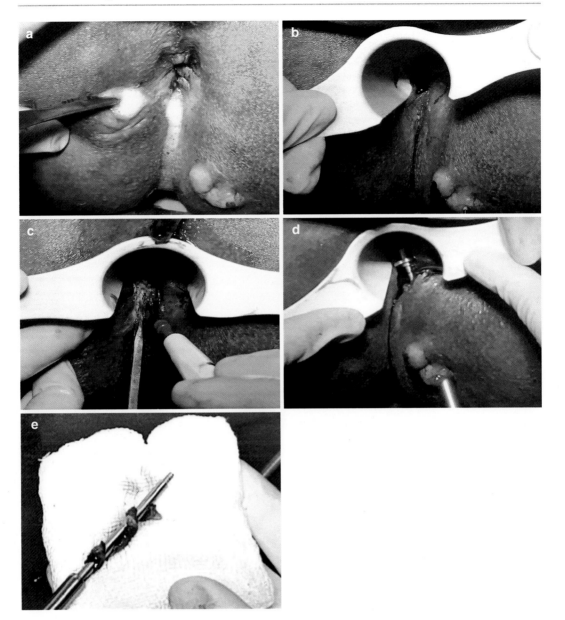

Fig. 16.5 (**a–e**) Steps of distal coring and proximal fistulotomy in a fistula with multiple external openings and a single internal opening. (**a**) Hydrogen peroxide injected through the external opening showing bubbles in other communicating tracts. Bubbles seen coming out of single internal opening at 6 o'clock. (**b**) Methylene blue injected through the external opening for demarcation of fistula tracts. (**c**) Excision of internal opening along with fistulotomy done from the shortest fistula tract leading to separation of all other communicating tracts. (**d**) Coring out of the fistula tract. (**e**) Cored-out fistula tract

answer is simple. A large fistulotomy wound creates a large raw area that takes a long time to heal. As recurrence is always from the primary source, laying open, the long distal tract offers no advantage. Hence, distal coring with proximal fistulotomy is a better option. However, there is a limitation of the fistula tract length that can be cored out with FiXcision. The distal tract can be curetted and laser ablated in longer tracts.

16.10.4.2 Why Do I Prefer Coring of the Distal Fistula Tract?

Coring the distal tract helps eradicate the cryptoglandular infection in the distal tract. As mentioned above, the concept is based on Park's technique of excision of the internal opening followed by surgical coring of the fistula tract [3]. In my opinion, this is the only hybrid procedure where the primary source of infection is eliminated from the intersphincteric space.

16.10.5 Results of Histopathology Examination of Fistula Tracts

In all cases, the curetted necrotic material was sent for a histopathology examination. At our center, less than 1% granulomatous inflammation was reported to suggest tuberculosis. The rest showed an inflammatory infiltrate comprising lymphomononuclear cells, suggesting chronic inflammatory pathology. The findings were consistent with cryptoglandular infection as etiopathogenesis.

16.11 Anal Glands: Pathological Insight!

16.11.1 Does Epithelialization of the Tract or Anal Glands Have Any Role in Persistent Fistula!

As surgeons, we are constantly disturbed by recurrences. It is a well-known fact that the anal gland is infected in most cases, leading to a fistula or an abscess formation [17]. The excision of the internal opening and the epithelized fistula tract, as recommended by Park, made me dig into the literature to get an insight into the correlation between the fistula tract epithelium and its role in recurrence.

In one of the publications on "The pathogenesis and treatment of fistula in ano" in 1961 [3], Park advocated laying open the fistula tract. His lines read as follows:

> *Following the lay-open type of operation, it is necessary to prevent the mucosal edges from joining as a bridge over the wound because this will cause the fistula to form again. The classical reason for this is that any tract with an internal opening in an anal canal will form a fistula. If the views presented here are correct, the efficacy of a 'lay-open' is because the anal-gland epithelium lining the fistula is made to form part of the wall of the anal canal. If the mucosal edges join over the incised tract, the fistula recurs because this gland epithelium is still present and will line the new tract as it did the old one. Utilizing the technique described above, all anal-gland epithelium is removed, and hence the wound edges can unite without forming a recurrent fistula.*

He specified that the epithelium lining the anal gland could form a fistula again. Therefore, he recommended excising all the anal gland epithelium and preventing mucosa from joining as a bridge over the wound.

Lunniss et al. in 1995 [18], discovered the epithelium lining the intersphincteric fistula tract in patients having lower perianal fistula. Although the effect of epithelialization on the healing of a fistula has not been yet studied, the researchers speculate that it may contribute to the persistence of a fistula. However, according to other researchers, epithelium proliferation in perianal fistulas is a delayed process that has little bearing on the fistula's healing rate. This hypothesis is still widely accepted, and numerous papers and textbooks quote this study [19–24].

The crux of the discussion is that it is pertinent to remove the epithelialized tissue to prevent recurrence or persistence. Whether one opts for excision or curettage is an individual's choice.

As I have already stated, I excise the internal opening, mucosa, submucosa, and surrounding tissue and open the intersphincteric space to remove the primary focus of infection. The margins of the excised tissue are marsupialized to avoid the bridging effect.

16.12 How to Select a Hybrid Procedure

16.12.1 What to Do and When to Do It?

There is always a tailor-made approach for fistula management. The different hybrid techniques adopted for the different fistulas are discussed below.

Fig. 16.6 (**a, b**) Intersphincteric fisula. (**a**) Intersphincteric tract type A1. (**b**) Diagrammatic representation showing fistulotomy for A1 type of fistula

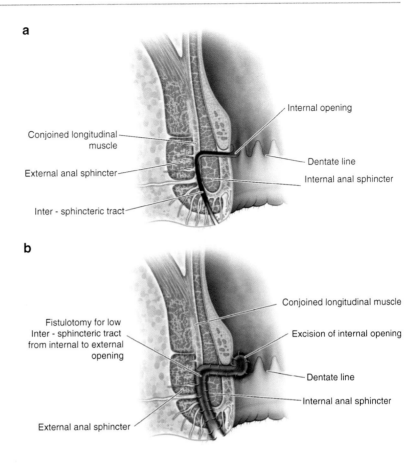

a

Internal opening

Conjoined longitudinal muscle

Dentate line

External anal sphincter

Internal anal sphincter

Inter - sphincteric tract

b

Conjoined longitudinal muscle

Fistulotomy for low Inter - sphincteric tract from internal to external opening

Excision of internal opening

Dentate line

Internal anal sphincter

External anal sphincter

16.12.1.1 Intersphincteric Tract

Assess whether the tract is simple or complex, high or low. If the fistula is simple and the tract is less than 3 cm, excision of the primary source of infection followed by fistulotomy and marsupialization of the margins is the choice (Fig. 16.6a, b).

In the intersphincteric fistula with long tracts associated with a high blind tract or a rectal opening (type A2 or A3), proximal fistulotomy is done from the excised internal opening to the anal verge, followed by curettage and laser ablation of the distal tract. The mucosa, submucosa, and the surrounding tissue are excised, followed by an incision over the fibers of the internal anal sphincter to explore the intersphincteric and deep intersphincteric space. I prefer to excise the internal opening in an oval shape by giving an incision 5 mm above the internal opening. The fibers of the internal sphincter are white, running transversally. Once the internal opening is tackled, the extensions, if any, get separated from the primary source of infection. These extensions are curetted and laser-ablated. Coring of the distal tract can also be done from the excised internal opening to the external perianal opening (Fig. 16.7a–d).

In intersphincteric fistulas without any external openings and extensions going upwards toward the rectum or pelvis (types A4 and A5), the first step remains excision of the internal opening through the transanal approach. The deep intersphincteric space is entered, and the primary focus of infection is removed. The intersphincteric extensions are identified, curetted, and irrigated, followed by laser ablation of the unhealthy granulation tissue. Fistulotomy is carried out from the internal opening to the anal verge at 6 o'clock for drainage purposes, as shown in Fig. 16.8a–e.

The combination of laser and fistulotomy gives excellent results. There is a low probability of incontinence as only the lower part of the internal sphincter and the subcutaneous part of the external sphincter are cut. This procedure dif-

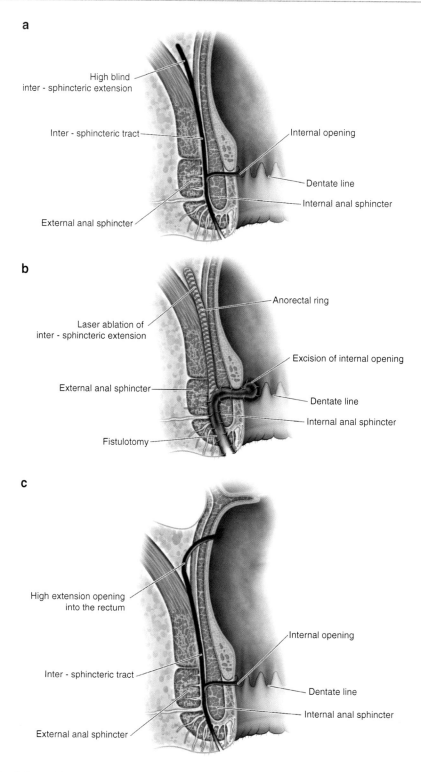

Fig. 16.7 (**a–d**) Intersphincteric fistula types A2 and A3. (**a**) Type A2 with upward extension in the intersphincteric space. (**b**) Internal opening excised, fistulotomy done, and the upward extension laser ablated. (**c**) Type A3 fistula with upward extension opening into the rectum. (**d**) Laser ablation of upward extension after fistulotomy and excision of the internal opening. In long tracts, fistulotomy is done up to anal verge

d

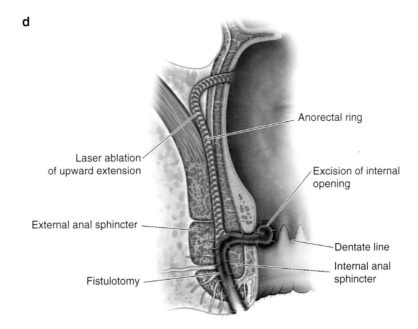

Fig. 16.7 (continued)

fers from what has been mentioned in the original publication of Park, wherein for types A2 to A5, the laying open of the entire intersphincteric space was recommended [3].

The pelvic drainage technique is better in the intersphincteric fistula of type A6 as this tract is not an actual fistula but only an extension from the pelvis (Fig. 16.9a, b). The intersphincteric part can be curetted and laser-ablated. However, as the primary pathology is in the pelvis, managing the source of primary infection is a must.

One should remember that the infection in the intersphincteric space through the infected anal gland is responsible for A1 to A5 types of intersphincteric fistulas. In contrast, pelvic infection is responsible for A6.

16.12.1.2   Trans-sphincteric Tract

A trans-sphincteric fistula is simple if less than 30% of the external anal sphincter is involved and complex if more than 30% is involved [25]. Abscesses that extend through both the internal and exterior sphincters cause these fistulas. Such fistulas are challenging to treat with standard surgical techniques as there are chances of recurrence and incontinence (Fig. 16.10a–d).

In a long and low trans-sphincteric fistula tract (type B1), I prefer proximal fistulotomy. The internal opening is excised, and the intersphincteric and deep intersphincteric spaces are opened to eliminate the primary source of infection. The distal tract is cored out after laser ablation. It is always better to restrict fistulotomy wounds from internal opening up to the anal verge. There is no point in opening the entire tract. In a shorter tract, an alternative to coring is a simple fistulotomy, as shown in Fig. 16.10a, b. In fistulotomy, along with the lower part of the internal anal sphincter, the subcutaneous and the superficial parts of the external anal sphincter are also incised.

In type B2 of trans-sphincteric fistula with extensions, carrying out proximal fistulotomy will lead to separation of the extensions that can be curetted and laser-ablated, as shown in Fig. 16.10c, d.

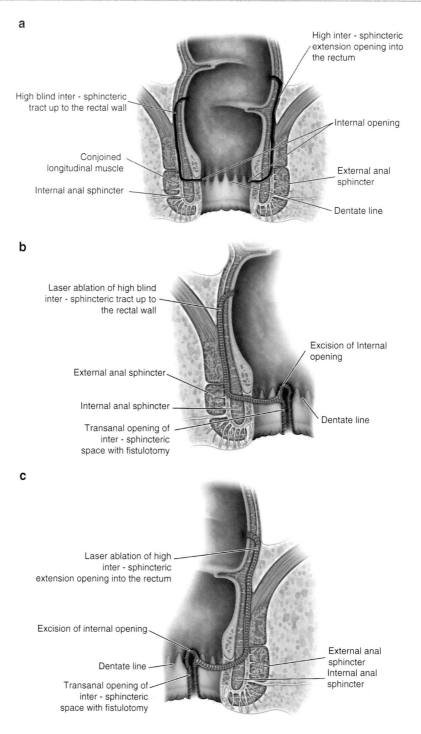

Fig. 16.8 (**a–e**) Intersphincteric fistula types A4 and A5. (**a**) Type A4 intersphincteric fistula showing high blind extension up to the rectal wall, without external opening. (**b**) Transanal opening of intersphincteric space with fistulotomy at 6 o'clock position. Upward extension is laser ablated. (**c**) Transanal opening of intersphincteric space with fistulotomy at 6 o'clock position for high rectal opening. Extension of rectal opening laser ablated. (**d**) A5 type of intersphincteric fistula with pelvic extension, without external opening. (**e**) Transanal opening of intersphincteric space with fistulotomy at 6 o'clock position for pelvic extension in A5 type. The intersphincteric tract laser ablated. The pelvic extension curetted

d

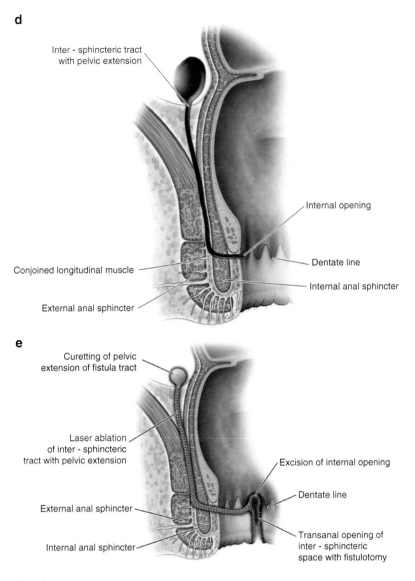

Inter - sphincteric tract with pelvic extension

Internal opening

Conjoined longitudinal muscle

Dentate line

Internal anal sphincter

External anal sphincter

e

Curetting of pelvic extension of fistula tract

Laser ablation of inter - sphincteric tract with pelvic extension

Excision of internal opening

Dentate line

External anal sphincter

Internal anal sphincter

Transanal opening of inter - sphincteric space with fistulotomy

Fig. 16.8 (continued)

In a high trans-sphincteric tract, one can adopt the following hybrid procedures, depending upon one's expertize:

- Laser with VAAFT
- Distal laser proximal fistulotomy (My preference)
- Distal coring proximal fistulotomy (My preference)
- Distal laser proximal SLOFT
- Distal laser with proximal LIFT

Fistulotomy with primary sphincter repair can also be done. It is an extensive surgical procedure creating a sizable raw area. One should have the expertize to carry out primary sphincter repair.

Fig. 16.9 (a, b)
Intersphincteric fistula.
(a) Intersphincteric
fistula type A6 showing
the pelvic extension. (b)
Laser ablation of the
tract done after removal
of primary infection of
pelvic origin

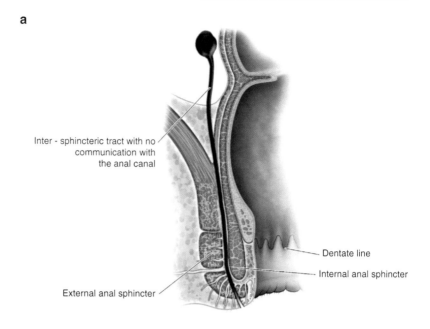

a

Inter - sphincteric tract with no
communication with
the anal canal

Dentate line

Internal anal sphincter

External anal sphincter

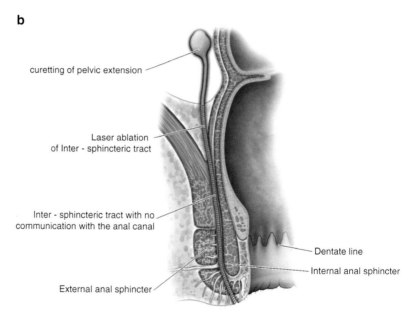

b

curetting of pelvic extension

Laser ablation
of Inter - sphincteric tract

Inter - sphincteric tract with no
communication with the anal canal

Dentate line

Internal anal sphincter

External anal sphincter

I would like to emphasize that no matter which procedure one opts for, removing the primary source of infection is crucial.

16.12.1.3 Suprasphincteric Fistulas

These fistulas are pretty challenging to treat. Their incidence, however, is very low. In these fistulas, the primary source of infection is first eliminated. As suggested by Park, the intersphincteric part of the tract can be opened. The rest of the tract forming a loop over the sphincter complex and extending toward the perineum can be curetted and laser-ablated. Fistulotomy at 6 o'clock helps drainage

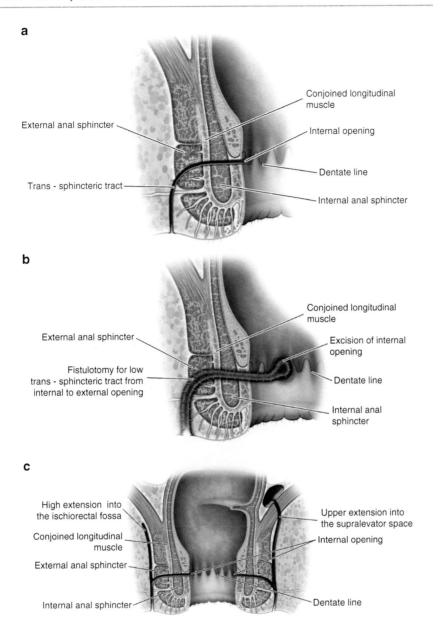

Fig. 16.10 (**a–e**) Trans-sphincteric fistula types B1 and B2 with short distal tracts (less than 4 cm). (**a**) Simple trans-sphincteric fistula type B1. (**b**) Diagrammatic representation of fistulotomy involving the lower part of internal anal sphincter, subcutaneous and superficial parts of the external anal sphincter. (**c**) Trans-sphincteric fistula type B2 showing an upward extension into the ischiorectal fossa. (**d**) Laser ablation of upward extension with fistulotomy. (**e**) Fistulotomy with laser ablation of supralevator extension

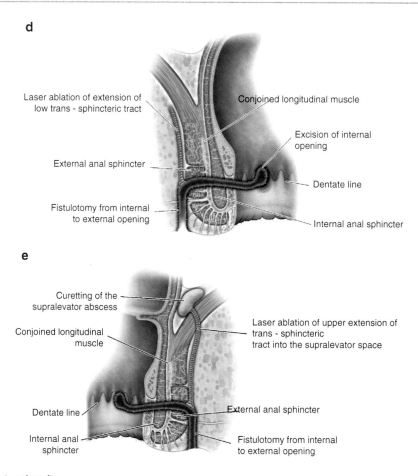

d

Laser ablation of extension of
low trans - sphincteric tract

Conjoined longitudinal muscle

Excision of internal
opening

External anal sphincter

Dentate line

Fistulotomy from internal
to external opening

Internal anal sphincter

e

Curetting of the
supralevator abscess

Conjoined longitudinal
muscle

Laser ablation of upper extension of
trans - sphincteric
tract into the supralevator space

Dentate line

External anal sphincter

Internal anal
sphincter

Fistulotomy from internal
to external opening

Fig. 16.10 (continued)

(Fig. 16.11a–c). Alternatively, a seton can be placed.

16.12.1.4   Extrasphincteric Fistula

In an extrasphincteric fistula, VAAFT with laser ablation can be considered. Overall, the results will depend upon the type of etiology one is dealing with (Fig. 16.12a, b).

16.12.1.5   Horseshoe Fistula

In a horseshoe fistula with two trans-sphincteric tracts and a single internal opening, it is essential to tackle the internal opening and the primary source of infection (Fig. 16.13). A fistulotomy can be done from 6 o'clock to the anal verge, separating the two horseshoe tracts. Both the tracts can be curetted and laser-ablated, followed by coring.

Fig. 16.11 (a–c) Suprasphincteric fistula. (**a**) Suprasphincteric fistula. (**b**) Diagrammatic representation of laser ablation of the suprasphincteric tract. (**c**) Diagrammatic representation of opening of intersphincteric space up to the anorectal ring with laser ablation of the tract (Preferred approach)

a

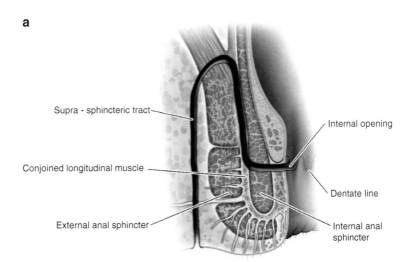

b

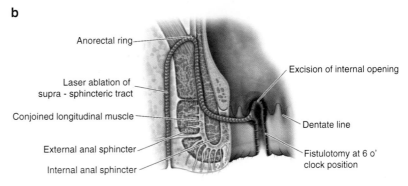

c

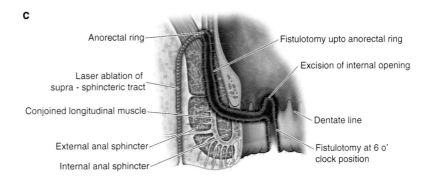

Fig. 16.12 (a, b)
Extrasphincteric tract.
(**a**) Extrasphincteric
fistula. (**b**)
Diagrammatic
representation of laser
ablation of the tract

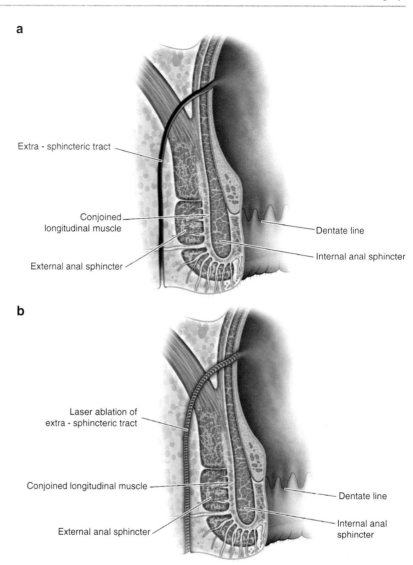

a

Extra - sphincteric tract

Conjoined
longitudinal muscle

Dentate line

Internal anal sphincter

External anal sphincter

b

Laser ablation of
extra - sphincteric tract

Conjoined longitudinal muscle

Dentate line

External anal sphincter

Internal anal
sphincter

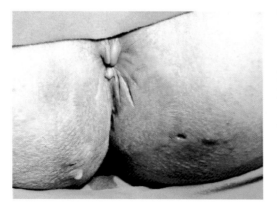

Fig. 16.13 Horseshoe fistula with multiple external openings at 5 and 7 o'clock position

16.13   Core Tips While Performing Fistula Surgery

I would like to share a protocol that I always follow in my practice while operating a fistula.

- Always identify the internal opening preoperatively by digital rectal examination. Failure to identify the internal opening is associated with 80% recurrence of fistulas [26].
- Get an MRI fistulogram for appropriate anatomical representation of the tracts, especially in a complex fistula. Plan your procedure

before the surgery but be prepared for any change in procedure as perioperative findings may differ from MRI.

- Never probe the tract forcefully, as this may create an iatrogenic opening.
- Always send the pus for culture sensitivity and the curetted necrotic material from the fistula tract for histopathology.
- While operating, demarcate the tract with methylene blue and hydrogen peroxide. Staining the tracts with methylene blue helps identify the extensions if any.
- Due to fibrosis near the internal opening or an hourglass deformity, sometimes the dye cannot be seen coming out of the internal opening. In such a situation, insert a lacrimal probe or infant feeding tube through the internal opening to trace the course.
- For fistula surgery with laser, radial fiber is used. Collateral injury is minimized due to the shallow penetration depth (2–3 mm beyond the fistula tract) [27].
- Thorough irrigation of the tract with normal saline is mandatory after curetting or laser ablation to remove the debris.
- Consider the cost-effectiveness of the procedure and explain the chances of recurrence.
- Explain the postoperative wound care management to the patients and call the patients for regular follow-ups.

16.14   Your Queries! My Answers!

1. **How to proceed when there is no internal opening?**

   A fistula is difficult to cure when it has no orifice, is blind, and has many windings.—Paulus

   Rarely may one not find an internal opening during a digital rectal examination or surgery. When methylene blue is injected through the external opening, it cannot be seen coming out of the internal opening. Instead, the fistula tract and surrounding tissue swell when the dye or hydrogen peroxide is injected. In such

cases, gently insert the probe from the external opening and see the extent to which it goes smoothly. Give a nick over the tip of the probe and bring it out. Apply Allis forceps towards the medial part of the opened tract and give traction downwards and outwards. If one can see the pull over the mucosa inside, it invariably indicates the internal opening site. Alternatively, saline can be injected into the mucosa at the dentate line posteriorly. The part of mucosa which does not lift indicates the fibrotic part of the tract.

Still, if the internal opening cannot be identified, leave the incised part of the tract as such. It may be a case of a sinus rather than a fistula. When the internal opening or a part of the duct that opens at the anal crypt becomes fibrosed, a sinus is formed (Fig. 16.14) [28].

In my practice, if I cannot find the internal opening, which is rare, I prefer to give a nick over the probe at the tip and bring it out as near the dentate line as possible and separate the tract, followed by curetting and laser ablation.

Sometimes, the anal fistula tract is narrow and takes the shape of an hourglass in the intersphincteric space, making probing impossible. Even when hydrogen peroxide is injected through the external opening, the internal opening may not be identified. It is better to use a lacrimal probe used by ophthalmologists to probe the tract.

2. **What to do if one cannot probe the tract at all?**

   It can happen when the tract is narrow, obstructed, kinked, branched, or has stenotic segments [26]. Such tracts can be dealt with fistulectomy [26]. The probing of the tract can be attempted under vision using the VAAFT scope. However, it is not an easy procedure. If the probing from an external opening fails, try to probe from an internal opening, as in a railroad method. If the dissection is done in the wrong plane and a tract is opened, the presence of necrotic tissue would right away alert the surgeon to find the proper plane.

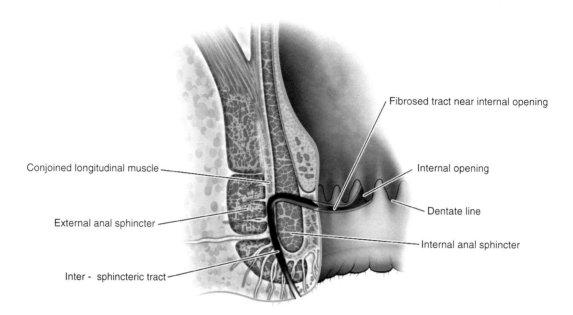

Conjoined longitudinal muscle

External anal sphincter

Inter - sphincteric tract

Fibrosed tract near internal opening

Internal opening

Dentate line

Internal anal sphincter

Fig. 16.14 Fibrosed tract near internal opening

3. **How to deal with fistulas having an external opening at the scrotal base?**

In such cases, there is always a fear of damaging the urethra. One must catheterize such patients before surgery. Any hybrid procedure may be carried out irrespective of the length of the tract. The most important aspect is identifying the internal opening. A VAAFT scope can be inserted from an external opening to locate the internal opening. One can see bright light near the internal opening. A combination of LIFT with laser ablation of the tract may be done at 12 o'clock. Alternatively, a proximal fistulotomy with distal coring or laser ablation of the distal tract can be done.

If the internal opening is at the 6 o'clock position and a tract has extended up to the scrotal base due to anterior and upward extension, then the tract is curvilinear. In such cases, a probe is inserted from the external opening at the base of the scrotum, and the tip can be seen on the anal verge at 6 o'clock. A nick is given over the tip, and the probe is brought out, separating the distal tract. The probe is reinserted from the separated tract and brought out through the internal opening (hockey J-shaped tract). A

proximal fistulotomy is carried out over the probe. The separated distal tract is curetted and laser-ablated. There is no need to create large raw areas. Since the tract is large and tissue debris is sometimes present after laser ablation, a seton can be placed for drainage for a week.

4. **What can be done to prevent bleeding during FiXcision?**

Sometimes, FiXcision can cause bleeding. The bleeding is from the surrounding adipose tissue rather than the tract itself. The chances of bleeding are more in recurrent fistulas as the vessels may retract due to fibrosis. The ideal way to control the bleeding is to insert the VAAFT scope to visualize the bleeder and cauterize it.

5. **What are the precautions to be taken after coring the tract?**

It is always advisable to insert the guide through the cored-out tract and take a circum-ambulation stitch using 2-0 Polyglactin to avoid fecal matter entering the wound. Remember, after coring, a tunnel is left behind with internal communication with the anal canal. The liquid part of the fecal matter can enter this tunnel and lead to infection.

6. **How to deal with supralevator induration?**

The identification of the supralevator induration requires expertize [29]. On digital rectal examination, one can feel bogginess or induration above the anorectal ring. The supralevator induration is either an upward extension of the cryptoglandular infection or a downward extension from pelvic disease. The management will depend upon the type of pathology.

7. **How to manage a fistula when there is no external opening?**

Managing a fistula where the external opening is absent is challenging for a surgeon. A fistula may be present with no external opening [26]. The external opening position is related to the complexity level of the tract [30]. The intersphincteric fistulas of types A4 and A5, with cephalad and high extension up to puborectalis muscle level, do not have any external openings [31]. In most cases, it can be linked to a high supralevator or intersphincteric abscess [31]. In such cases, the entire internal sphincter up to the anorectal sling can be divided through the transanal approach without incontinence.

8. **Sometimes the patient complains of pain near the site of the almost healed fistula? What can it be?**

Such complaints should never be ignored, as the patient will be the first to know of any discomfort. He should be examined thoroughly. I had operated on a patient with a recurrent fistula, which had nearly healed. After 12 weeks of surgery, the patient complained of pain on and off and pus discharge. On examination, I could not find any abscess or pus discharge. I could see only a small unhealed part of the fistulotomy wound. I curetted the tract hoping it would heal. A few days later, the patient again came to me with the same complaints. I could see active pus discharge this time. I sent the patient for MRI, which revealed a low intersphincteric tract approximately 2.5 cm in length. I took the patient for surgery and subsequently laid open the unhealed tract, which healed well. The patient would have had a persistent fistula if I had not listened to his complaint.

In my clinical practice, I have realized that many patients postoperatively are left in the hands of inexperienced staff for dressings or have no proper follow-ups. Regular follow-ups are a must till the fistula heals completely. During the healing process, care must be taken to relieve the bowels properly. Adding a laxative in the postoperative period will ultimately render good healing.

16.15 Case Presentations

Case 1

A 50-year-old gentleman came to OPD with the complaint of pus discharge from an opening near the scrotal region. He was a known case of HIV on antiviral therapy. There were two external openings on examination, one at the root of the scrotum and second at the penoscrotal junction, approximately 3 cm apart. The total length of the tract was approximately 10 cm. A single internal opening was present at 12 o'clock (Fig. 16.15a). His MRI revealed a low intersphincteric fistula extending anteriorly and superiorly. His CD4 count was within normal limits. Medical fitness was taken from the attending physician before surgery. All the necessary precautions were taken as per HIV protocol.

As the patient was immunocompromised, I planned for a minimally invasive procedure, Distal Laser Proximal SLOFT (DLPS). The tracts and the openings were demarcated by injecting diluted methylene blue from the external opening. The dye could be seen coming out from the internal opening. The whole tract was curetted, the necrotic material was removed and sent for a histopathology examination. Submucosal ligation of the fistula tract was performed, followed by laser ablation of the distal tract. The wound was irrigated from the scrotal opening with normal saline. Normal saline could be seen coming out of the separated tract (Fig. 16.15b). The small tract between the two external openings was laid open.

Discussion

The patient with an external opening near the scrotum should always be catheterized before

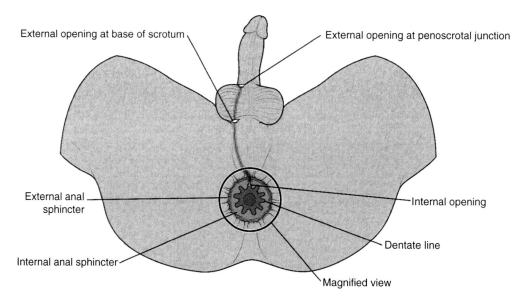

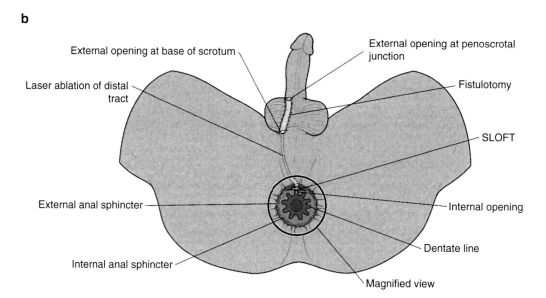

Fig. 16.15 (**a**) Two external openings, one at the penoscrotal junction and second at the base of scrotum. Internal opening at 12 o'clock position. (**b**) SLOFT at 12 o'clock with separation of distal tract. A small fistulotomy at the site of two external openings

surgery to prevent urethral injury. As the patient was immunocompromised, the least invasive procedure was performed. The part of the tract near the penoscrotal junction was spared from laser ablation because of its proximity to the urethra.

Case 2

Mr. Y, a young male, was very much disturbed with pus discharge in the anal area. He was from a village and consulted a local physician for his disease. He was given some medication, but there was no relief. He then consulted me about his problem. On examination, two fistula tracts were seen, one anterior and another posterior, with two internal openings. The anterior tract was transsphincteric, about 4–5 cm long, with an internal opening at 12 o'clock and an external opening at 1 o'clock. The posterior tract was intersphincteric, approximately 2.5 cm long, with an external opening at 7 o'clock and an internal opening at 6 o'clock. It was a case of synchronous fistula, a rare but known presentation. The condition was explained to the patient, and routine investigations for the surgery were done.

The patient was taken for surgery. I decided to operate on the anterior tract first. Methylene blue was injected from the external opening at 1 o'clock and could be seen coming out from 12 o'clock. The tract was laser-ablated, and the deep intersphincteric space was explored to remove the primary source of infection, followed by coring out the distal tract using FiXcision.

The second part of the surgery was to deal with the posterior tract. The posterior tract had an internal opening at 6 o'clock and an external opening at 7 o'clock. A dye was injected at 7 o'clock and was seen coming out at 6 o'clock. Fistulotomy followed by marsupialization was done after excising the internal opening. The patient was discharged the next day (Fig. 16.16a, b).

Discussion

A synchronous fistula is a tract with two external and two separate internal openings. One must differentiate it from a complex fistula as the latter may have multiple external openings, but the internal opening is single. It was not as easy a case as it initially appeared. Performing fistulotomy for both the tracts was impossible because it would have caused incontinence, even if transient. As I was not comfortable cutting the internal and external sphincters, both anteriorly and posteriorly, and wanted to create the least raw area, I decided on a hybrid procedure for the anterior tract, a combination of coring and proximal fistulotomy without cutting the external sphincter. The laser ablation before coring out caused shrinkage of the tract, making it easier to core. As the posterior tract was small, fistulotomy was an ideal procedure.

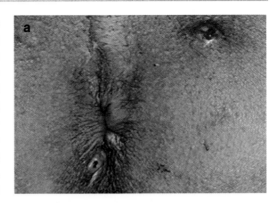

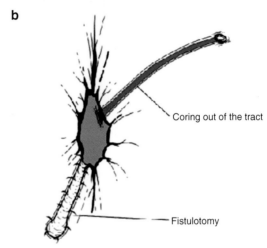

Coring out of the tract

Fistulotomy

Fig. 16.16 (**a**, **b**) Synchronous fistula. (**a**) External openings at 1 o'clock and 7 o'clock positions. (**b**) Coring for the long tract at 1 o'clock and fistulotomy for small tract at 7 o'clock

Case 3

Mr. F, an army personnel, who had been operated on twice for fistula, came for consultation. The patient had a recurrence and wanted another opinion. His complaints were pain and pus discharge from the anus. He was in despair. There was an external opening at the penoscrotal junction and an internal opening at the 12 o'clock position (Fig. 16.17a). His MRI revealed an intersphincteric fistula with an internal opening at 12 o'clock, extending superiorly with an external opening at the base of the penile shaft. The length of the tract was approximately 9 cm. After getting all the preoperative investigations, surgery was planned. The procedure I planned was a distal laser with proximal LIFT. The tract was identified and demarcated with diluted methylene blue. A probe was inserted through the external opening and brought out from the internal opening at 12 o'clock. LIFT procedure was carried out. The distal tract was curetted and laser-ablated. The laser ablation of the tract near the penoscrotal junction was not done due to the proximity to the urethra (Fig. 16.17b).

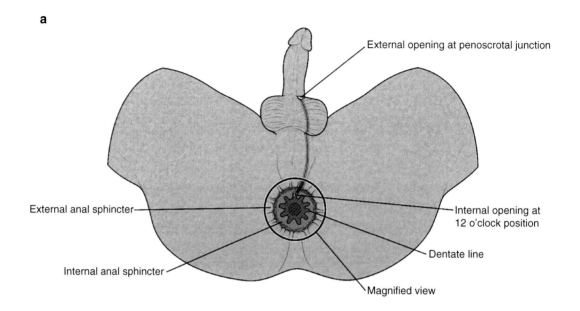

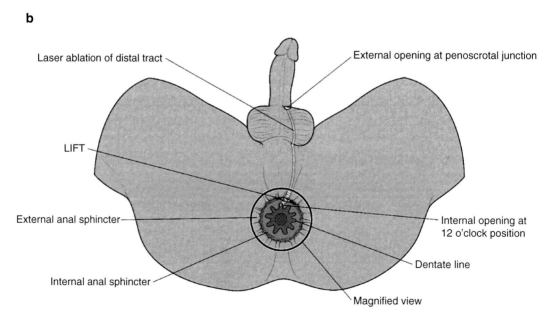

Fig. 16.17 (**a**) External opening at the penoscrotal junction and internal opening at 12 o'clock position. (**b**) LIFT done at 12 o'clock position with laser ablation of distal tract

Discussion

The patient had a fistula tract extending from the deep anterior anal space. As the internal opening was easily identified, there was no point in doing VAAFT. The laser ablation of the distal tract after curetting helps in faster healing. LIFT is another technique that is used as a sphincter-saving procedure. LIFT is not routinely done in our practice. However, as a colorectal surgeon, I feel that one should be aware of all the modalities available for the surgical management of a fistula.

Case 4

A 40-year-old gentleman was operated on for fistula thrice, but he had a recurrence each time. Subsequently, a diversion colostomy was done by a colleague. A few months later, he still had pus discharge from two openings in the ischiorectal region. On examination, there were two external openings in the gluteal region, 12 cm and 15 cm from the anal verge. An internal opening was present at the 6 o'clock position at the dentate line. The patient was anxious as he had been told that the fistula tracts would collapse after a colostomy, but the discharge persisted even after a year. The patient got an MRI, which revealed a complex trans-sphincteric fistula with inter-sphincteric, right ischiorectal, and gluteal collections with multiple external openings (St. James University Hospital classification (grade 4)) (Fig. 16.18a).

Undoubtedly the case was challenging. I decided on a hybrid procedure, a combination of VAAFT with laser ablation of the distal fistula tract and proximal fistulotomy. The fistulous tracts were demarcated by methylene blue, and hydrogen peroxide was injected from an external opening. Bubbles could be seen coming out of a single internal opening at 6 o'clock. A probe was

Fig. 16.18 (**a**) Two external openings in the gluteal region. Internal opening at 6 o'clock position at the dentate line. (**b**) Postoperative wound

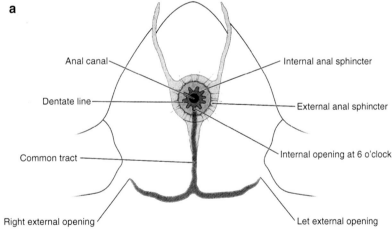

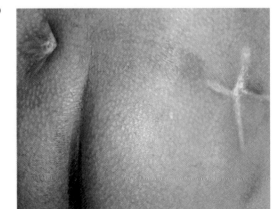

inserted through the external opening at 5 o'clock. It came out of the external opening at 7 o'clock, indicating a communicating horizontal tract, as shown in the above image. VAAFT scope was inserted but could not be tilted through the T-shaped junction. Then the scope was inserted through the internal opening. Although VAAFT is an excellent diagnostic tool, it did not add to the diagnosis already made on MRI. The tract from 5 o'clock to 7 o'clock was curetted, irrigated, and laser-ablated. Then, through an internal opening, a laser fiber was inserted, and the vertical extension of the tract was ablated. A fistulotomy was done starting from the internal opening up to the anal verge after performing an excision of the internal opening. Finally, marsupialization was carried out at the fistulotomy site.

There was complete healing of the tract in 4 weeks. After 9 months, the colostomy reversal was done. On deep analysis, I was convinced that the key to success, in this case, was a good fistulotomy and laser ablation of the distal tracts. A larger fistulotomy would have resulted in extensive raw areas with prolonged healing time (Fig. 16.18b).

Case 5

One of my colleagues referred a 60-year-old male patient to me. Two years ago, a surgeon operated on him for Fournier's gangrene. He remained well for 2 years. For the last 2 months, he had pus discharge from the perianal area, for which he consulted my colleague.

Two external openings were seen on examination, one at 9 o'clock and the other at 6 o'clock. They were approximately 6 and 10 cm from the anal verge. On DRE, a single internal opening was seen at 6 o'clock. The MRI showed a complex trans-sphincteric fistula tract extending superiorly along the right lateral wall of the sphincter complex involving the external sphincter and then coursing along the right posterior lateral wall to open at the dentate line. A hybrid procedure comprising distal coring with proximal fistulotomy was planned.

After preoperative investigations, he was taken for surgery. Methylene blue was injected from the internal opening and seen coming out

from the external opening at 9 o'clock and the internal opening at 6 o'clock, showing intercommunication between the two tracts (Horseshoe fistula).

Proximal fistulotomy followed by marsupialization was done. Both the tracts were cored out using FiXcision after laser ablation. The patient recovered well.

Discussion

Fistulotomy at 6 and 9 o'clock would have resulted in large wounds with prolonged healing time. The principle behind the procedure was to create the least raw area. Simple modifications can lead to excellent results if the surgical principles are not compromised.

Case 6

Mr. Q, 45-year man, was referred to me by one of my colleagues. The patient suddenly developed a painful swelling in the perianal area. The pain was severe and continuous. He went to my colleague, who treated him symptomatically. The pain subsided, and Mr. Q was alright for a week. After that, he again had pain and pus discharge, for which he was referred to me. He was apprehensive and wanted me to prescribe medicines without examining him. Somehow, I was able to convince him for examination. I was surprised to see three external openings; the first was at 1 o'clock at the root of the scrotum, the second at 3 o'clock, and the third at 9 o'clock, with a single internal opening at the 12 o'clock position on the dentate line. It was an inverted Y-shaped tract (Fig. 16.19). I explained the case and advised him for surgery. He was not keen but eventually agreed. I recommended an MRI, but he refused.

After getting all the prerequisites, I shifted him to the operation theatre. Hydrogen peroxide and methylene blue were injected from an external opening at 1 o'clock. The dye came out from the internal opening at 12 o'clock at the dentate line. Fistulotomy with marsupialization was done at 12 o'clock from the dentate line to the anal verge after exploring the deep intersphincteric space. All the intercommunicating tracts got separated after fistulotomy. All the tracts were cored out after laser ablation, and the external openings

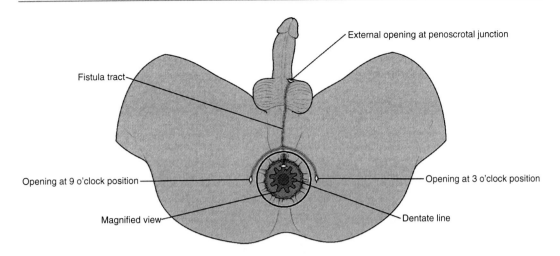

Fig. 16.19 Y-shaped fistula tract. Three external openings, one at the penoscrotal junction, the second at 3 o'clock, and the third at 9 o'clock position with an internal opening at 12 o'clock

were widened. The patient was discharged the next day. When he came for a follow-up, he was pleased and appreciated my decision.

Discussion

It was an inverted Y-shaped tract, and I combined FiXcision with proximal fistulotomy. FiXcision helped to core the entire tract, and fistulotomy helped remove the nidus of infection and separate the communicating Y-shaped tracts. The procedure could be completed without creating large wounds.

16.16 Conclusion

After attempting different hybrid procedures, the most reliable procedure remains distal coring and proximal fistulotomy with laser ablation of the distal tract. The recurrence rate after this procedure is minimal as the primary source of infection is completely removed. With the advent of the laser, it has become effortless to manage the distal tract. I must admit that I have been highly inspired by Park's technique, which I follow very religiously.

Take-Home Message

A paradigm shift from traditional to sphincter-saving methods has emerged as a boon for patients and surgeons. As a surgeon, I feel that

there is always a fear of failure in whatever procedure one follows. Still, in this evidence-based era, I advise my colleagues to evaluate the literature, the reported data, and the evidence supporting the procedure before adopting it. The Cochrane database, randomized trials, and cohort studies can be excellent guides for using a technique.

References

1. Pathak DU, Agrawal V, Taneja VK. Submucosal ligation of fistula tract (SLOFT) for anorectal fistula: an effective and easy technique. Ambulatory Surg. 2014;20(3):42–3.
2. Gupta K, Mital K, Gupta R, Bakshi T. Distal laser proximal fistulotomy-a new sphincter-saving technique a comparative study with other sphincter-saving procedures. Int J Recent Sci Res. 2020;11(03):37892–4.
3. Parks AG. Pathogenesis and treatment of fistula-in-ano. Br Med J. 1961;1(5224):463.
4. Kasiri MM, Riss S, Stift A, Binder AD, Kogovšek U, Huth M, Kronberger IE. Optimized fistulectomy using the novel FiXcision® device: a technical feasibility study and evaluation of short-term healing rates. Tech Coloproctol. 2019;23(6):579–82.
5. FiXcision AMI. https://www.ami.at/en/produkt/fixcision.
6. Giamundo P. Laser treatment for anal fistulas: what are the pitfalls? Tech Coloproctol. 2020;24(7):663–5.
7. Rojanasakul A. LIFT procedure: a simplified technique for fistula-in-ano. Tech Coloproctol. 2009;13(3):237–40. https://doi.org/10.1007/s10151-009-0522-2.

8. Ellis CN, Rostas JW, Greiner FG. Long-term outcomes with the use of bioprosthetic plugs for the management of complex anal fistulas. Dis Colon Rectum. 2010;53:798–802.

9. Hong KD, Kang S, Kalaskar S, et al. Ligation of inter-sphincteric fistula tract (LIFT) to treat anal fistula: systematic review and meta-analysis. Tech Coloproctol. 2014;18:685–91.

10. Lehmann J-P, Graf W. Efficacy of LIFT for recurrent anal fistula. Colorectal Dis. 2013;15(5):592–5.

11. Meinero P, Mori L. Video-assisted anal fistula treatment (VAAFT): a novel sphincter-saving procedure for treating complex anal fistulas. Tech Coloproctol. 2011;15(4):417–22. https://doi.org/10.1007/s10151-011-0769-2.

12. Emile SH, Elfeki H, Shalaby M, Sakr A. A systematic review and meta-analysis of the efficacy and safety of video-assisted anal fistula treatment (VAAFT). Surg Endosc. 2018;32(4):2084–93. https://doi.org/10.1007/s00464-017-5905-2.

13. Romaniszyn M, Walega PJ. Are two better than one? VALIFT: video-assisted ligation of the inter-sphincteric fistula tract—a combination of two minimally invasive techniques for treatment of trans-sphincteric perianal fistulas. Tech Coloproctol. 2019;23(3):273–6.

14. Weledji EP. Idiopathic anal fistula: fistulotomy or fistulectomy? Adv Res Gastroentero Hepatol. 2018;11(4):555817.

15. Pfefer, T. J., Choi, B., Vargas, G., McNally-Heintzelman, K. M., & Welch, A. J. (1999). Mechanisms of laser-induced thermal coagulation of whole blood in vitro. In Rox Anderson R et al Lasers in surgery: advanced characterization, therapeutics, and systems IX (Vol. 3590, pp. 20-31). SPIE.

16. Hill MR, Shryock EH, Rebell FG. Role of the anal glands in the pathogenesis of anorectal disease. J Am Med Assoc. 1943;121(10):742–6.

17. McColl I. The comparative anatomy and pathology of anal glands. Arris and Gale's lecture was delivered at the Royal College of Surgeons of England on Feb 25, 1965. Ann R Coll Surg Engl. 1967;40(1):36.

18. Lunniss PJ, Sheffield JP, Talbot IC, Thomson JP, Phillips RK. Persistence of idiopathic anal fistula may be related to epithelialization. Br J Surg. 1995;82(1):32–3.

19. Buchanan GN, Sibbons P, Osborn M, et al. Experimental model of fistula-in-ano. Dis Colon Rectum. 2005;48:353–8. https://doi.org/10.1007/s10350-004-0769-7.

20. Jun SH, Choi GS. Anocutaneous advancement flap closure of high anal fistulas. Br J Surg. 1999;86:490–2. https://doi.org/10.1046/j.1365-2168.1999.01077.x.

21. Williams JG, Farrands PA, Williams AB, et al. The treatment of anal fistula: ACPGBI position statement. Colorectal Dis. 2007;9:18–50. https://doi.org/10.1111/j.1463-1318.2007.01372.x.

22. Safar B, Jobanputra S, Sands D, Weiss EG, Nogueras JJ, Wexner SD. Anal fistula plug: initial experience and outcomes. Dis Colon Rectum. 2009;52:248–52. https://doi.org/10.1007/DCR.0b013e31819c96ac.

23. Van Koperen PJ, Ten Kate FJW, Bemelman WA, Slors JFM. Histological identification of epithelium in perianal fistulae: a prospective study. Colorectal Dis. 2010;12:891–5. https://doi.org/10.1111/j.1463-1318.2009.01880.x.

24. Mitalas LE, van Onkelen RS, Monkhorst K, Zimmerman DD, Gosselink MP, Schouten WR. Identification of epithelialization in high trans-sphincteric fistulas. Tech Coloproctol. 2012;16(2):113–7. https://doi.org/10.1007/s10151-011-0803-4.

25. Bubbers EJ, Cologne KG. Management of complex anal fistulas. Clin Colon Rectal Surg. 2016;29(1):43–9. https://doi.org/10.1055/s-0035-1570392.

26. Abou-Zeid AA. Anal fistula: intraoperative difficulties and unexpected findings. World J Gastroenterol. 2011;17(28):3272–6. https://doi.org/10.3748/wjg.v17.i28.3272.

27. Wilhelm A, Fiebig A, Krawczak M. Five years of experience with the FiLaC™ laser for fistula-in-ano management: long-term follow-up from a single institution. Tech Coloproctol. 2017;21(4):269–76. https://doi.org/10.1007/s10151-017-1599-7.

28. Parks AG, Gordon PH, Hardcastle JD. A classification of fistula-in-ano. Br J Surg. 1976;63(1):1–12. https://doi.org/10.1002/bjs.1800630102.

29. Tozer P, Philips RKS. Fistulotomy and lay open technique. In: Abcarian H, editor. Anal fistula: principles and management. New York: Springer; 2014. p. 56–7.

30. Becker A, Koltun L, Sayfan J. Simple clinical examination predicts complexity of perianal fistula. Colorectal Dis. 2006;8(7):601–4.

31. Van Onkelen RS, Gosselink MP, Schouten WR. Treatment of anal fistulas with high inter-sphincteric extension. Dis Colon Rectum. 2013;56(8):987–91. https://doi.org/10.1097/DCR.0b013e3182908be6.

17

"All sinuses heal unless something keeps them open."

Lord and Miller

Key Concepts
- Pilonidal sinus is a cavity or tract in the sacro-coccygeal region caused by recurring infection and persistent inflammation.
- Pilonidal sinus disease is attributed to the entry of the hair through a primary opening called the pit.
- Minimally invasive techniques like endoscopic pilonidal sinus treatment (EPSiT) and video-assisted laser ablation of the pilonidal sinus (VALAPS) have gained popularity.
- Pit picking combined with VALAPS gives good results with a low recurrence.

17.1 Introduction

Pilonidal sinus disease (PSD) is a sacrococcygeal cavity or tract formed by recurrent infection and persistent inflammation [1]. In 1847, A.W. Anderson published a paper on "hair extracted from an ulcer" [2, 3]. Warren later documented three instances in 1854, making the first case series in "Pilonidal sinus disease" [4]. R.M Hodges invented the word "Pilonidal disease" in 1880 [5]. The word is a combination of Pilus and Nidus; Pilus means "hair," and Nidus means "nest." In 1883, O.H. Mayo described the condition for the first time [6]. This condition is often called jeep disease, as many U.S soldiers riding jeeps were affected by the pilonidal disease during the wars [2]. Over 79,000 soldiers in the American army had surgery for pilonidal sinus disease. Two thousand soldiers during the Vietnamese war were operated on for pilonidal sinus every year [7].

17.2 Epidemiology

The prevalence of pilonidal sinus is 26 people per 100,000 [8]. In a 2.2:1 ratio, men are more often infected than women [2]. Each year, an estimated 70,000 Americans are afflicted by this disease [9]. According to Kazim Duman et al., pilonidal sinus is more common in the Turkish community than in other groups [7]. In studies on pilonidal disease in south India, P. Rajasekharan et al. found that most individuals were in the age category of 16–25 years, with a male-to-female ratio of 2.98:1 [10]. After the age of 40, PSD is uncommon.

17.3 Location

The most typical location is the natal cleft (94%) [10]. A study conducted by N. Sion-Vardy reported some ectopic locations of the pilonidal

K. Gupta, *Lasers in Proctology*, https://doi.org/10.1007/978-981-19-5825-0_17

sinus, including the penis, abdomen, scalp, groin, axilla, and neck [11]. Another location is interdigital, seen in the hands of the barbers as an occupational hazard [12].

17.4   Risk Factors of Pilonidal Sinus

According to Hralak et al., pilonidal sinus disease is the second most prevalent condition among soldiers [13]. It affects white males more than any other in the young age group [13]. Although there is not much information in the literature to analyze the risk factors, the following are some of the most prevalent ones [13]:

- Obesity
- Sedentary lifestyles
- Hirsute
- Male gender
- Occupations requiring prolonged sitting like long-distance drivers
- Deep natal cleft
- Local trauma
- Poor personal hygiene
- Excessive sweating

17.5   Etiology

Many surgeons and clinicians considered pilonidal disease congenital in origin [2]. Harlak et al. found a family history of pilonidal disease in roughly 15% of patients [13]. Patey et al. hypothesized in 1946 that pilonidal disease resulted from the hair sucked from the adjacent soft tissue, causing an inflammatory reaction. Hence it was considered an acquired disease [14].

There are three main theories to support the acquired origin of pilonidal disease.

17.5.1   Bascom Theory

In 1980, Bascom provided histological evidence with a series of stages in the disease progression to support the acquired theory. The skin of the natal cleft is stretched and lifted away from the sacrococcygeal fascia while sitting or bending during physical activity. A negative pressure is created, and a suction effect is produced due to gluteal movements that draw hair into the cavity, causing folliculitis and a small subdermal abscess. This small subdermal abscess grows over time, eventually becoming a large abscess cavity [14].

17.5.2   Karydakis Theory

Karydakis described three main factors for the formation of pilonidal disease

- The invader, loose hair "H." "H" represents the number of hair, kind of hair (whether tough or silky), and shape.
- A force resulting in hair penetration "F"—depends upon the depth and shape of the natal cleft.
- Skin vulnerability "V"—depends upon whether the skin is soft, macerated, excoriated, or has wide pores.

When hair is implanted in the natal cleft, it bores deeper and deeper into the subcutaneous tissue like a screw motion effect. The hair always inserts on its root end, and hence, only loose hair can get inserted. The hair's keratin flakes allow the hair follicle to move unidirectional [1, 15]. As a result, the hair burrows deep in the pit. The sinus tracts may spread laterally, forming secondary openings with unhealthy granulation tissue. Based on findings, a formula was designed for pilonidal sinus disease

$$PSD = {}^{\prime}H{}^{\prime} \times {}^{\prime}F{}^{\prime} \times {}^{\prime}V^{2\,\prime}$$

If all the above three factors are present, pilonidal sinus develops [15]. Loose hair has scales on it. When the hair falls, the friction causes the hair to enter the depth of the natal cleft in the center. Insertion of one hair allows other hair to enter the natal cleft. The point of entry of the hair is the primary sinus, and the point of exit is the secondary sinus [1, 15]. Karydakis suggests that if only new hair entry could be stopped, many pilonidal sinuses could be self-cured [15]. According to Karydakis, folliculitis, although common, does not lead to pilonidal sinus [15].

17.5.3   Stelzner Theory

Stelzner advocated the pilonidal sinus as a retention dermopathy of an acquired origin, suggesting that the folds of the deep skin, body hair stiffness, and the rolling action push hair like a pin into the skin. When hair is rubbed, it moves in the direction of its root, with the hair scales pointing outwards toward the surface [16].

17.6   Pathophysiology

Activities like sitting and bending cause the breaking of hair follicles and the formation of pits. The buttock friction and the shearing forces allow the hair in the natal cleft to enter the pits by suction effect. These pits may get filled with debris, followed by a tract or sinus formation. The mechanical forces generated during sitting and bending result in the penetration of hair deeper into the tissue [1]. This leads to the formation of an acute pilonidal abscess.

Follicular occlusion tetrad is a complex involving; acne conglobata, dissecting cellulitis of the scalp, hidradenitis suppurativa, and pilonidal sinus. All these conditions have the same pathophysiology [17]. Because of follicular occlusion, several authors consider pilonidal disease part of "follicular occlusion tetrad" [17]. Stelzner et al. (1984) observed a hook-shaped hair follicle in the pits and hypothesized that hair migration was unidirectional [17]. Studies further supported the hook morphology by Dahl et al., who also proposed that sharp ends of the hair contributed to piercing of the skin [18].

In their study "hair in the sinus," Friederike et al. identified short hairpieces with the rootless sharp cut ends inside pilonidal sinus canals. The fragments were morphologically like the free short hair instead of intact hair. Short head hair penetrates the pilonidal canal more readily than long hair [19]. Davage, in 1954, observed that the hair found in the pilonidal cavity originated from the neighboring overlying tissue, and there were no follicles within the cyst's wall [20].

17.7   Histopathology

On histopathology examination, the pilonidal cyst wall comprises of vascular pyogenic granulation tissue [20]. Stratified squamous epithelium lines the sinus tract [2]. There are anaerobic and aerobic bacteria in an infected pilonidal sinus, making it polymicrobial [21].

17.8   The Direction of the Sinus Tract

In most cases, the pilonidal sinus tract is cephalad and rarely caudal, corresponding to the direction of hair follicle growth. The presence of sinus toward the caudal direction is often mistaken as fistula-in-ano.

17.9   Clinical Presentation of the Disease

A complete clinical evaluation should be done. It includes:

- A detailed history
- Physical examination

17.9.1   History

The patients are usually young, with jobs requiring prolonged sitting. The commonest symptoms are:

- Painful or painless swelling at the base of the tail bone
- Pus or blood-stained discharge from the cavity
- Redness of the skin around the area
- Intermittent swelling and spontaneous drainage with a foul-smelling discharge
- Formation of one or more holes lateral to the midline or in the midline
- Hair protruding from the lesion

17.9.2 Physical Examination

Physical examination may reveal

- Painful swelling posterior to the anal orifice in the sacrococcygeal region (Fig. 17.1a) [20].
- Single or multiple openings near the coccyx or off the midline (Fig. 17.1b, c).

- Single or multiple pits with hair (Fig. 17.1d–f).
- Abscesses associated with the pits.
- A long sinus tract.

There may be warmth, redness, and tenderness if the pilonidal abscess is present. On palpation, there may be fluctuant swelling in the midline or lateral to the midline at the intergluteal

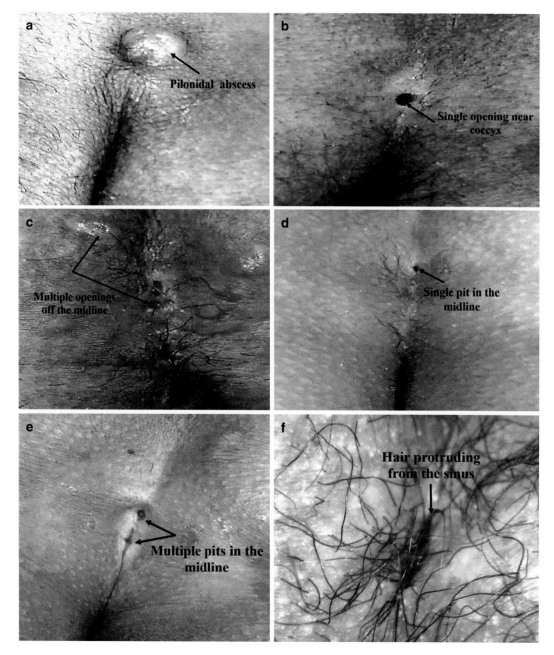

Fig. 17.1 (**a**) Swelling posterior to the anal orifice in the sacrococcygeal region. (**b**) Single opening near the coccyx. (**c**) Multiple openings near the coccyx or off the midline. (**d**) Single pit. (**e**) Multiple pits. (**f**) Pits with protruding hair

cleft. In some cases, loose hair can protrude from the sinus (Fig. 17.1f). A fistula-in-ano must be ruled out if the sinus tract is going caudally.

17.10 Navicular Area

The navicular area lies between the natal cleft's lateral edges and their posterior extensions [22] (Fig. 17.2). The posterior border of the anal tri-

angle marks the posterior border of the navicular cleft. The patient is placed in a jackknife position to mark the navicular area. The buttocks are drawn together, and the outer contact lines mark the natal cleft's lateral edges. Before releasing the buttocks, the edges are marked with a pen. This reveals a ship-like shaped area referred to as a navicular area [22].

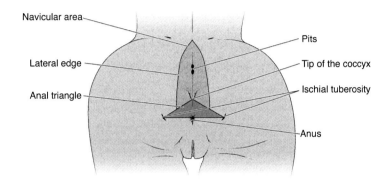

Fig. 17.2 Navicular area

17.11 Classification of Pilonidal Sinus

Tezel proposed a new classification for the pilonidal sinus based on the navicular area's representation of symptoms [22]. The diagrammatic representation of the classification is shown in Fig. 17.3a–e. A detailed description of Tezel's classification and how to manage pilonidal sinus are shown in Table 17.1.

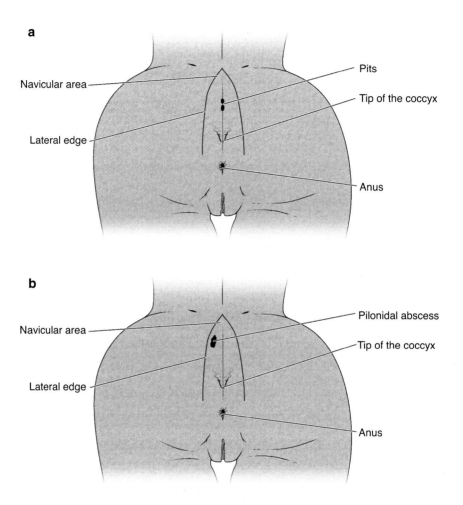

Fig. 17.3 (**a**–**e**) Tezel's classification. (**a**) Type 1: presence of pit (asymptomatic). (**b**) Type 2: acute pilonidal abscess. (**c**) Type 3: pits restricted in the navicular area with abscess drainage. (**d**) Type 4: extensive sinus disease with sinus opening outside the navicular area. (**e**) Type 5: recurrent pilonidal sinus disease after surgical treatment

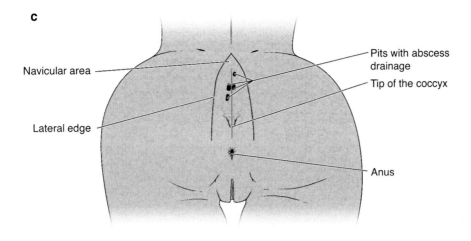

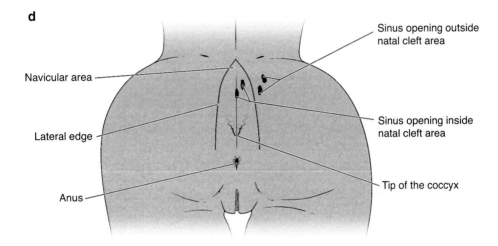

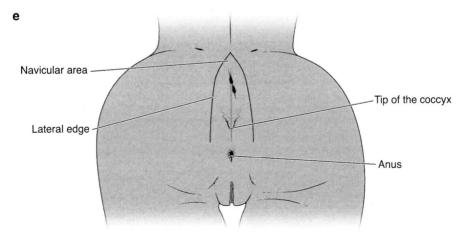

Fig. 17.3 (continued)

Table 17.1 Tezel's classification of pilonidal sinus

Type of pilonidal sinus	Presentation	Surgical recommendation
Type I	Asymptomatic pit(s) with no history of drainage or abscess	• No surgical intervention • Removal of local hair • Maintain hygiene
Type II	Acute pilonidal abscess	• Drainage using a lateral incision
Type III	Pit(s) in the navicular part with an abscess or prior drainage history	• Bascom's procedure
Type IV	A severe condition in which one or more sinus openings are located outside the navicular region	• Outside of the navicular region, the Bascom treatment is coupled with separate excision of pits
Type V	Recurrent pilonidal sinus	• Bascom procedure

17.12 Imaging

If the patient has inflammatory bowel disease, anorectal fistula, pelvic sepsis, or neoplastic lesion, an MRI can provide a definitive diagnosis [23]. MRI findings in individuals with pilonidal sinus may sometimes resemble perianal and deep-seated sepsis or anal fistula. However, the lack of intersphincteric sepsis or any enteric opening helps distinguish the two entities on MRI [23].

17.13 Differential Diagnosis

Pilonidal sinus disease should always be differentiated from other conditions present in the sacrococcygeal region, as shown in Table 17.2.

Some authors believe that the pilonidal sinus and anal fistula can co-exist and communicate. In a study by Pankaj Garg, 9 individuals out of 1284 had a co-existing fistula and pilonidal sinus disease [24]. The pathophysiology explained in his study was as follows:

Table 17.2 Differential diagnosis

Disease	Features
Abscess	• Pilonidal sinus is associated with abscesses, but not all abscesses can be defined as pilonidal abscesses • Location of the abscess
Hidradenitis suppurativa	• Primary lesions are deep-seated nodules approximately 0.5–2 cm • On rupturing, the tract is formed subcutaneously • The disease often affects the groin, axillary, perianal, and perineal regions
Fistula-in-Ano	• Position of the external opening • Communication with the anal canal • Tract palpation • Internal opening • MRI
Epidural abscess	• Percussion tenderness • Local or radiating back pain • Fever • Worsening of pain during recumbency
Furuncles	• Infection of hair follicles that goes deep into the skin • It may have a small pus pocket
Sacral osteomyelitis	• Infection of the sacrum • Associated with fever, chills, and rigors • X-ray of the spine shows osteomyelitis
Carbuncles	• Group of the infected hair follicles with pus • Usually associated with diabetes
Folliculitis	• Inflammation of hair follicles
Pyoderma gangrenosum	• Ulcerative lesions • Associated with other comorbidities • The patients are in their late forties

• Both these diseases existed independently.
• The pilonidal sinus was a primary condition, but it progressed to the point where it developed into a fistula with an anorectal opening.
• One of the anal fistula tracts traveled posteriorly and opened in the lower back [24].

17.14   Management of Pilonidal Sinus Disease

The removal of diseased tissue remains the mainstay of surgical management. In the case of an asymptomatic pilonidal sinus, hair removal, either by shaving the area or laser epilation, is recommended [25]. Incision and drainage are the first-line therapies for pilonidal sinus with acute abscess [25]. Pilonidal sinus without an abscess can be treated with surgical excision [25]. The conventional surgical procedures vary from limited or wide excisions of pilonidal sinus followed by primary closure or healing by secondary intention. The most commonly used procedure is the Bascom technique which involves the removal of midline pits followed by closure along with draining and curetting of the associated abscess cavity [26]. Many other procedures, including Z-Plasty, Rhomboid excision (Limberg flap), V-Y fasciocutaneous flap, Karydakis procedure, and advancement flaps, have been described [27]. These procedures are associated with large wounds, pain, discomfort, and a recurrence rate ranging from 3% to 40% [28]. Phenol installation, sinusotomy, and sinusectomy, which involves circumferential incision of the pilonidal sinus, are other management modalities [29, 30]. The flap procedure requires preserving the vitality of the flap tissues [31].

17.14.1   Minimally Invasive Techniques for Pilonidal Sinus: Newer Surgical Modalities

Minimally invasive surgical procedures have gained popularity in treating pilonidal sinus in the last decade. Meinero et al. [32] and Milone et al. [29] developed the concept of endoscopic treatment for pilonidal sinus. Having succeeded in fistula surgery using video-assisted anal fistula

treatment (VAAFT), Meinero et al. successfully tried a similar technique in treating the pilonidal sinus and named it "Endoscopic pilonidal sinus treatment (EPSiT) [32]." The principle is, to destroy the pilonidal sinus tract with monopolar cautery under direct vision. In Milone's technique, the pilonidal sinus is treated by removing a minor elliptical wedge of subcutaneous and inflammatory tissue while the overlying skin remains intact [29]. The use of the endoscope provided direct visualization of the tract. Milone et al. [29] reported faster healing of the pilonidal sinus tract due to a small elliptical incision 2 mm deep and 5 mm wide.

The procedure I do in my practice is a hybrid procedure combining pit excision, Video endoscopy and Laser ablation.

17.15   Video-Assisted Laser Ablation of the Pilonidal Sinus (VALAPS)

VALAPS is a minimally invasive procedure done under spinal anesthesia. It involves removing hair and necrotic material from the sinus tract by sharp curettage under vision followed by laser ablation. The laser emits controlled energy at 65–80 °C, whereas in cautery, the energy emitted is 300–400 °C. Moreover, the conduction pathways in cautery cannot be controlled. The laser has better soft-tissue ablation and hemostatic qualities and is more effective than electrocautery.

17.15.1   Principle

The video endoscope offers direct visibility of the sinus tract. The laser energy destroys the sinus epithelium while simultaneously obliterating the tract. The necrotic material and hair are removed under direct vision, reducing the chances of recurrence.

17.15.2   Device for Video-Assisted Endoscopy

- Fistuloscope 8°, outer diameter 3.3 × 4.7 mm, working length handle 18 cm, angled eyepiece (Fig. 17.4)
- Obturator
- Handle
- Endoscopic seal for working channel
- Wire tray for cleaning, storage, and sterilization
- Coagulation electrode
- Brush
- Grasping forceps 2 mm diameter, length 30 cm with double action jaws
- Plastic handle
- Outer sheath
- Camera

17.15.3   Device for Pit Excision

- Dermatology biopsy forceps (Fig. 17.5). Different sizes are available.

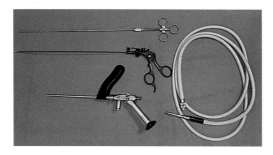

Fig. 17.4 VAAFT scope equipment

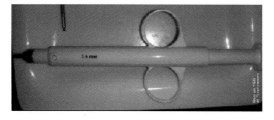

Fig. 17.5 Pit biopsy forceps

17.15.4   Energy! Dosage! Fiber!

- **Energy**: Total energy delivered depends on the length of the tract.
- **Dosage**: 10 W per second per mm in continuous mode using 1470 nm wavelength.
- **Fiber**: 360° radial fiber.

17.15.5   Technique

Preoperatively, a circular area of 6–10 in. around the opening of the sinus is shaved. The patient is placed in a prone position under spinal anesthesia. After cleaning and draping, the pits are excised using punch biopsy forceps (Fig. 17.6a). In the absence of a secondary opening, the sinus tract is converted into a tunnel using a metal probe inserted through the sinus opening and brought out through an iatrogenic opening created 3–4 mm wide and 1–1.5 cm lateral to the midline (Fig. 17.6b). Converting a sinus into a tunnel helps visualize the tract and remove the necrotic material. In the presence of a secondary opening, the VAAFT scope is inserted through this to visualize the entire tract (Fig. 17.6c, d). The hair and necrotic material are identified and removed with sharp curetting followed by irrigation of the sinus tract (Fig. 17.6e–g). Alternatively, the necrotic material can be removed with a brush and forceps provided with the VAAFT equipment. The necrotic material is sent for histopathology.

Corona 360° radial laser 600 μm with distal and outer diameters of 1800 μm is introduced into the sinus through the working channel of the video endoscope. The entire tract is then ablated using laser equipment of 1470 nm wavelength. The energy is released in a dosage of 10 W per second per mm, continuous mode (Fig. 17.6h). While releasing the energy, make sure there is a distance of at least 1 cm between the laser fiber tip and the video endoscope lens. Otherwise, the scope's tip can be damaged with thermal energy.

The tract is again curetted and irrigated to remove the burnt-out necrotic material. The final

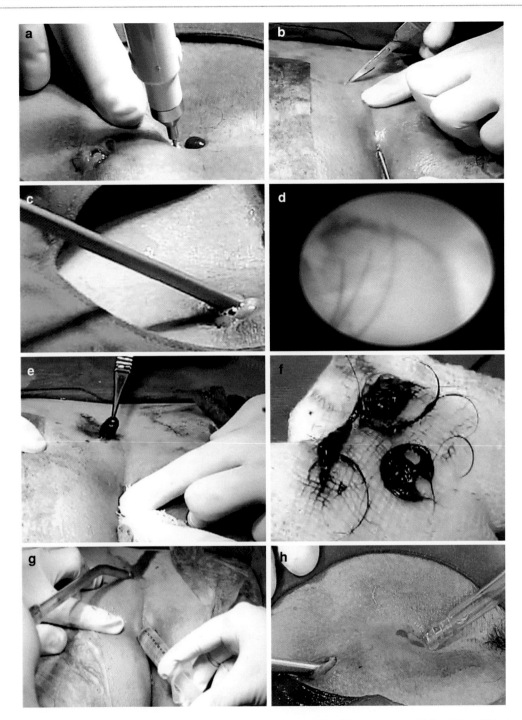

Fig. 17.6 (**a–i**) Steps of video-assisted laser ablation of pilonidal sinus technique. (**a**) Excision of pits using pit excision forceps. (**b**) Creation of an iatrogenic opening 1–1.5 cm away from the midline (optional). (**c**) Insertion of the VAAFT scope through the secondary opening of pilonidal sinus. (**d**) Presence of necrotic material and hair as seen under video endoscope. (**e**) Curetting of the sinus tract. (**f**) Tuft of hair as seen after curetting the sinus tract. (**g**) Irrigation of the tract. (**h**) Laser ablation of the sinus tract using radial fiber. (**i**) Closing of pits after excision (optional)

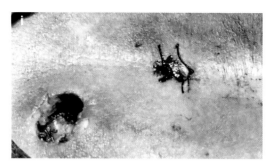

Fig. 17.6 (continued)

step of the procedure is the closure of pits, which is optional (Fig. 17.6i). The wound is finally dressed using nanosilver gel ointment. At the time of discharge, saline irrigation of the wound is carried out to remove any leftover debris. Patients are taught to dress the wound using sterile bandages and ointment. Follow-up of patients is done after 1 week.

17.15.6   Postoperative Care

- Diclofenac sodium as an analgesic and Amoxycillin with Clavulanic acid 625 mg twice daily as an antibiotic are prescribed for 5–7 days.
- Of late, the wound is dressed with hemoglobin spray containing 10% carbonylated hemoglobin, 0.9% sodium chloride, 0.7% phenoxyethanol, and 0.05% N-acetylcysteine. The spray is inserted into the sinus tract using a nozzle. It improves oxygen availability by binding oxygen from the environment and dif-

fusing it into the wound bed. This accelerates the recovery process [33]. A study on Hb spray in wounds has shown a reduction in wound size by 63% after 4 weeks [33].
- Micronized amniotic membrane provides an excellent environment for cell proliferation [34]. Micronized granules of dehydrated human amnion chorion membrane coated with 0.5% (w/w) broad-spectrum antimicrobial biocide, PHMB (polyhexamethylene biguanide), can also be inserted into the sinus tract. The dressing is required twice a week.
- Instructions are also given to keep the surrounding area clean and maintain personal hygiene. The patients are advised to shave the surrounding area every 2 weeks.

17.15.7   Results of VALAPS

At our center, an efficacy study was undertaken of 38 participants with PSD, 35 (92.10%) of whom were males, and 3 (7.90%) were females. The participants were between 18 and 34 years (only 1 patient was 45-year-old). There were 16 (42.10%) students, 13 (34.21%) I.T. professionals, and 9 (23.68%) drivers by profession. None of the patients had diabetes, hypertension, and dyslipidemia.

The mean operational time was 25.2 ± 6.23 min. The mean VAS pain score at 1 h from surgery was 3.5 ± 0.5, at 6 h, it was 2.2 ± 0.3, and at 24 h of surgery was 1.1 ± 0.2 (Fig. 17.7).

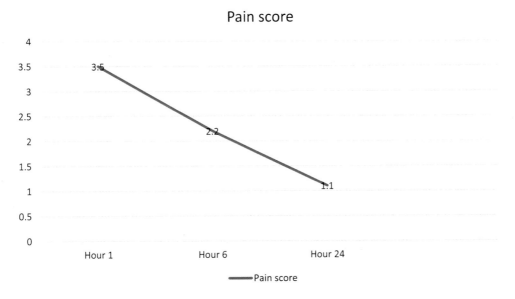

Fig. 17.7 Pain score on first, third, and seventh day

It took an average of 3 ± 1.2 days to return to work. The mean duration for recovery was 21 days. Out of 38, 12 patients complained of discharge from the wound site for about 7–8 days. Two patients were lost in follow-up. Seven patients had a recurrence in whom the procedure was repeated. The overall success rate was 95.3%. The success rate of video-assisted procedures is shown in Table 17.3.

A summary of the various procedures showing technical steps, complications, and recurrence rates is shown in Table 17.4.

Table 17.3 Success rate of video-assisted laser ablation of pilonidal sinus

Journal	Success rate (%)
Epub Clinical trial 2014 [35]	96.3
Epub Comparative study 2019 [36]	92.5
International Journal of Current Advanced Research Research article [37]	95.3

Table 17.4 Recurrence rate of various surgical procedures in pilonidal sinus

Type of procedure	Technical steps	Complications	Recurrence rate (%)
V-Y advancement flap [1]	• Creation of full-thickness V-shaped incision down to the gluteal fascia • It is closed to form a postrepair suture line in the shape of a Y [1]	• Wound site infection 0–10.2% • Wound dehiscence 10.2% • Seroma 0–4.6% [38–40]	• 0–11% [38–40]
Z plasty [41]	• Excision of the affected part with the placement of lateral flaps incised down to the level of the fascia [41]	• Wound infection 60% • Seroma 56% • Wound dehiscence 48% • Hematoma 52% [42]	32% [42]
Bascom procedure [26]	• Midline follicle excision and lateral drainage [26]	–	15% [26]
Bascom cleft lift closure [43]	• Excision of the sinus tracts with the placement of a full-thickness skin flap across the cleft and closed off-midline [43]	Minor complications 34.5% [43]	4.7% [43]
Karydakis [15]	• Elliptical excision of the affected part with fixation of the flap base to the sacral fascia • The flap is closed by suturing the edge off-midline [15]	Infection 1.8%	0.9–4.4% [15]
Limberg flap [38]	• A midline rhomboid incision to the presacral fascia [38]	Minor complications 16.7% [44]	7.1% [44]

Table 17.5 Results of EPSiT

Journal	Author	Success rate
Journal of the Society of Laparoscopic and Robotic surgeons 2017 [45]	Gabriella Giarrantano	97%
Int J Colorectal Disease 2019 [46]	Piercarlo Meinero	95%
Journal of Coloproctology 2020 [47]	Elias Saikaly	Complete wound healing in all the patients

17.15.8 Results of Minimally Invasive Procedures

The results of EPSiT are shown in Table 17.5.

17.16 Discussion

While treating pilonidal sinus, one is dealing with four parts of the disease:

• The pits—which are the primary source
• The sinus cavity—the tract
• The lateral midline tract or abscess, and
• The hair

Any procedure that takes care of these disease characteristics and has low recurrence should be considered an ideal treatment.

Complete excision can be midline or off-midline. Midline excisional methods are associated with higher recurrences and, therefore, not recommended. Off-midline excisional techniques are the most commonly employed, e.g., the Limberg flap or Karydaki's procedure.

Soll et al. proposed sinusectomy as a minimally invasive procedure for pilonidal sinus with low recurrence rate and faster return to work after surgery [48]. Meinero et al. revolutionized this field by employing a fistuloscope that allowed better visualization of the sinus tract [32]. Gips et al. 2008 performed minimally invasive surgeries employing trephines [49], video-assisted ablation of the pilonidal sinus (VAAPS), and endoscopic pilonidal sinus treatment (EPSiT). Prosthetic plugs were employed by Milone et al. Their minimally invasive approach did not leave any surgical scar [30]. Pappas et al. in 2018 described a minimally invasive procedure for PSD using a diode laser [50].

The technique I use for my patients is a hybrid procedure where the pits are removed by punch biopsy forceps followed by video-assisted laser ablation of the pilonidal sinus. The recurrence will be high unless the primary source of infection is removed. The sinus cavity will not heal unless all the hair is removed that can be better managed under vision. The cavity can be curetted, and hemostasis achieved using a laser. It can be ablated using a fan-shaped technique. Dressing the wound after the surgery is an essential aspect that increases the cure rate. Patients should be taught to take proper care of the area.

Minimally invasive techniques in pilonidal sinus provide many advantages. They have shorter operative time, shorter hospital stay, less postoperative pain, faster healing rates, and early return to work.

Several studies have been cited by Peter C Minneci et al., 2018 to establish the effectiveness of laser hair epilation in minimizing PSD recurrence [51]. Wagih Mommtaz Ghanam et al. published a study in 2011 that found a very low recurrence rate of 2.3% in individuals who had laser epilation as an adjunct to pilonidal sinus surgery. Lavelle et al. recorded a decrease in recurrence rate following laser hair epilation [52].

International guidelines have included the role of minimally invasive procedures in pilonidal sinus management. In 2019, the "American Society of Colon and Rectal Surgeons (ASCRS)" issued a weak set of guidelines for minimally invasive treatments in chronic and acute pilonidal diseases involving endoscopic or video-assisted procedures for PSD. The grade of recommendation is 2B, as shown in Table 17.6 [53]. Italian Society of Colorectal Surgery has also included minimally invasive procedures in its guidelines for managing PSD in 2021. The grade of recommendation is 1B [54]. According to guidelines, minimally invasive treatments are validated techniques that should be the treatment of choice in limited pilonidal disease (single pit or multiple pits on the midline).

Table 17.6 Operative management of pilonidal sinus disease. Grade of recommendation by ASCRS [53]

Presentation of the disease	Operative management	Grade of recommendation
Presence of an abscess	I&D regardless of whether it is a primary or recurring episode	Strong recommendation based on moderate-quality evidence, 1B
Chronic pilonidal disease	Excision and primary repair (with consideration for off-midline closure)	Strong recommendation based on moderate-quality evidence, 1B
Complex and recurrent chronic pilonidal disease	Flap-based procedure	Strong recommendation based on moderate-quality evidence, 1B
Acute and chronic pilonidal disease	Minimally invasive techniques	Weak recommendation based on moderate-quality evidence, 2B

17.17 Case Presentation

Mr. C, a 25-year-old male patient, complained of pain at the base of the tailbone and difficulty in sitting since 5 months. He occasionally noticed wetness in the tailbone area. He was prescribed antibiotics by a general physician but had no relief. When the patient consulted me, on local examination, a small pit could be seen in the midline. There was no secondary opening. He was diagnosed to be a case of pilonidal sinus. The patient was taken for surgery, and a hybrid procedure combining Video Assisted Laser Ablation of Pilonidal Sinus (VALAPS) and pit excision was performed. The wound was dressed with octenidine for 2 days, followed by dressing with Amnion Chorion granules and hemoglobin spray from the third postoperative day onwards. The patient was given instructions to keep the area clean and shaved. Postoperative wound care was explained. The wound fully healed after 2 weeks of surgery (Fig. 17.8a–d).

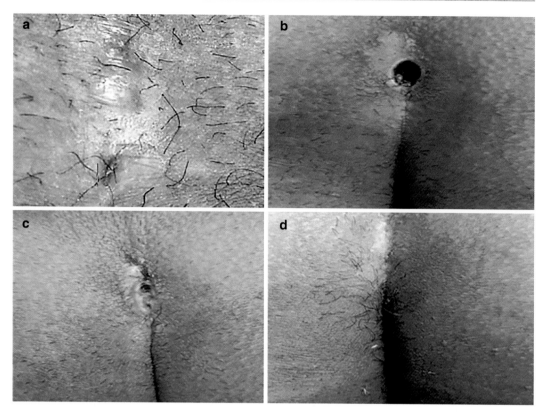

Fig. 17.8 (**a**) Presence of primary pit in anococcygeal region. (**b**) Pit excision done using skin biopsy forceps. (**c**) Postoperative wound after 1 week. (**d**) Complete healing of the wound after 2 weeks

17.17.1   Opinion

VALAPS is a minimally invasive procedure with good results in pilonidal sinus disease. Formation of a large wound secondary to removal of the primary opening is common. The best results are achieved with hemoglobin spray and PHMB Amnion Chorion granules. The same can be injected into the sinus tract.

17.18   Your Queries, My Answers

1. **Why recurrence after Pilonidal sinus surgery?**

   "The term 'recurrence' is used when symptoms of the disease reappear after complete wound healing" [55]

Recurrence may be due:

(a) Omission of the tracts.
(b) Infection.
(c) Dead and necrotic tissue—Recurrence might be triggered by the collection of dead or necrotic tissue in the intergluteal cleft, poor hygiene, or excessive sweating.
(d) Midline suture—A suture placed in the midline is under significant tension.
(e) Depth of natal cleft—One of the prominent reasons for recurrence is the deep natal cleft.
(f) Inappropriate wound care.

Recurrence in individuals with excisional wounds is also caused by poor wound management and a lack of depilation [56].

2. Is there a role of Vacuum-Assisted Closure (VAC) in pilonidal sinus?

VAC after pilonidal sinus excision reduces the healing time and promotes wound closure. In a study, Tomasz Banasiewiz et al. found that VAC treatment reduces wound healing time, postoperative pain, and job absenteeism [57].

3. What is the role of pit excision in pilonidal sinus?

The term "pit" refers to a small opening in the natal cleft through which hair can enter. The pits are seen in the midline and are treated by excision. These pits may form the primary root of infection or entry point of the hair.

4. Is there any role of laser removal of hair in pilonidal sinus treatment?

Entrapped hair in the pilonidal sinus cavity remains the primary etiologic factor in the formation of the disease. Keeping the area free from hair can prevent a recurrence. Therefore, shaving the natal cleft is advised as a routine, postoperatively. Some authors do recommend laser epilation.

5. Is there the role of FiXcision in pilonidal sinus surgery?

Sometimes I wonder, can fixcision be used in treating pilonidal sinus tracts, especially with secondary openings? FiXcision is an instrument that is routinely used in coring out the fistula tracts. A fixcision instrument measuring 3–4 mm in diameter can be used to core out the pilonidal sinus tracts. The advantage of the coring of the pilonidal sinus tract is that all the hair and necrotic material can be removed. The procedure is minimally invasive and looks promising.

Take-Home Message

The video-assisted laser ablation of the pilonidal sinus (VALAPS) technique is viable for managing the pilonidal sinus. It allows the surgeon to examine the sinus tract directly, and the hair, which is the primary cause of pilonidal sinus disease, can be removed under vision. Laser ablation helps to ablate the necrotic material and shrink the tract. Low postoperative discomfort and a quick return to work are advantages of this technique. Results so far look promising.

References

1. Khanna A, Rombeau JL. Pilonidal disease. Clin Colon Rectal Surg. 2011;24:46–53.
2. Nixon AT, Garza RF. Pilonidal cyst and sinus. StatPearls; 2020.
3. Anderson AW. Hair extracted from an ulcer. Boston Med Surg J. 1847;36:64–76.
4. Warren JM. Abscess containing hair on the nates. Am J Med Sci. 1854;28:113.
5. Hodges RM. Pilonidal sinüs. Boston Med Surg J. 1880;103:485–6.
6. Mayo OH. Observations on injuries and diseases of the rectum. London: Burgess and Hill; 1833. p. 45–6.
7. Duman K, Gırgın M, Harlak A. Prevalence of sacrococcygeal pilonidal disease in Turkey. Asian J Surg. 2017;40(6):434–7.
8. Søndenaa K, Andersen E, Nesvik I, Søreide JA. Patient characteristics and symptoms in chronic pilonidal sinus disease. Int J Color Dis. 1995;10(1):39–42.
9. Johnson EK, Vogel JD, Cowan ML, Feingold DL, Steele SR, Clinical Practice Guidelines Committee of the American Society of Colon and Rectal Surgeons. The American Society of Colon and Rectal Surgeons clinical practice guidelines for the management of pilonidal disease. Dis Colon Rectum. 2019;62(2):146–57.
10. Rajasekharan D, Nagaraja JB, Subbarayappa S. Pilonidal sinus in South India: a retrospective review. Indian J Colorectal Surg. 2019;2(3):71.
11. Sion-Vardy N, Osyntsov L, Cagnano E, Osyntsov A, Vardy D, Benharroch D. Unexpected location of pilonidal sinuses. Clin Exp Dermatol. 2009;34(8):e599–601. https://doi.org/10.1111/j.1365-2230.2009.03272.x.
12. Patel MR, Bassini L, Nashad R, Anselmo MT. Barber's interdigital pilonidal sinus of the hand: a foreign body hair granuloma. J Hand Surg Am. 1990;15(4):652–5. https://doi.org/10.1016/s0363-5023(09)90031-4.
13. Harlak A, Mentes O, Kilic S, Coskun K, Duman K, Yilmaz F. Sacrococcygeal pilonidal disease: analysis of previously proposed risk factors. Clinics (Sao Paulo, Brazil). 2010;65(2):125–31. https://doi.org/10.1590/S1807-59322010000200002.
14. Patey DH, Scarff RW. Pathology of postanal pilonidal sinus; its bearing on treatment. Lancet. 1946;2(6423):484–6. https://doi.org/10.1016/s0140-6736(46)91756-4.
15. Karydakis GE. Easy and successful treatment of pilonidal sinus after explanation of its causative process. Aust N Z J Surg. 1992;62(5):385–9.
16. Stelzner F. Die Ursache des pilonidal sinus und der Pyodermia fistulans sinifica [Causes of pilonidal sinus and pyoderma fistulans sinifica]. Langenbecks Arch Chir. 1984;362(2):105–18. German. https://doi.org/10.1007/BF01254185.
17. Vasanth V, Chandrashekar BS. Follicular occlusion tetrad. Indian Dermatol Online J. 2014;5(4):491–3. https://doi.org/10.4103/2229-5178.142517.
18. Dahl HD, Henrich MH. [Light and scanning electron microscopy study of the pathogenesis of piloni-

dal sinus and anal fistula]. Langenbecks Arch Chir. 1992;377(2):118–24.

19. Bosche F, Luedi MM, van der Zypen D, Moersdorf P, Krapohl B, Doll D. The hair in the sinus: sharp-ended rootless head hair fragments can be found in large amounts in pilonidal sinus nests. World J Surg. 2018;42(2):567–73. https://doi.org/10.1007/s00268-017-4093-5.

20. Davage ON. The origin of sacrococcygeal pilonidal sinuses based on an analysis of four hundred sixtythree cases. Am J Pathol. 1954;30(6):1191–205.

21. Oh HB, Abdul Malik MH, Keh CH. Pilonidal abscess associated with primary actinomycosis. Ann Coloproctol. 2015;31(6):243–5. https://doi.org/10.3393/ac.2015.31.6.243.

22. Tezel E. A new classification according to navicular area concept for sacrococcygeal pilonidal disease. Colorectal Dis. 2007;9(6):575–6. https://doi.org/10.1111/j.1463-1318.2007.01236.x.

23. Taylor SA, Halligan S, Bartram CI. Pilonidal sinus disease: M.R. imaging distinction from fistula in ano. Radiology. 2003;226(3):662–7.

24. Garg P. Anal fistula and pilonidal sinus disease coexisting simultaneously: an audit in a cohort of 1284 patients. Int Wound J. 2019;16(5):1199–205. https://doi.org/10.1111/iwj.13187.

25. Steele SR, Perry WB, Mills S, Buie WD. Practice parameters for the management of pilonidal disease. Dis Colon Rectum. 2013;56(9):1021–7.

26. Bascom J, Bascom T. Utility of the cleft lift procedure in refractory pilonidal disease. Am J Surg. 2007;193(5):606–9.

27. Lim J, Shabbir J. Pilonidal sinus disease-a literature review. World J Surg Surg Res. 2019;2019(2):1117.

28. Sohn N, Martz J. Pilonidal disease. In: Cameron JL, editor. Current surgical therapy. 8th ed. Philadelphia, PA: Elsevier Mosby; 2004. p. 280–4.

29. Milone M, Sosa Fernandez LM, Milone F, De Palma GD. Endoscopic pilonidal sinus: how far have we come? Dis Colon Rectum. 2018;61(6):e343. https://doi.org/10.1097/DCR.0000000000001100.

30. Priyadarshi S, Dogra BB, Nagare K, Rana KV, Sunkara R, Kandari A. A comparative study of open technique and Z-plasty in management of pilonidal sinus. Medical J Dr DY Patil Univ. 2014;7(5):574.

31. Isik A, Ramanathan R. Approaches to the treatment of pilonidal sinus disease, clinical practice in 2019. Int Wound J. 2020;17(2):508–9. https://doi.org/10.1111/iwj.13265.

32. Meinero P, Mori L, Gasloli G. Endoscopic pilonidal sinus treatment (E.P.Si.T.). Tech Coloproctol. 2014;18(4):389–92. https://doi.org/10.1007/s10151-013-1016-9.

33. Hunt SD, Elg F. Clinical effectiveness of hemoglobin spray (Granulox®) as adjunctive therapy in the treatment of chronic diabetic foot ulcers. Diabetic Foot Ankle. 2016;7:33101. https://doi.org/10.3402/dfa.v7.33101.

34. Life cell. https://www.lifecell.in/amchoplast-flo.

35. Milone M, Musella M, Di Spiezio Sardo A, Bifulco G, Salvatore G, Sosa Fernandez LM, Bianco P, Zizolfi B, Nappi C, Milone F. Video-assisted ablation of pilonidal sinus: a new minimally invasive treatment—a pilot study. Surgery. 2014;155(3):562–6. https://doi.org/10.1016/j.surg.2013.08.021.

36. Milone M, Velotti N, Manigrasso M, Milone F, Sosa Fernandez LM, De Palma GD. Video-assisted ablation of the pilonidal sinus (VAAPS) versus sinusectomy for treatment of chronic pilonidal sinus disease: a comparative study. Updat Surg. 2019;71(1):179–83. https://doi.org/10.1007/s13304-018-00611-2.

37. Gupta K, Mital K, Gupta R. Video-assisted laser ablation of pilonidal sinus VALAPS—a combined minimally invasive approach for management of pilonidal sinus. IJCAR. 2019;8(09):19789–93.

38. Tavassoli A, Noorshafiee S, Nazarzadeh R. Comparison of excision with primary repair versus Limberg flap. Int J Surg. 2011;9:343–6.

39. Berkem H, Topaloglu S, Ozel H, Avsar FM, Yildiz Y, Yüksel BC, et al. V-Y advancement flap closures for complicated pilonidal sinus disease. Int J Colorectal Dis. 2005;20:343–8.

40. Öz B, Akcan A, Emek E, Akyüz M, Sözüer E, Akyıldız H, et al. A comparison of surgical outcome of fasciocutaneous V-Y advancement flap and Limberg transposition flap for recurrent sacrococcygeal pilonidal sinus disease. Asian J Surg. 2017;40:197–202.

41. Nursal TZ, Ezer A, Calişkan K, et al. Prospective randomized controlled trial comparing V-Y advancement flaps with primary suture methods in pilonidal disease. Am J Surg. 2010;199:170–7.

42. Kayal A, Hussain A, Choudhary A, Meghwal A. A comparative study between Karydakis flap reconstruction and double Z-plasty patients with sacrococcygeal pilonidal disease. Int Sch Res Notices. 2014;2014:523015.

43. Hatch Q, Marenco C, Lammers D, Morte K, Schlussel A, McNevin S. Postoperative outcomes of Bascom cleft lift for pilonidal disease: a single-center experience. Am J Surg. 2020;219(5):737–40. https://doi.org/10.1016/j.amjsurg.2020.03.005.

44. Karaca AS, Ali R, Capar M, Karaca S. Comparison of Limberg flap and excision and primary closure of pilonidal sinus disease, quality of life. J Korean Surg Soc. 2013;85(5):236–9.

45. Giarratano G, Toscana C, Shalaby M, Buonomo O, Petrella G, Sileri P. Endoscopic pilonidal sinus treatment: long-term results of a perspective series. J Soc Laparoendosc Surg. 2017;21(3):e2017.00043. https://doi.org/10.4293/JSLS.2017.00043.

46. Meinero P, La Torre M, Lisi G, Stazi A, Carbone A, Regusci L, Fasolini F. Endoscopic pilonidal sinus treatment (EPSiT) in recurrent pilonidal disease: a prospective international multicenter study. Int J Colorectal Dis. 2019;34(4):741–6. https://doi.org/10.1007/s00384-019-03256-8.

47. Saikaly E, Saad MK. Modified endoscopic piloni-
    dal sinus treatment (EPSiT): personal experience. J
    Coloproctol (Rio de Janeiro). 2020;40:233–236s.
48. Soll C, Dindo D, Steinemann D, Hauffe T, Clavien
    PA, Hahnloser D. Sinusectomy for primary pilonidal
    sinus: less is more. Surgery. 2011;150(5):996–1001.
    https://doi.org/10.1016/j.surg.2011.06.019.
49. Gips M, Melki Y, Salem L, et al. Minimal surgery for
    pilonidal disease using trephines: description of a new
    technique and long-term outcomes in 1,358 patients.
    Dis Colon Rectum. 2008;51:1656–1662; discussion
    1662–3.
50. Pappas AF, Christodoulou DK. A new minimally
    invasive treatment of pilonidal sinus disease with
    the use of a diode laser: a prospective large series
    of patients. Colorectal Dis. 2018;20(8):O207–14.
    https://doi.org/10.1111/codi.14285.
51. Minneci PC, Halleran DR, Lawrence AE, Fischer BA,
    Cooper JN, Deans KJ. Laser hair depilation for the
    prevention of disease recurrence in adolescents and
    young adults with pilonidal disease: study protocol for
    a randomized controlled trial. Trials. 2018;19(1):599.
    https://doi.org/10.1186/s13063-018-2987-7.
52. Lavelle M, Jafri Z, Town G. Recurrent pilonidal sinus
    treated with epilation using a ruby laser. J Cosmet
    Laser Ther. 2002;4:45–7.
53. Johnson EK, Vogel JD, Cowan ML, Feingold DL,
    Steele SR. The American Society of Colon and Rectal
    Surgeons clinical practice guidelines for the man-
    agement of pilonidal disease. Dis Colon Rectum.
    2019;62(2):146–57.
54. M. Milone, L. Basso, M. Manigrasso,
    R. Pietroletti, A. Bondurri, M. La Torre, G. Milito,
    M. Pozzo,·D. Segre, R. Perinotti, G. Gallo. Consensus
    statement of the Italian Society of Colorectal Surgery
    (SICCR): management and treatment of pilonidal dis-
    ease. Tech Coloproctol 2021;25(12):1269-1280.
55. Guner A, Boz A, Ozkan OF, Ileli O, Kece C, Reis
    E. Limberg flap versus Bascom cleft lift techniques
    for sacrococcygeal pilonidal sinus: a prospective, ran-
    domized trial. World J Surg. 2013;37:2074–80.
56. Yoldas T, Karaca C, Unalp O, Uguz A, Caliskan
    C, Akgun E, Korkut M. Recurrent pilonidal sinus:
    lay open or flap closure; does it differ? Int Surg.
    2013;98(4):319–23.   https://doi.org/10.9738/
    INTSURG-D-13-00081.1.
57. Banasiewicz T, Bobkiewicz A, Borejsza-Wysocki
    M, Biczysko M, Ratajczak A, Malinger S, Drews
    M. Portable VAC therapy improve the results of the
    treatment of the pilonidal sinus—randomized prospec-
    tive study. Pol Przegl Chir. 2013;85(7):371–6. https://
    doi.org/10.2478/pjs-2013-0056. PMID: 23945113

Role of Lasers in Anal Fissures

18

"Such extreme pain in the patient like no other with such tiny spatial dimensions"
Peters, 1920

Key Concepts

- An anal fissure is a linear tear extending from the mucocutaneous junction to the dentate line.
- An anal fissure may be acute or chronic, depending upon the duration.
- The majority of anal fissures are either posterior or anterior midline.
- An acute anal fissure can be treated with topical application and dietary modifications.
- The gold standard for treating fissures is the "lateral internal sphincterotomy."
- Using lasers to treat anal fissures involves cutting the internal anal sphincter.

18.1 Introduction

A linear tear in the anal canal that may stretch from the mucocutaneous junction to the dentate line is known as an anal fissure [1]. It is a painful anorectal condition predisposed to nonhealing and persistence [2]. Anal fissures are usually the result of constipation and diarrhea. Despite being a painful condition, its etiopathogenesis remains obscure [3].

18.2 Historical Aspect

Anal fissure was first mentioned in 1689 by Louis Lemonnier in "Traité de la fistule de l'anus ou du fondement" [4] In 1818, Boyer first described the treatment of anal fissure by sphincterotomy [3]. Later in 1824 Raphael B. Sabatier described anal fissures in his "De la Médecine opératoire" [4]. In 1920 Peter described this as a severely painful condition in which the pain is not only restricted to the anal region but also radiates to the back [4].

18.3 Epidemiology

It is common in both sexes and affects people of all age groups [5]. Women are most affected in the childbearing age or at parturition. Chaudhary et al. in a study, found that 18 percent of patients with anorectal symptoms had anal fissures [6]. The prevalence of 1.1/1000 persons a year equates to a lifetime risk of 7.8%, indicating that anal fissures are common [7]. Anterior anal fissures affect women more than men, approximately 25%:8% [8]. Approximately 235000 new cases of anal fissures are reported in U.S every year and 40% of them persist for months and even years [9].

18.4   Etiology of Anal Fissure

The etiology of the fissure depends upon whether the fissure is primary or secondary.

The causes of a primary fissure include:

- Diarrhea
- Passage of hard stools
- Injury due to trauma or anal sex
- Vaginal delivery [10]

A secondary fissure may be due to:

- Inflammatory bowel diseases like Crohn's [10]
- Granulomatous diseases like tuberculosis, sarcoidosis
- Surgical procedures in the anorectal region
- Malignancy
- Infections like HIV and syphilis [10]

18.5   Risk Factors

- Women in adolescence and childbearing age
- Constipation
- Low-fiber diet
- Obesity

Literature Digging into Various Causes of Anal Fissure
- Delley, in 1855 described that during childbirth, as the head of the fetus advances, the perineum is pushed back, which causes lengthening of the anal opening resulting in anal fissure. Injury to the anus can be caused by enemas, cannulas, and an unnatural sexual urge [11].
- Rick, in 1924 listed hemorrhoidal disease, burns, rashes, sweat, and fecal remains as the causes of anal fissure [12].
- Willemsen, in 1958, described iron deficiency as one of the reasons for the formation of anal fissures, similar to the formation of angular stomatitis [13].

- Lund et al. in 1996 considered constipation as one of the major causes of anal fissures [10].
- Elía Guedea M et al. in 2008, considered bariatric surgery in obese patients to cause anal fissures [14].
- Garg P. in 2010 identified a water stream in a bidet-toilet as a source of anterior fissure-in-ano [15].

18.6   Pathophysiology of Anal Fissure

Straining during defecation, trauma, and passage of hard stool can lead to tearing. Once there is tearing of anal canal mucosa (anoderm), there is pain and internal anal sphincter spasm. A high resting pressure of the anal canal develops, causing increased anal tone. As a result, the blood flow to the local area is reduced, leading to ischemia and poor healing. This results in a vicious cycle, and the fissure does not heal till the cycle is broken, as shown in Table 18.1 [16].

Other theories which are related to the formation of anal fissures are:

- Tearing of the anal valves due to passage of hard stool.
- Anal infection theory related to the cryptoglandular origin.
- Loss of elasticity due to infection and fibrosis.
- Straining during parturition and chronic constipation.
- Iatrogenic—As a complication of any inappropriate anal surgery [17]. Anal stenosis after hemorrhoidectomy can lead to a chronic anal fissure.

Lockhart—Mummery postulated that anal mucosa is best supported laterally and weakest posteriorly due to the external sphincter structure. The fibers of the external anal sphincter are not circular but elliptical that split around the anus. Further, the external anal sphincter's length

Table 18.1 Pathophysiology of anal fissure

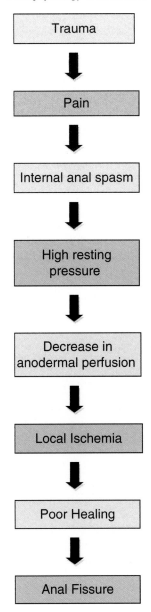

rectal arteries [19]. Because of this, the posterior commissure of the anal canal is less profused in approximately 85% of cases. Once the anal fissure is formed, the internal sphincter spasm further restricts the blood flow to the fissure site since the internal pudendal vessels run vertically upwards through the internal anal sphincter [20]. It leads to delayed healing resulting in a chronic ischemic ulcer. Using Doppler flowmetry, Schouten and colleagues evaluated microvascular perfusion of the anoderm. They concluded that anodermal blood circulation was much lower at the posterior commissure. Reduction of anal pressure by internal sphincterotomy improved anodermal blood flow, resulting in fissure healing [20, 21].

Goligher proposed that the internal anal sphincter below the dentate line was spastic. Hence, fissures are always limited to the dentate line, except those linked with inflammatory bowel illness [17].

18.7   Types of Anal Fissures

An anal fissure may be acute or chronic.

- An acute fissure is formed as a linear tear that heals within 6 weeks and has fresh mucosal edges [22].
- A chronic anal fissure heals after 6 weeks and may be associated with sentinel piles, hypertrophic anal papillae, and internal sphincter fibrosis at the fissure site [22].

Studies have revealed that 40% of the patients suffering from acute anal fissures advance to chronic anal fissures [23].

is half in females compared to males, leading to decreased anterior support [18]. This is believed to cause approximately 10% of anterior fissures in females [18].

Klosterhalfen et al. observed an absence of collaterals between the left and right inferior

18.8   Classification of Anal Fissures Based on Morphology

Anal fissures may be superficial or deep.

18.8.1 Characteristics of Superficial Anal Fissure

- Severe pain and bleeding.
- Anoderm separation on the surface with sharp edges.
- The internal anal sphincter is not breached at the base of the fissure.
- Heals spontaneously within days or weeks after conservative treatment [22, 24].

18.8.2 Characteristics of Deep Anal Fissure

- The internal anal sphincter fibers are often visible.
- Wide pear-shaped ulcer.
- A triad of indurated ulcer edges, sentinel pile, and proximal hypertrophic anal papillae is present [22, 24].

Most chronic anal fissures have three components; some have two, whereas others may present with only a persistent fissure (Fig. 18.1) [25].

18.9 Grading of Anal Fissures

Grading of anal fissures is shown in Fig. 18.1a–e.
Grade 1: Superficial linear tear
Grade 2: A deep linear tear with a small sentinel pile
Grade 3: Deep linear tear with fibrosed margin and sentinel pile
Grade 4: A wide tear with visible fibers of the internal anal sphincter and sentinel pile
Grade 5: A wide pear-shaped tear with visible fibers of the internal anal sphincter with hypertrophic anal papillae with sentinel piles

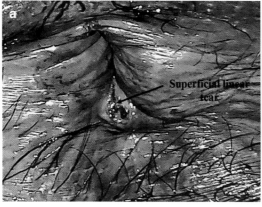
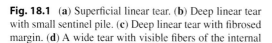
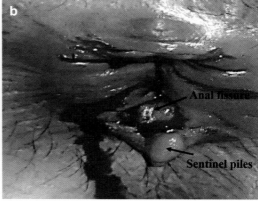

Fig. 18.1 (**a**) Superficial linear tear. (**b**) Deep linear tear with small sentinel pile. (**c**) Deep linear tear with fibrosed margin. (**d**) A wide tear with visible fibers of the internal anal sphincter. (**e**) A wide pear-shaped tear with visible fibers of the internal anal sphincter with hypertrophic anal papillae with sentinel piles

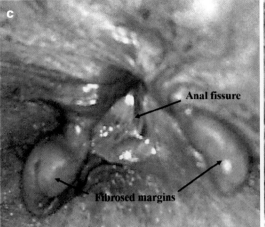

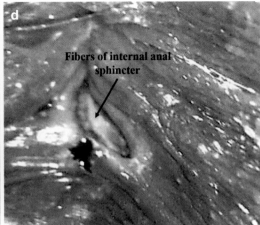

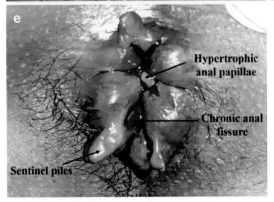

Fig. 18.1 (continued)

18.10 Location of Anal Fissure

The anal fissure may be located at

- Midline posterior—approximately in 70% (Fig. 18.2a)
- Midline anterior—25% in women and 8% in men (Fig. 18.2b)
- Both anterior and posterior—3% [26, 27] (Fig. 18.2c)

Fissures that are located laterally [22] may indicate an underlying etiology of:

- Ulcerative colitis
- Crohn's illness
- HIV and syphilis
- Tuberculosis
- Malignancy
- Leukemia

The anal fissure is located distal to the dentate line. Most anal fissures occur at the posterior or anterior midline, the posterior midline being most common [8]. The reason may be attributed to the fact that:

- The posterior commissure has a lesser blood flow than the rest of the anal canal [28].
- The external sphincter is elliptical in arrangement posteriorly, which causes less support to the anal canal [2].

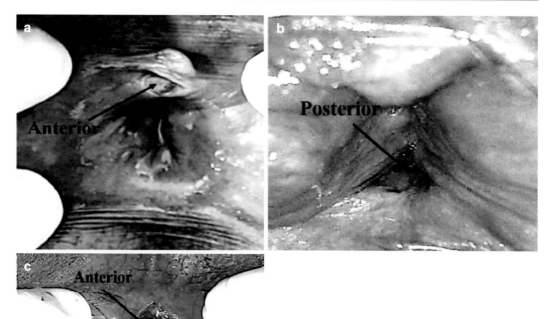

Fig. 18.2 (**a**) Anterior fissure. (**b**) Posterior fissure. (**c**) Presence of both anterior and posterior fissure

- The anal canal perfusion is inversely proportional to sphincter spasm or increased anal tone [2]. More the sphincter spasm, less is the perfusion.

18.11 Anatomical Considerations: Why Anal Fissures Are Painful?

The intermediate zone between the dentate line and mucocutaneous junction is innervated by the pudendal nerve, rendering fissures painful. Due to internal anal sphincter spasm, there is present increased anal tone leading to painful defecation.

The anal papillae may become hypertrophic due to constant irritation [29].

18.12 Why Does a Sentinel Pile Form in an Anal Fissure?

Sentinel means "to guard." When a fissure is formed, it causes inflammation and pain. As a response to the inflammation, reactive stromal hyperplasia may form at the proximal end of the lesion [30]. This is histologically identical to a fibroepithelial polyp. If healing does not occur across the defect produced by the fissure, the body attempts to heal it through the overgrowth of the proximal and distal ends of the defect, leading to "Sentinel piles" or "Sentinel tags."

18.13   Clinical Evaluation of Anal Fissure

The patient is often constipated. Sometimes the patient may complain of an irreducible mass outside the anal region that may often be confused with hemorrhoids.

18.13.1   History

- Anal fissures cause moderate to severe pain in the anal area. The pain starts during defecation and continues for hours. It is sharp cutting in nature.
- Due to the trauma caused by hard stool, painful bleeding is usually present. The blood is bright red and in the form of a streak.
- Chronic anal fissures are not always associated with bleeding.

18.13.2   Physical Examination

The patient is placed in the left lateral position. The buttocks are pulled apart gently. Due to pain, the patient may resist examination.

18.13.3   Inspection

- A longitudinal superficial tear is seen extending up to the dentate line.
- It may or may not be associated with bleeding.
- There may be tenderness at the fissure site.
- The tear in a chronic fissure can be deep enough to expose the internal anal sphincter's muscular fibers.
- Sentinel piles may be seen at the distal end of the fissure.

18.13.4   Palpation

- Presence of sentinel tags
- Induration, and fibrosis in chronic wounds
- Hypertrophic anal papillae
- Visible internal sphincter fibers

18.13.5   Digital Rectal Examination (DRE)

In acute fissure, the anal tone is increased due to spasm. It is mandatory to perform a thorough rectal examination to assess the exact etiology of anal fissures. It may be painful to examine the patient. The patient may have a vasovagal attack if a forceful insertion of the finger is attempted. In such cases, 5% Lidocaine jelly can be inserted in the anal canal with a nozzle or a Foley catheter and left for 15 to 20 min. The patient can be taken for DRE after that. Still, if the examination is painful, conservative management with calcium channel blockers, laxatives, and a sitz bath can be started. The patient can be called after 5 days for DRE and proctoscopy.

18.13.6   Proctoscopy

Proctoscopy is a must to rule out other associated anorectal disorders. It may not be possible to do it initially as the patient has severe pain.

18.14   Role of Anal Manometry in the Diagnosis of Anal Fissure

Anal manometry is employed to measure the resting anal pressure. Anal fissure patients have a higher resting pressure [31].

- Normal resting anal pressure 40–60 mmHg [32]
- Increased anal tone >80 mmHg
- Decreased anal pressure <40 mmHg [32]

18.15 Differential Diagnosis of Anal Fissure

- Thrombosed external hemorrhoids
- Perianal abscess
- Perianal ulceration in inflammatory bowel disease, tuberculosis, and sexually transmitted diseases

18.16 Complications of Anal Fissure

If left untreated, the fissure may cause:

- Pain
- Infection
- Bleeding
- Fistula formation

The anal glands at the fissure site may get infected, forming an intersphincteric fistula (Fig. 18.3a). The margins of the sentinel piles sometimes heal from the sides with an unhealed fissure underneath, forming a subcutaneous fistula (Fig. 18.3b).

18.17 Why Is an Anal Fissure Described as an Ischemic Ulcer?

A chronic fissure is a type of ischemic ulcer [33]. Due to the internal anal sphincter spasm, the patients with anal fissures have an increased anal tone leading to increased resting anal canal pressure [33]. Hence, blood vessels feeding the distal anal mucosa are compressed, resulting in chronic anal fissure. The posterior commissure is less profused and further responsible for ischemia.

18.18 Management of Anal Fissures

The management of fissure include

- Dietary modifications
- Sitz bath
- Medical management
- Surgical management

18.18.1 Dietary Modification

The patient is advised to increase dietary fiber and fluid intake to keep the stool soft. The recommended dose of fiber intake is about 38 g in men and 28 g in women. The water intake should be 2 to 3 L/day. Strong recommendations are based on moderate-quality evidence, 1B [34].

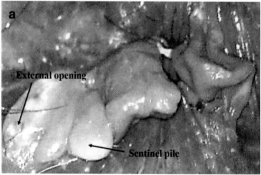
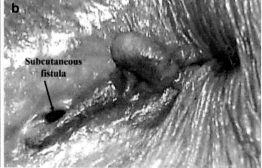

Fig. 18.3 (**a**) Chronic fissure-in-ano with intersphincteric fistula. (**b**) Subcutaneous fistula formation

18.18.2   Sitz Bath

A Sitz bath reduces the sphincter spasm and increases the blood flow, leading to pain relief. This is more effective than topical anesthetics and topical hydrocortisone [34].

18.18.3   Medical Management

Medical management includes the use of laxatives and topical agents. The osmotic laxatives are used as they soften the stools. The most typical used laxatives include lactulose and polyethylene glycol. The common topical ointments used are nitroglycerine (GTN) and calcium channel blockers (diltiazem, nifedipine). Botulinum toxin can also be used in the management of fissures.

18.18.3.1   Laxatives

Constipation is one of the most common causes of anal fissure. If dietary changes do not help relieve constipation, laxatives are used. Commonly used laxatives are osmotic. Bulk-forming laxatives should be avoided.

Mechanism of Action of Laxatives
Bulk-Forming Laxatives These types of laxatives help keep fluid in the stool and enhance the weight and consistency of the stool [35, 36]. If used in anal fissures, they will further aggravate the pain. Examples are psyllium and methylcellulose.

Osmotic Agents These agents draw water into the stool, making stools soft for easy evacuation. Lactulose, milk of magnesia, polyethylene glycol (PEG), and sorbitol [35, 36] are few examples.

18.18.3.2   Topical Agents and Their Mechanism of Action

Topical agents act as a chemical sphincterotomy [37]. They cause a reduction in the internal sphincter spasm, leading to decreased anal tone and promoting healing [37–39].

Nitroglycerine (GTN)
The neurotransmitter nitroglycerine relaxes the internal anal sphincter [40]. It provides abundant nitrous oxide in the muscle tissue leading to the healing of anal fissures [38]. Studies have reported that 40% of the patients suffer from headaches when they use GTN. The headaches sometimes are so severe that patients discontinue their use [39]. Another drawback is a significantly higher recurrence rate than observed with surgical treatment [41].

Calcium Channel Blockers
They act by decreasing the intracellular availability of calcium [42]. The topical nifedipine reduces anal sphincter tone, which helps in promoting blood flow and faster healing. Nifedipine combined with 2% lidocaine jelly produces a dual effect as lidocaine causes numbness of the area but does not heal the fissure. Diltiazem promotes muscular sphincter relaxation by inhibiting calcium channels in smooth muscles [8]. According to studies, topical nifedipine has a greater healing rate than diltiazem [43].

18.18.3.3   Botulinum Toxin (Botox)

Clostridium botulinum generates botulinum toxin type A, which works by preventing acetylcholine from being released at the neuromuscular junction [44]. It blocks sympathetic nerve function and the myogenic tone of the internal anal sphincter. Hence, it helps in reducing the sphincter's increased tone and increasing the local tissue perfusion leading to healing of the chronic anal fissure [45]. It can cause local paralysis, lasting for months [45, 46]. Botox has a similar action as that of lateral sphincterotomy [47]. Botulinum toxin injection is linked with greater healing rates when compared to other topical treatments. As per the practice parameters of "The American Society of Colon and

Rectal Surgeons," the evidence is 1C (Strong recommendation based on low- to very-low quality) [48].

Technique
The patient is positioned in the left lateral or lithotomy position. An insulin syringe with a needle is used for injecting. The injection is given into the internal anal sphincter at 5 and 7 o'clock on both sides of the fissure [45]. The total dose given is 30–40 units.

Results
Radwan et al. found an 89% success rate in their trial [45]. Botulinum toxin should be considered a minimally invasive procedure for anal fissure, according to a comprehensive review by Yiannakopoulou [49].

Complications
- Heart block
- Skin allergic reactions
- Increased urinary residual volume
- Postural hypotension
- Tachycardia
- Muscle weakness [50]
- Temporary incontinence in 18%
- Perianal hematomas in 20% [2]

18.18.4   Surgical Management

Any fissure that fails to respond to conservative management is an indication of surgical intervention. Surgical management aims to reduce anal spasms and hence increases the blood flow.

Indications
- Chronic anal fissure
- Lack of response to medical management
- An increase in anal tone associated with fissures
- Fissure associated with underlying fistula
- Presence of persistent pain, bleeding
- Relapsing or refractory fissures

Contraindications
- Fecal incontinence, which might become worse following surgery

- Elderly patients with laxed anal tone (weaker sphincter complex)
- Multiparous women

Techniques of Surgical Management
- Anal dilatation
- Fissurectomy
- Lateral internal sphincterotomy
- Advancement flap (Anoplasty)

18.18.4.1   Anal Dilatation
Stretching of the anal canal was the first treatment proposed for anal fissures. However, this procedure is obsolete because of a high incontinence rate [51].

18.18.4.2   Fissurectomy
Fissurectomy is another technique practiced by surgeons to treat chronic anal fissures.

Principle
It aims to successfully "freshen" the fissure margins and convert a chronic fissure into an acute one [52].

Indications
Patients who are at risk of incontinence like:

- Elderly patients with laxed anal tone
- Multiparous female patients
- Refractory fissure

Technique
The fissure is excised using a scalpel or scissors. Hence, an acute wound is created without scar tissue and is left to heal by secondary intention [52].

Nowadays, this technique is not commonly practiced. The results of fissurectomy are shown in Table 18.2.

Table 18.2   Results of fissurectomy

Journal	Incontinence
Bara, B. K [53] Cureus	Flatus—40%
	Liquid—32.5%
Kongressbd Dtsch Ges Chir Konge J Meier Zu Eissen [54]	Fecal spotting in 3.1%

Complications of Fissurectomy
- Keyhole deformity due to continuous see page of the fecal matter [55]
- Transient incontinence

18.18.4.3 Lateral Internal Sphincterotomy
It is deemed the gold standard [56].

Principle
Sphincter tone is minimized by dividing the internal anal sphincter. There are two techniques to execute a lateral internal sphincterotomy:

- Open method
- Closed method

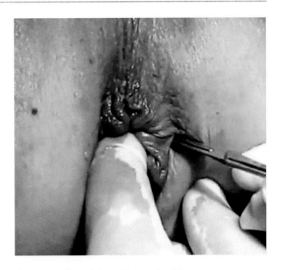

Fig. 18.4 Closed lateral internal sphincterotomy

Open Lateral Internal Sphincterotomy
Between the index finger and the thumb, the intersphincteric groove is palpated. A lateral incision through the anoderm is made across the intersphincteric groove at 3 o'clock. The internal anal sphincter muscle fibers are identified. The internal anal sphincter is divided up to the dentate line with electrocautery or scissors. If the division is made using a sharp instrument, adequate hemostasis must be maintained. The anoderm is left open to heal by secondary intention [2].

Closed Lateral Internal Sphincterotomy (CLIS)
It was first introduced by Notaras in 1969 and was named "lateral subcutaneous sphincterotomy" [56].

The intersphincteric groove is palpated at the left lateral position. A finger is placed in the anal canal, and a surgical scalpel with 15 no. blade is inserted into the intersphincteric plane. The blade is then rotated medially, and the internal sphincter fibers are divided in a sawtooth manner up to the dentate line. The small wound, approximately 3 to 4 mm, is left open to heal by secondary intention (Fig. 18.4) [2, 57, 58].

The internal sphincter is divided up to the dentate line in both open and closed procedures minimizing the resting pressure without affecting the physiology of the anal canal. A small wound is created with the closed approach, but both techniques are equally effective.

18.18.4.4 Advancement Flap (Anoplasty)
Anoplasty is a procedure that involves curettage of the fissure followed by placement of a flap [59].

Indications
Chronic anal fissure with lax anal tone in multiparous women and elderly patients.

Technique
Anoplasty is performed by elevating a 1 cm thick subcutaneous cellular tissue and local skin flap [59]. The flap is sutured to the rectal mucosa covering the fissure [59]. The procedure is similar to the flap technique raised to cover the internal opening discussed under sphincter-saving techniques.

Advantages
- Wound healing is quicker [59].
- Reduction in risk of anal stenosis.

Complications
- Dehiscence
- Necrosis
- Infection

The results of the anal advancement flap are mentioned in Table 18.3.

However, many surgeons have combined techniques or modified anoplasty to enhance effectiveness [61].

Table 18.3 Results of advancement flap

Journal	Author	The outcome of the study
Cirugía Española (English Edition) 2018 [59]	Giordano et al. and Chambers et al.	98% cure rate
		0–3.3% risk of incontinence
		5.9% dehiscence
Zhong Xi Yi Jie He Xue Bao RCT 2011 [60]	Zhen-Yi—Wang	Faster wound healing
		Relief in wound pain

18.19 Laser Lateral Internal Sphincterotomy

Lateral internal sphincterotomy with laser can be performed either by open or closed technique. The principle and the basic technique remains the same as in open or closed lateral internal sphincterotomy. The only difference is that instead of scissors or cautery, a laser fiber is used for sphincter division. The cutting by laser is precise and immediate hemostasis is achieved.

Type of Fiber: Bare

Dose: 10 W continuous mode

Technique

The intersphincteric groove is palpated. In an open technique, an incision using bare laser fiber is made over the intersphincteric groove at the 3 o'clock position through the anoderm (Fig. 18.5a). The fibers of

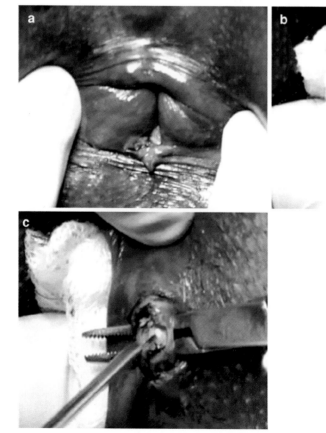

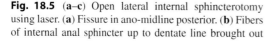

Fig. 18.5 (**a–c**) Open lateral internal sphincterotomy using laser. (**a**) Fissure in ano-midline posterior. (**b**) Fibers of internal anal sphincter up to dentate line brought out through the intersphincteric groove at 3 o'clock position. (**c**) Cutting of sphincter fibers with a bare fiber

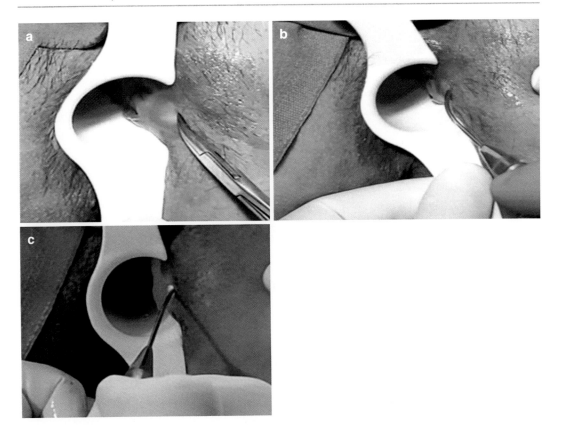

Fig. 18.6 (**a–c**) Closed lateral internal sphincterotomy using laser. (**a**) Identification of intersphincteric groove. (**b**) Insertion of bare fiber through the groove. (**c**) Cutting of fibers of internal anal sphincter up to dentate line

the internal anal sphincter up to the dentate line are brought out of the small incision of around 4 mm using a fine artery forceps (Fig. 18.5b). The sphincter fibers are divided using bare laser fiber (Fig. 18.5c). The fissure's base is then curetted. The anoderm is left open to heal by secondary intention. Alternatively, the bare fiber can be introduced through the intersphincteric groove and rotated medially to cut the fibers of the internal anal sphincter, just like in closed internal sphincterotomy (Fig. 18.6a–c). However, the chances of partial sphincterotomy are pretty high in a closed procedure using laser.

Advantages of Using Lasers
- Bloodless field.
- No lateral spread of current as seen with electrocautery.
- No chances of partial sphincterotomy if the procedure is performed under vision.

18.20 How Much Sphincter Should Be Divided?

According to studies, in females, dividing the internal sphincter up to 1 cm or less than 25% is safe while doing lateral internal sphincterotomy [57]. Many surgeons feel that the internal sphincterotomy should be done as follows:

- If there is a marked spasm or hypertonia, cut the sphincter up to the dentate line.
- In case there is a mild spasm, cut the sphincter up to the length of the fissure.

However, according to "American Society of Colon and Rectal Surgeons practice parameters," the lateral internal sphincterotomy should always be performed up to the dentate line, irrespective of the length of the fissure [34].

- If the anal tone is normal, sphincterotomy should never be performed. The treatment of choice is the anal advancement flap.

18.21   Why Should Posterior Sphincterotomy Not Be Done?

The complications associated with posterior sphincterotomy are

- **Incontinence**

  According to a study conducted by Poisson in 1977 [62] and Orsay et al. in 2004 [63], incontinence is worse following posterior sphincterotomy. Anatomically, a weak triangular region of loose tissue between the internal and external sphincters can cause anal incontinence.
- **Delayed wound healing and keyhole deformity**

  Because the posterior commissure is less profuse, the wound healing may take 3 to 4 weeks. Delayed wound healing may also be because of seepage of the liquid part of fecal matter from the posterior sphincterotomy site. Moreover, once the healing occurs, it may lead to keyhole deformity.

18.22   Results of Closed Versus Open Lateral Internal Sphincterotomy

- In a study comparing open versus closed lateral internal sphincterotomy, Gupta et al. discovered that 4.4% of open lateral sphincterotomy patients had delayed postoperative recovery. The closed method resulted in a lower mean pain score and a short stay in the hospital [58].
- M Wiley et al. reported that the pain score did not vary significantly between closed and open internal sphincterotomy. The success rate was 96% [64].
- In a study by El Sanabani et al. on open versus closed, 6% of patients in a closed technique developed low perianal fistula. The open

group had a recurrence rate of 0.015%, whereas the closed group had 1.9% [65].
- A study by Hareesh Mahabala Mukri et al. reported significantly less bleeding, constipation, and postoperative pain in the patients who underwent closed lateral sphincterotomy [66].

Some Interesting Facts About Sphincterotomy

- Miles, in 1919 treated fissures by "pectenotomy," which was a division of the pecten band area between the dentate line and white line of Hilton [67].
- Morgan and Milligan (1934) and Gabriel (1948) treated fissures by excising anal fissures and dividing the spastic, subcutaneous part of the external sphincter [68].
- Later, Eisenhammer in 1951 and Goligher in 1955 stated that the fibrous band was the spastic lower margin of the internal sphincter and was wrongly identified as the inferior verge of the external sphincter [67–69].

The credit for treating anal fissures by internal sphincterotomy goes to Eisenhammer [70]. The lower half of the internal sphincter was incised in the posterior midline of the anal canal, across the fissure. The wound was left to heal by secondary intention. However, this technique was associated with side effects; cutting of the sphincter posteriorly caused seepage of the liquid part of stool leading to keyhole deformity, and secondly, it was associated with a high incidence of incontinence. Later, in 1955, Goligher proposed lateral internal sphincterotomy as a therapeutic option for anal fissures [67, 68].

Today's technique of lateral internal sphincterotomy is a combination of Eisenhammer and Goligher procedures, i.e., dividing the internal anal sphincter, laterally.

18.23 Anal Fissure in Crohn's Disease

Multiple fissures, asymptomatic fissures, and nonhealing fissures should raise the suspicion of Crohn's disease. Skin tags that are large, edematous, and painful are prevalent [71]. The commonest presentations [72] are:

- Low anal fistula (26.7%)
- Anal fissure (27.6%)
- Perianal abscess (29.5%)

18.23.1 Management

Surgery is contraindicated as it may lead to postoperative incontinence and nonhealing wounds. Patients should be treated conservatively.

18.24 Management of Anal Fissure in HIV

The mainstay of treatment is the control of CD4 count [73]. Lateral internal sphincterotomy results are approximately 92%.

18.25 A Word About Relapsing and Refractory Fissures

Failure of medical management is the most typical problem one can encounter while treating anal fissures conservatively. The word relapsing fissure means recurrence after a certain period of disease management, and refractory means that the fissure has stopped responding to the treatment. In cases of recurrence following topical ointments or Botox, LIS is the preferred alternative. If the patient has a relapsing fissure following lateral internal sphincterotomy at 3 o'clock, a counter sphincterotomy can be performed at 9 o'clock. In female patients, one should proceed with caution while undergoing an internal sphincterotomy due to the shorter length of the anal canal.

18.26 Discussion

It is widely accepted that lateral internal sphincterotomy is the best modality for treating anal fissures. The mainstay of anal fissure is less blood supply in the posterior commissure. As a result, an ischemic ulcer is formed, which does not heal. Medical management with laxatives and topical applications using GTN or calcium channel blockers is effective. Most of the fissures heal within 6 weeks. However, the fissures may relapse.

Eisenhammer initially recommended internal anal sphincterotomy in 1951 for anal fissure treatment [66]. Later in 1959, he recommended that the extent of the sphincterotomy should be limited to the dentate line. This was based on his observation that a fissure was formed at the internal sphincter base instead of the subcutaneous part of the external anal sphincter [74]. This formed the basis of the currently followed technique.

Internal sphincterotomy, if performed posteriorly, causes keyhole deformity, and the wound healing is delayed due to the seepage of the stool. Hence, the most preferred treatment is a lateral internal anal sphincterotomy [55].

Anal fissures are associated with internal anal sphincter spasm. The lateral internal sphincterotomy reduces the spasm with relatively minor complications. Although the recurrence rate is less with this procedure, a mild incidence of incontinence can be there (Table 18.4) [75]. It is vital to remember that lateral internal sphincterotomy incontinence is transient, with permanent disability in less than 1% of the patients [75]. Performing transanal electrostimulation of the internal anal sphincter may reduce incontinence [76]. As a treatment for chronic incontinence, injecting bulking substances into the internal sphincter may be an option (Solesta, PTQ, GateKeeper, Durasphere, or Coaptite) [77].

The early studies report laser lateral internal sphincterotomy to be less painful than open. Table 18.5 summarizes the "American Society of Colon and Rectal Surgeons" recommendations for anal fissure treatment.

Table 18.4 Incidence of anal incontinence after lateral internal sphincterotomy

Journal	Author	Incontinence
Dis Colon Rectum 1999 [78]	D.C Nyman	Flatus 6%
		Fecal soiling 8%
		Loss of solid stool!%
		Incontinence 3%
Disease of the Colon and Rectum [79] 2004	Hyman	Incontinence 8%
Dis Colon Rectum 2005 [80]	Sergio Casillas	Temporary incontinence-31%
		Persistent incontinence 30%
European Surgical Research 2011 [81]	Kement et al.	Incontinence 11.7%
Asian Journal of Surgery 2019 [82]	Turan Acar et al.	Incontinence 1.9%
Asian Journal of Surgery 2022 [83]	Marie Shella De Robes	Liquid incontinence 2%
		Gas incontinence 3%
		Solid incontinence 1%

Table 18.5 Practice parameters of The American Society of Colon and Rectal Surgeons

Procedure	Recommendations
Lifestyle modification and dietary changes in acute anal fissures: Laxatives, high-fiber diet, sitz bath [48, 60]	1B—strongly recommended evidence-based on moderate quality
Topical nitrates	1A—strongly recommended evidence-based on high quality
Calcium channel blockers	1A—strongly recommended evidence-based on high quality
Botulinum toxin	1C—strongly recommended evidence-based on low and very low-quality
Lateral internal sphincterotomy	1A—strongly recommended evidence-based on high quality

18.27 Case Presentation

Mr. B, 52, a male patient, presented with pain during defecation and pus discharge from the anal area. To start with, the patient had only pain during defecation. He was diagnosed to be a case of fissure in ano and treated conservatively by one of my colleagues. Later, the pus started coming out from the fissure site, and a diagnosis of acute fissure in ano with suppuration was made. The conservative management was continued, but the patient had no relief. After a month-long treatment, he came to me for consultation as the pain worsened. Local examination revealed a chronic fissure with a small perianal abscess at 6 o'clock. On digital rectal examination, there was noticeable discomfort at 6 o'clock, and pus could be seen oozing out when the finger was inserted. It was a case of fissure in the ano (midline posterior) with a small perianal abscess and a communicating low intersphincteric fistula. Proctoscopy was not significant. The MRI revealed a fistulous tract with an internal opening at 6–7 o'clock. The patient was taken for surgery. To my surprise, when methylene blue and hydrogen peroxide were injected through the abscess, the dye could be seen coming out of the two internal openings, one below the dentate line and the other at the dentate line. As the patient had a fissure with a small perianal collection and a communicating low intersphincteric fistula, a fistulectomy was done, with excision of the fissure and the abscess (Fig. 18.7a–f). Marsupialization of the margins of the fistulectomy wound was done.

18.27.1 Opinion

The patient's presenting complaints were pain during defecation which was due to an anal fissure. A thorough examination revealed perianal collection with communicating intersphincteric fistula. As already mentioned, the anal gland lying below the fissure can become infected, leading to a fistula. Moreover, it is known that sphincterotomy at 6 o'clock can lead to a keyhole deformity. However, in this case, there was no option except to do a low-end fistulectomy at the 6 o'clock position due to the presence of both fistula and fissure.

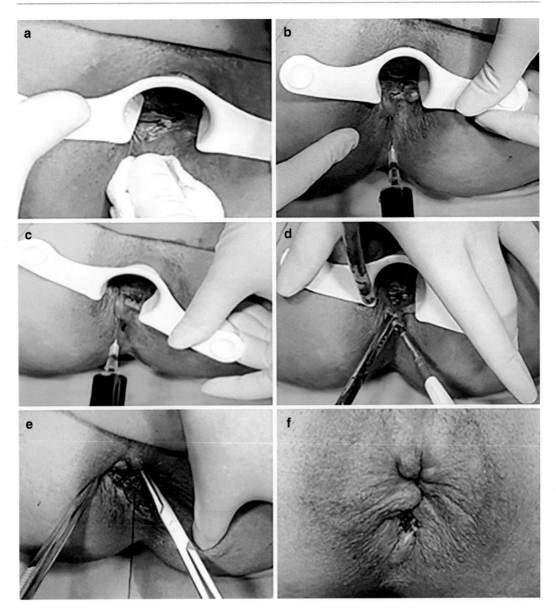

Fig. 18.7 (a) Presence of a small perianal abscess with fissure in ano at 6 o'clock. (b, c) Injecting methylene blue through the abscess. Two openings are seen, one below the dentate line and the other at the dentate line. (d) Fistulectomy being done with excision of fissure and the abscess. (e) Marsupialization of the margins of the fistulectomy wound. (f) Final image at the end of the surgical procedure

18.28 Your Query, My Answer

1. **Why is a lateral internal sphincterotomy advised instead of a fissurectomy in the anal fissure with increased anal tone?**

    As mentioned in the text, a fissurectomy is associated with a keyhole deformity. Moreover, there is loose areolar tissue in the midline posteriorly between the internal and external sphincters, and mild anal incontinence may occur after fissurectomy and sphincterotomy if done posteriorly. Please remember that a few authors have observed that even after lateral internal sphincterotomy, there can be anal incontinence.

Take-Home Message

In acute anal fissures, the typical presentation is painful bleeding. Anal fissures are usually managed with medical treatment. Individuals with recurring anal fissures or who do not respond to medication should be subjected to surgery. The lateral internal sphincterotomy is deemed the gold standard in surgical management of anal fissures. Nowadays, anal dilatation has no role. Adopting the closed or open method is the surgeon's choice. The posterior sphincterotomy should be avoided. The use of laser in sphincterotomy provides good hemostasis and less postoperative pain.

References

1. Abcarian H, Lakshmanan S, Read DR, Roccaforte P. The role of the internal sphincter in chronic anal fissures. Dis Colon Rectum. 1982;25(6):525–8. https://doi.org/10.1007/BF02564159.
2. Beaty JS, Shashidharan M. Anal fissure. Clin Colon Rectal Surg. 2016;29(1):30–7. https://doi.org/10.1055/s-0035-1570390.
3. McNamara MJ, Percy JP, Fielding IR. A manometric study of anal fissure treated by subcutaneous lateral internal sphincterotomy. Ann Surg. 1990;211(2):235–8. https://doi.org/10.1097/00000658-199002000-00017.
4. Wienert V, Raulf F, Mlitz H. Historical aspects of anal fissure pathology. In: Anal fissure. Cham: Springer; 2017. p. 91–8.
5. Popat A, Pandey CP, Agarwal K, Srivastava VP, Sharma SM, Dixit A. A comparative study of the role of topical diltiazem 2% organic gel and lateral internal sphincterotomy for the management of chronic fissure in ano. Int J Contemporary Med Res. 2016;3(5):1363–5.
6. Chaudhary R, Dausage CS. Prevalence of anal fissure in patients with anorectal disorders: a single-centre experience. J Clin Diagn Res. 2019;13(2):PC05–7.
7. Mapel DW, Schum M, Von Worley A. The epidemiology and treatment of anal fissures in a population-based cohort. BMC Gastroenterol. 2014;14(1):1–7.
8. Zaghiyan KN, Fleshner P. Anal fissure. Clin Colon Rectal Surg. 2011;24(1):22–30. https://doi.org/10.1055/s-0031-1272820.
9. Barton J. Nitroglycerin and Lidocaine topical treatment for anal fissure. RxTriad. 2002;5(4):1–2.
10. Lund JN, Scholefield JH. Etiology and treatment of anal fissure. Br J Surg. 1996;83:1335–44. https://doi.org/10.1002/BJS.1800831006.
11. Delley LA. Die Fissura ani und ihre rationelle Behandlung [dissertation]. Bern: Universität Bern; 1855.
12. Rick J. Fissura ani [dissertation]. Bonn: Universität Bonn; 1922.
13. Willemsen C. Ursachen von Analfissuren [dissertation]. Düsseldorf: Universität Düsseldorf; 1963.
14. Elía Guedea M, Gracia Solanas JA, Royo Dachary P, Ramírez Rodríguez JM, Aguilella Diago V, Martínez DM. Prevalence of anal diseases after Scopinaro's biliopancreatic bypass for super-obese patients. Cir Esp. 2008;84:132–7.
15. Garg P. Water stream in a bidet-toilet as a cause of anterior fissure-in-ano: a preliminary report. Color Dis. 2010;128:601–2.
16. Madalinski MH. Identifying the best therapy for chronic anal fissure. World J Gastrointest Pharmacol Ther. 2011;2(2):9–16. https://doi.org/10.4292/wjgpt.v2.i2.9.
17. Goligher J. Surgery of anus, rectum, and colon. London: Baillière Tindall; 1975.
18. Lockhart-Mummery JP. Diseases of the rectum and colon and their surgical treatment. London: Baillere; 1934.
19. Klosterhalfen B, Vogel P, Rixen H, Mittermayer C. Topography of the inferior rectal artery: a possible cause of chronic, primary anal fissure. Dis Colon Rectum. 1989;32(1):43–52.
20. Schouten WR, Briel JW, Auwerda JJ. Relationship between anal pressure and anodermal blood flow. The vascular pathogenesis of anal fissures. Dis Colon Rectum. 1994;37:664–9.
21. Schouten WR, Briel JW, Auwerda JJ, De Graaf EJ. Ischaemic nature of anal fissure. Br J Surg. 1996;83:63–5.
22. Jahnny B, Ashurst JV. Anal fissures. In: StatPearls. Treasure Island, FL: StatPearls Publishing; 2020.
23. Choi YS, Kim DS, Lee DH, Lee JB, Lee EJ, Lee SD, Song KH, Jung HJ. Clinical characteristics and incidence of perianal diseases in patients with ulcerative colitis. Ann Coloproctol. 2018;34(3):138–43.
24. Nelson RL. Anal fissure (chronic). BMJ Clin Evid. 2014;2014:0407.
25. Arslan K, Erenoğlu B, Doğru O, Kökçam S, Turan E, Atay A. Effect of chronic anal fissure components on isosorbide dinitrate treatment. World J Surg. 2012;36(9):2225–9. https://doi.org/10.1007/s00268-012-1604-2.
26. Gordon PH, Nivatvongs S. Principles and practice of surgery for the colon, rectum, and anus. 2nd ed. St. Louis, MO: Quality Medical Publishing, Inc.; 1999.
27. Ricciardi R, Dykes SL, Madoff RD. Anal fissure. In: Beck DE, et al., editors. The ASCRS manual of colon and rectal surgery. New York: Springer; 2014. p. 235–44. https://doi.org/10.1007/978-1-4614-8450-9_12.
28. Schouten WR, Briel JW, Auwerda JJ, Boerma MO. Anal fissure: new concepts in pathogenesis and treatment. Scand J Gastroenterol Suppl. 1996;218:78–81. https://doi.org/10.3109/00365529609094734.

29. Gupta PJ. Hypertrophied anal papillae and fibrous anal polyps, should they be removed during anal fissure surgery? World J Gastroenterol. 2004;10(16):2412–4. https://doi.org/10.3748/wjg.v10.i16.2412.

30. Yang E, Palefsky JM. Diseases of the anus. In: Crum CP, Lee KR, Nucci MR, Granter SR, Howitt BE, Parast MM, Boyd T, Peters III WA, editors. Diagnostic gynecologic and obstetric pathology. Philadelphia, PA: Elsevier; 2018. p. 224–57.

31. Parker SC, Madoff RD. Diagnosis and management of fecal incontinence. In: Yeo CJ, editor. Shackelford's surgery of the alimentary tract. 7th ed. Philadelphia, PA: Elsevier; 2013.

32. Lee JT, Vogler SA, Madoff RD. Diagnosis and management of fecal incontinence. In: Yeo CJ, editor. Shackelford's surgery of the alimentary tract, 2 volume set. 8th ed. Philadelphia, PA: Elsevier; 2019. p. 1721–32.

33. Madalinski M, Chodorowski Z. Why the most potent toxin may heal anal fissure. Adv Ther. 2006;23(4):627–34. https://doi.org/10.1007/BF02850051.

34. Stewart DB Sr, Gaertner W, Glasgow S, Migaly J, Feingold D, Steele SR. Clinical practice guideline for the management of anal fissures. Dis Colon Rectum. 2017;60(1):7–14.

35. Liu LW. Chronic constipation: current treatment options. Can J Gastroenterol. 2011;25(Suppl B):22B–8B.

36. Bashir A, Sizar O. Laxatives. In: StatPearls. Treasure Island, FL: StatPearls Publishing; 2020.

37. Haq Z, Rahman M, Chowdhury RA, Baten MA, Khatun M. Chemical sphincterotomy—first line of treatment for chronic anal fissure. Mymensingh Med J. 2005;14(1):88–90.

38. Mustafa NA, Cengiz S, Türkyilmaz S, Yücel Y. Comparison of topical glyceryl trinitrate ointment and oral nifedipine in the treatment of chronic anal fissure. Acta Chir Belg. 2006;106(1):55–8. https://doi.org/10.1080/00015458.2006.11679834.

39. Scholefield JH, Bock JU, Marla B, Richter HJ, Athanasiadis S, Pröls M, et al. A dose-finding study with 0.1%, 0.2%, and 0.4% glyceryl trinitrate ointment in patients with chronic anal fissures. Gut. 2003;52(2):264–9.

40. Bacher H, Mischinger HJ, Werkgartner G, Cerwenka H, El-Shabrawi A, Pfeifer J, Schweiger W. Local nitroglycerin for treatment of anal fissures: an alternative to lateral sphincterotomy? Dis Colon Rectum. 1997;40(7):840–5. https://doi.org/10.1007/BF02055444.

41. Carapeti EA, Kamm MA, McDonald PJ, Chadwick SJ, Melville D, Phillips RK. Randomised controlled trial shows that glyceryl trinitrate heals anal fissures, higher doses are not more effective, and there is a high recurrence rate. Gut. 1999;44(5):727–30. https://doi.org/10.1136/gut.44.5.727.

42. Cook TA, Brading AF, Mortensen NJ. Differences in contractile properties of anorectal smooth muscle and the effects of calcium channel blockade. Br J Surg. 1999;86(1):70–5.

43. Jabbar L. The comparative study between the topical preparations of diltiazem versus the nifedipine in treatment of anal fissure. J Int Pharm Res. 2018;45(1):21–4.

44. Nigam PK, Nigam A. Botulinum toxin. Indian J Dermatol. 2010;55(1):8–14. https://doi.org/10.4103/0019-5154.60343.

45. Radwan MM, Ramdan K, Abu-Azab I, Abu-Zidan FM. Botulinum toxin treatment for anal fissure. Afr Health Sci. 2007;7(1):14–7. https://doi.org/10.5555/afhs.2007.7.1.14.

46. Brin MF. Botulinum toxin: chemistry, pharmacology, toxicity, and immunology. Muscle Nerve Suppl. 1997;6:S146–68.

47. Sajid MS, Vijaynagar B, Desai M, Cheek E, Baig MK. Botulinum toxin vs glyceryl trinitrate for the medical management of chronic anal fissure: a meta-analysis. Color Dis. 2008;10:541–6.

48. Rosen L, Abel ME, Gordon PH, Denstman FJ, Fleshman JW, Hicks TC, Huber PJ, Kennedy HL, Levin SE, Nicholson JD, et al. Practice parameters for the management of anal fissure. The Standards Task Force American Society of Colon and Rectal Surgeons. Dis Colon Rectum. 1992;35(2):206–8. https://doi.org/10.1007/BF02050683.

49. Yiannakopoulou E. Botulinum toxin and anal fissure: efficacy and safety systematic review. Int J Color Dis. 2012;27(1):1–9. https://doi.org/10.1007/s00384-011-1286-5.

50. Chaptini C, Casey G, Harris AG, Wattchow D, Gordon L, Murrell DF. Botulinum toxin A injection for chronic anal fissures and anal sphincter spasm improves quality of life in recessive dystrophic epidermolysis bullosa. Int J Womens Dermatol. 2015;1(4):167–9. https://doi.org/10.1016/j.ijwd.2015.08.002.

51. Pinsk I, Czeiger D, Lichtman D, Reshef A. The long-term effect of standardized anal dilatation for chronic anal fissure on anal continence. Ann Coloproctol. 2021;37(2):115–9. https://doi.org/10.3393/ac.2020.03.16.

52. Zeitoun JD, Blanchard P, Fathallah N, Benfredj P, Lemarchand N, de Parades V. Long-term outcome of a fissurectomy: a prospective single-arm study of 50 operations out of 349 initial patients. Ann Coloproctol. 2018;34:83–7.

53. Bara BK, Mohanty SK, Behera SN, Sahoo AK, Swain SK. Fissurectomy versus lateral internal sphincterotomy in the treatment of chronic anal fissure: a randomized control trial. Cureus. 2021;13(9):e18363. https://doi.org/10.7759/cureus.18363.

54. Meier zu Eissen J. Chronische Analfissur, Therapie [Chronic anal fissure, therapy]. Kongressbd Dtsch Ges Chir Kongr. 2001;118:654–6. . German. https://doi.org/10.1007/978-3-642-56458-1_231.

55. Mazier WP. Keyhole deformity. Fact and fiction. Dis Colon Rectum. 1985;28(1):8–10. https://doi.org/10.1007/BF02553897.

56. Notaras MJ. Lateral subcutaneous sphincterotomy for anal fissure—a new technique. Proc R Soc Med. 1969;62(7):713.

57. Murad-Regadas SM, Fernandes GOS, Regadas FSP, et al. How much of the internal sphincter may be divided during lateral sphincterotomy for chronic anal fissure in women? Morphologic and functional evaluation after sphincterotomy. Dis Colon Rectum. 2013;56(5):645–51.

58. Gupta V, Rodrigues G, Prabhu R, Ravi C. Open versus closed lateral internal anal sphincterotomy in the management of chronic anal fissures: a prospective randomized study. Asian J Surg. 2014;37(4):178–83. https://doi.org/10.1016/j.asjsur.2014.01.009.

59. Giordano P, Gravante G, Grondona P, Ruggiero B, Porrett T, Lunniss PJ. Simple cutaneous advancement flap anoplasty for resistant chronic anal fissure: a prospective study. World J Surg. 2009;33(5):1058–63. https://doi.org/10.1007/s00268-009-9937-1.

60. Wang ZY, Liu H, Sun JH, Mao XM, Xu WX, Wu YG, Zhang HY, Zhu LJ, Jin W, Wu J, Li Y, Wu C, Jiang ZL, Shi L, Li Y, Dong W. Mucosa advancement flap anoplasty in treatment of chronic anal fissures: a prospective, multicenter, randomized controlled trial. Zhong Xi Yi Jie He Xue Bao. 2011;9(4):402–9. . Chinese. https://doi.org/10.3736/jcim20110409.

61. Kenefick NJ, Gee AS, Durdey P. Treatment of resistant anal fissure with advancement anoplasty. Color Dis. 2002;4(6):463–6. https://doi.org/10.1046/j.1463-1318.2002.00373.x.

62. Poisson J. Anal fissure. Can J Surg. 1977;20:417–21.

63. Orsay C, Rakinic J, Perry WB, Hyman N, Buie D, Cataldo P, Newstead G, Dunn G, Rafferty J, Ellis CN, Shellito P, Gregorcyk S, Ternent C, Kilkenny J 3rd, Tjandra J, Ko C, Whiteford M, Nelson R, Standards Practice Task Force; American Society of Colon and Rectal Surgeons. Practice parameters for the management of anal fissures (revised). Dis Colon Rectum. 2004;47(12):2003–7. https://doi.org/10.1007/s10350-004-0785-7.

64. Wiley M, Day P, Rieger N, Stephens J, Moore J. Open vs. closed lateral internal sphincterotomy for idiopathic fissure-in-ano: a prospective, randomized, controlled trial. Dis Colon Rectum. 2004;47(6):847–52. https://doi.org/10.1007/s10350-004-0530-2.

65. Al Sanabani J, Al Salami S, Al Saadi A. Closed versus open lateral internal anal sphincterotomy for chronic anal fissure in female patients. Egypt J Surg. 2014;33(3):178.

66. Mukri HM, Kapur N, Guglani V. Comparison of open versus closed lateral internal sphincterotomy in the management of chronic anal fissure. Hell J Surg. 2019;91(2):91–5.

67. Hoffmann DC, Goligher JC. Lateral subcutaneous internal sphincterotomy in the treatment of anal fissure. Br Med J. 1970;3(5724):673–5. https://doi.org/10.1136/bmj.3.5724.673.

68. Eisenhammer S. The surgical correction of chronic internal anal (sphincteric) contracture. S Afr Med J. 1951;25:486.

69. Eisenhammer S. The evaluation of the internal anal sphincterotomy operation with special reference to anal fissure. Surg Gynecol Obstet. 1959;109:583.

70. Villanueva Herrero JA, Henning W, Sharma N, Deppen JG. Internal anal sphincterotomy. In: StatPearls. Treasure Island, FL: StatPearls Publishing; 2022.

71. Safar B, Sands D. Perianal Crohn's disease. Clin Colon Rectal Surg. 2007;20(4):282–93. https://doi.org/10.1055/s-2007-991027.

72. Platell C, Mackay J, Collopy B, Fink R, Ryan P, Woods R. Anal pathology in patients with Crohn's disease. Aust N Z J Surg. 1996;66(1):5–9. https://doi.org/10.1111/j.1445-2197.1996.tb00690.x.

73. Elroy Patrick W. Human immunodeficiency virus and the anorectum. Alexandria J Med. 2013;49(2):163–7.

74. Ray JE, Penfold JCB, Gathright BJ Jr, Roberson SH. Lateral subcutaneous internal anal sphincterotomy for anal fissure. Dis Colon Rectum. 1974;17(2):139–44.

75. Verma R, Kumar S, Mishra V, Kumar N. Early outcome of internal laser sphincterotomy versus open internal sphincterotomy in the treatment of anal fissures. Indian J Appl Res. 2021;11(9):55–9. https://doi.org/10.36106/ijar/7913551.

76. Aho Fält U, Lindsten M, Strandberg S, Dahlberg M, Butt S, Nilsson E, Zawadzki A, Johnson LB. Percutaneous tibial nerve stimulation (PTNS): an alternative treatment option for chronic therapy-resistant anal fissure. Tech Coloproctol. 2019;23(4):361–5. https://doi.org/10.1007/s10151-019-01972-5.

77. Vaizey CJ, Kamm MA. Injectable bulking agents for treating fecal incontinence. Br J Surg. 2005;92(5):521–7. https://doi.org/10.1002/bjs.4997.

78. Nyam DC, Pemberton JH. Long-term results of lateral internal sphincterotomy for chronic anal fissure with particular reference to the incidence of fecal incontinence. Dis Colon Rectum. 1999;42(10):1306–10. https://doi.org/10.1007/BF02234220.

79. Hyman N. Incontinence after lateral internal sphincterotomy: a prospective study and quality of life assessment. Dis Colon Rectum. 2004;47(1):35–8. https://doi.org/10.1007/s10350-003-0002-0.

80. Casillas S, Hull TL, Zutshi M, Trzcinski R, Bast JF, Xu M. Incontinence after a lateral internal sphincterotomy: are we underestimating it? Dis Colon Rectum. 2005;48(6):1193–9. https://doi.org/10.1007/s10350-004-0914-3.

81. Kement M, Karabulut M, Gezen FC, Demirbas S, Vural S, Oncel M. Mild and severe anal incontinence after lateral internal sphincterotomy: risk factors, postoperative anatomical findings and quality of life. Eur Surg Res. 2011;47:26–31. https://doi.org/10.1159/000324902.

82. Acar T, Acar N, Güngör F, Kamer E, Güngör H, Candan MS, Bağ H, Tarcan E, Dilek ON, Haciyanli M. Treatment of chronic anal fissure: Is open lateral internal sphincterotomy (LIS) a safe and adequate option? Asian J Surg. 2019;42(5):628–33.

83. De Robles MS, Young CJ. Real-world outcomes of lateral internal sphincterotomy vs. botulinum toxin for the management of chronic anal fissures. Asian J Surg. 2022;45(1):184–8. https://doi.org/10.1016/j.asjsur.2021.04.027.

"The wound disrupts the normal continuity of a body structure."
Dorland's Medical Dictionary

Key Concepts

- Management of the postoperative wound is an essential aspect of preventing postoperative complications like dehiscence or infection.
- Anorectal wound management aims to promote wound healing and protect it from soiling by fecal matter.
- Normal wound healing involves four phases: hemostasis, inflammation, proliferation, and tissue remodeling.
- Cleaning the wound with normal saline maintains the viability of the tissue.
- A moist wound environment is required for healthy wound healing.

19.1 Introduction

Surgery is the leading cause of injuries, mortality, hospital infections, and disability in the worldwide healthcare system. Management of the postoperative wound is an essential aspect of preventing postoperative complications like wound dehiscence or surgical site infection.

19.2 Aims and Objectives

The aims and objectives of wound healing are:

- Promotion of healthy granulation tissue
- Protection of the wound from an unhealthy environment

- Decrease in the pain
- To avoid contamination of the wound from soiling with body fluids or waste [1]

19.3 Why Is Wound Care Necessary After Anorectal Surgeries?

- Continuous fecal soiling
- A large amount of pus discharge
- Difficult to dress the anorectal area
- Dressings may be required multiple times a day
- Vacuum-assisted closure of wound (VAC) cannot be applied easily
- The inability of the patient to see the anorectal wound himself

19.4 Healing Phases of Wound

Wound healing occurs either by primary or secondary intention [2]. In healing by primary intention, the wound is closed, and healing occurs by rapid epithelialization [3]. The scarring is minimal as the edges of the wound are well approximated. In healing by secondary intention, the wound is left open to heal. It undergoes a process of natural healing, and scars are more significant [3]. Irrespective of the type of wound, the healing process involves four phases: hemostasis, inflammation, proliferation, and tissue remodeling [4].

Wound healing is only achieved if all these phases occur appropriately and timely. Unfortunately, all the anorectal wounds heal by secondary intention.

19.5   Postoperative Wound Care After Anorectal Surgery

The most common postanorectal surgery complaints are pain and itching in the wound area. There are two patterns of pain reported following anorectal surgery: discomfort during resting and pain experienced during defecation [5]. The resting pain lasts for around 24 to 48 h after surgery and gradually decreases. Postsurgery, the internal anal sphincter spasm causes pain during defecation, which takes a few days to go away [5].

General principles to follow for healing the wounds after anorectal surgery include:

- Ice packs
- Sitz bath
- Topical ointments
- Laxatives

19.5.1   Ice Packs

19.5.1.1   The Principle Behind Using Ice Finger

The laser light targets the chromophore and is absorbed by the tissue at a specific temperature. The temperature rise produces a large amount of heat that can cause thermal damage. The postoperative use of an ice finger is beneficial in two ways: First, it helps lower the raised temperature after lasers; second, it reduces the edema caused by the lasers. To be precise, the ice finger prevents the mucosa from collateral thermal damage.

As mentioned earlier, laser hemorrhoidoplasty causes edema due to cellular injury. Therefore, immediately after the surgery, an ice finger is introduced into the anal canal to decrease the edema and counter the thermal effect of the lasers

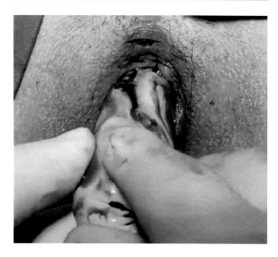

Fig. 19.1   Insertion of ice finger after laser hemorrhoidoplasty

(Fig. 19.1). This finger is removed after 8 to 10 min. The cold compressions can be given in the initial 24 h. One should refrain from keeping the ice finger for a long time or ice directly over the mucosa as it can cause crystallization in the arterioles leading to a condition like frostbite.

19.5.2   Sitz Bath

Hydrotherapy to relieve pain is one of the oldest treatments used and acts as a natural healer [5]. McConnell, in 1993 advocated the use of a sitz bath to relieve the pain. The sitz bath helps to promote blood flow, eliminate wound soiling, and relaxes the internal anal sphincter to expedite wound healing [6]. After anorectal surgery, a hot sitz bath significantly reduces postoperative pain [6].

The sitz bathtub is filled with lukewarm water [6]. The pelvic area and perineum are immersed for 15 to 20 min. The procedure can be repeated two to three times a day. It is advisable not to add potassium permanganate, povidone-iodine, or cetrimide (Savlon) and use plain water only. Before sitting in a sitz bathtub, one must feel the water with the finger to assess the temperature, which should not

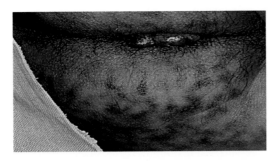

Fig. 19.2 Burns in the perianal area after hot sitz bath

exceed 40 °C to 42 °C. Hot water can cause perianal burns and excoriation of the perineal skin (Fig. 19.2).

Lafoy and Geden recommended a cold sitz bath to reduce perineal pain and post episiotomy pain [7]. A cold sitz bath causes local anesthesia, vasoconstriction, decreases spasm and muscle irritability [8]. According to Shafiq, the sitz bath relieves pain by a neural pathway causing the internal anal sphincter to relax [9]. Haus et al. reported a decrease in pain after using warm water spray [10].

19.5.3 Topical Ointments After Surgery

19.5.3.1 A Combination of Metronidazole, Sucralfate, and Lidocaine

These ointments relieve pain and swelling of the postoperative anorectal wounds. The patient is advised to apply the ointment 10 min before and after defecation.

Mechanism of Action

Metronidazole
Metronidazole is an antibiotic active against anaerobic bacteria [11].

Mechanism of Action
- Acts on anaerobic bacteria
- Promotes epithelialization
- Reduces the time for the tissue repair [12]

Sucralfate
Sucralfate is a cytoprotective agent that can combine with the mucoproteins and form a protective barrier at wound sites. Studies by Parvin J Gupta report a decrease in pain after the use of sucralfate topically after hemorrhoidectomy [13].

Mechanism of Action
- Increases local blood flow
- Stimulates prostaglandins, cell migration, and epithelial growth factors [14]

Studies by Mina Alvandipur et al. reported a decrease in the wound healing time [14].

Lidocaine
Lidocaine works as a local anesthetic that is capable of reducing pain.

Mechanism of Action
- Blocks sodium channels causing numbness.

The neurons of local tissue become incapable of signaling the brain of the sensations [2, 15].

Pedrotti P et al. reported a decrease in pain after applying lidocaine [16].

Commonest Uses
Postoperative wounds after anorectal surgery and anal fissure.

19.5.3.2 Calcium Dobesilate for Local Application in Hemorrhoids

Calcium dobesilate is a venotonic drug that improves the tonicity of the veins [17].

Mechanism of Action
- Reducing microvascular permeability
- Decreases platelet aggregation and hence the thickness of blood, leading to improved blood flow in veins [17]

A study conducted by Patel et al. reported a decrease in rectal bleeding with a success rate of

81.35% after 6 weeks of using calcium dobesilate [18].

After laser hemorrhoidoplasty, patients are advised to apply the ointment for a week.

19.5.3.3 A Combination of Lidocaine and Nifedipine and Diltiazem

Lidocaine is a local anesthetic, whereas nifedipine is a calcium channel blocker.

Mechanism of Action

As discussed above, lidocaine works by blocking signals to the brain. Nifedipine is a calcium channel blocker that blocks the action of calcium on the blood vessels and relaxes the smooth muscles of the internal anal sphincter. As a result, it promotes blood flow to the area, thus diminishing the pain and spasm [19].

Usually, these ointments have an applicator for local application. The applicator is inserted approximately 2.5 cm into the anal canal, and the medicine is released. However, postsurgery using a gloved finger for application can also be used [19]. Another calcium channel blocker is diltiazem (2%), with a similar mechanism of action as nifedipine.

Commonest Uses

Anal fissures. Postoperatively, after lateral internal sphincterotomy, the ointment can also be applied at the fissure site for faster healing.

19.5.4 Use of Laxatives

Another common problem faced after anorectal surgery is apprehension during defecation. There is always a fear of pain. Dietary modifications and toilet training remain the mainstay of management. Dietary changes include the use of a high-fiber diet. The laxatives are used to keep the stools soft and decrease the patient's discomfort.

Commonly used laxatives are:

- Bulk-forming
- Osmotic agents

19.5.4.1 Mechanism of Action of Bulk-Forming Laxatives

These laxatives act by retaining water in the stool and increasing the consistency and weight of the stool [20]. While using bulk laxatives, it is always advisable to increase water intake as lack of water can cause bloating and bowel obstruction [21, 22]. Usually, 2 to 3 litres of water intake is recommended per day.

Example: Methylcellulose, Polycarbophil, Psyllium

19.5.4.2 Mechanism of Action of Osmotic Agents

These work by drawing water from the lumen of the bowel [20, 22]. In my practice, I prefer to use osmotic laxatives.

Example: Polyethylene glycol, Lactulose

Dosage: The dosage prescribed is 35–40 mL of osmotic laxative twice a day, which can be tittered depending on the individual's need.

19.6 Wound Cleaning

After every anorectal surgery, proper wound cleaning is necessary to enhance healing and reduce discomfort.

19.6.1 The Best Cleansing Agent: Povidone-Iodine or Water!

Povidone-iodine is not recommended for cleansing wounds as it has the potency to destroy and damage the cells vital for the healing process [23]. The normal saline solution is used as it is an isotonic solution. It is noncytotoxic and does not interfere with healing [24, 25]. Moreover, it does not change the normal bacterial flora [25]. However, studies also report that simple tap water is an equally effective agent for wound cleaning [23]. Fernandez et al., in their study, have supported that water, when obtained from a supply of potable drinking water, can be used to clean the wounds [26].

19.6.2 Cleaning of the Wound After Fistula and Fissure Surgery

Keeping the wound clean after fistulotomy is mandatory. Fecal matter can cause contamination of the wound. After defecation, using a hand faucet to clean the area is the best option. However, everyone cannot afford it. Therefore, an economical way to clean the area is to fill water in an empty plastic water bottle and make multiple holes in the cap. The bottle is then pressed, and the area is thus cleaned with a significant amount of pressure. Rubbing of tissue paper or toilet roll should be avoided to prevent injury to the open wound. Soft and clean muslin cloth or towel can be used to dry the area. Cotton balls should be avoided for cleaning the area as the lint may get stuck in the wound margins and later cause irritation and itching.

Discharge is a common complaint of the patients postfistula surgery. Using sterile dressing pads after application of the ointments can avoid soiling and contamination of the clothes. In case seton has been placed, replacement of seton at regular intervals prevents the infection. The tunneling fistula wounds created after coring can be washed using an irrigation cannula (Fig. 19.3).

The presence of hyper granulation tissue indicates an underlying infection. Curetting can be done in OPD if hyper granulation tissue is present.

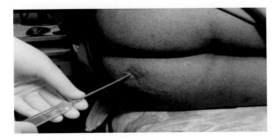

Fig. 19.3 Irrigation of fistula wounds using irrigation cannula

19.6.3 Cleaning of Wounds After Pilonidal Sinus

Educating the patients to manage the wound and peri-wound area is crucial [27]. The following must be explained to the patient and the attendants.

- Cleansing of the wound
- Change of dressings
- Hair removal—once in 2 weeks
- Avoiding prolonged sitting

19.7 Special Dressings for Anal Fistula and Pilonidal Sinus Wounds

The latest modalities of the wound care include the following:

19.7.1 Hemoglobin Spray

Hemoglobin spray comprises purified hemoglobin of bovine origin. The hemoglobin has been used for wound healing for 50 years [28]. A wound heals faster if the oxygen demand in the wound is met rapidly [29]. Hemoglobin spray is reported to cause wound size reduction, decrease in slough, and reduction in pain in chronic wounds [30].

19.7.1.1 Mechanism of Action

Oxygen is essential for wound healing. Hemoglobin spray binds atmospheric oxygen and diffuses it into the wound bed, increasing the oxygen concentration of the wound, and hence accelerating wound healing [31].

Oxygen is involved in various biological processes, protein synthesis, cell proliferation, and angiogenesis, responsible for tissue function and integrity [32]. In the initial stages of wound healing, the vascularity near the wounds is disrupted, causing hypoxia. If the oxygen supply to the wound is increased, the healing is hastened. Hemoglobin spray can be injected into the tunneling wound after coring of fistula tracts and in cases of pilonidal sinus after VALAPS. In open wounds, post fistulotomy, hemoglobin spray can be used for topical application.

19.7.2 Dried Amnion Chorion Granules with PHMB

The human amniotic membrane for wounds dates to the early 1900s [33]. The dried amnion chorion granules are micronized particulate forms of dehydrated human amnion chorion membrane. These are natural skin substances derived from the human placenta. They are impregnated with 0.5% (w/w) polyhexamethylene biguanide (PHMB) [34].

19.7.2.1 Mechanism of Action

- The amnion membrane provides growth factors and promotes angiogenesis, epithelialization, and crosses biofilms [35]. PHMB works by destroying the microbial cell membranes leading to cell death [36] (Fig. 19.4).

The micro size of the granules can be injected into the postoperative pilonidal sinus and cored-out fistula tracts. Studies have reported 50% wound size reduction after 2 weeks, with 83% complete wound healing within 12 weeks in chronic wounds [34] (Fig. 19.5a–c).

Fig. 19.4 Mechanism of action of PHMB

PHMB enters the bacterial cell → Arrests the cell division and condenses the bacterial chromosomes → Bacterial Cell death

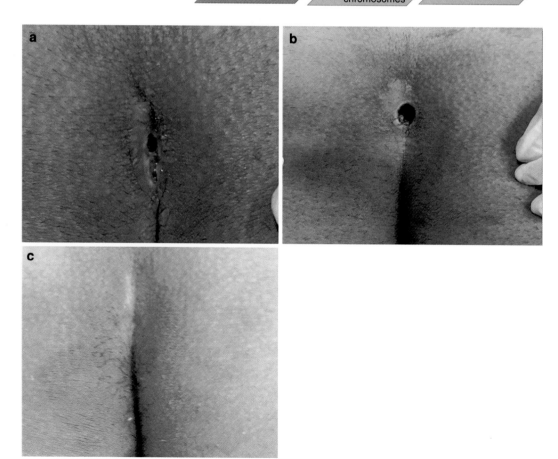

Fig. 19.5 (**a**) Postoperative wound. (**b**) Postoperative wound after 1 week of surgery. (**c**) Postoperative wound after 3 weeks of surgery

However, long-term studies are required to know the efficacy in fistula wounds.

19.7.3   Use of Silver Dressings for Pilonidal Sinus

An ideal dressing needed for proper wound healing must be able to absorb excess exudate, reduce bacterial load, fill cavities, maintain moisture, and enhance the blood supply. Silver reduces the bioburden of the wound, thus taking care of the biofilms [37].

19.7.3.1   Mechanism of Action

The silver ions have a bactericidal effect by acting in three ways: first on the bacterial proteins and DNA, second on enzymes involved in vital cellular processes, and third on a cell wall, or cell membrane, thus inhibiting the respiration process [38]. Studies have reported a rapid decrease in wound size after using silver ointments [39, 40]. The dressing is done twice a day.

19.8   Discussion

Successful wound management depends on the basic understanding of the physiological changes in the wound healing process, the type of surgery performed, the type of wound closure, and the optimal treatment of the resultant wound [37]. The cleaning of the wounds is done as a part of the wound managing regime. However, the choice of a cleansing agent remains controversial [38]. Role of povidone-iodine, is questionable as it is cytotoxic. An ideal wound cleansing agent should be nontoxic to human tissues, reduce the bioburden, and not cause sensitivity reactions [39]. Studies have reported that normal saline, simple tap water, sterile water, and even potable water can be used as cleansing agents for the wound [39].

There are two cleaning methods: scrubbing and irrigation [38]. Scrubbing or rubbing the wound should be avoided to minimize trauma. Irrigation is considered one of the best methods for cleansing the wound [38]. The cleansing of the postoperative fistula and pilonidal sinus wounds should be carried out with gentle irrigation with either normal saline or water.

Postoperative care involves the use of topical ointments that should be antimicrobial, maintain moisture, and enhance wound healing. Commonly used ointments include a mixture of lidocaine, metrogyl, and sucralfate. Using topical agents like PHMB on the wound promotes wound healing by targeting the bacteria [40]. It is noncytotoxic and is clinically proven superior to povidone-iodine and silver nitrate for treating wounds [38, 41, 42]. The principle behind using hemoglobin spray in chronic wounds is well documented. The topical hemoglobin spray transports oxygen from the surrounding air and increases oxygen availability in the wound bed. It has been documented that hemoglobin spray should not be used with certain disinfectants, like octenidine, as it may impair its effectiveness [30, 31]. We achieved excellent results with hemoglobin spray in pilonidal sinus and fistula wounds at our center. Although there was a considerable reduction in wound size after the spray, this evaluation was not conducted as a formal randomized clinical study. Therefore, more studies are required to evaluate the efficacy of the hemoglobin spray. After dressing, the wound should be inspected. A healthy granulation tissue is usually pink and is indicative of good wound healing. If hyper granulation tissue is present in the fistula or pilonidal sinus wounds, curetting can be done in the OPD. Curetting refreshes the wound bed and promotes wound healing.

A question most frequently asked by a patient is how many times one can use an ointment postoperatively? The ointments should be applied twice a day but can also be used after each motion.

The third most crucial postoperative care is the management of pain. The patients operated on for anorectal surgeries often complain of pain during defecation. Lidocaine ointment 5% can be applied before defecation to avoid pain.

Laxatives, antibiotics, sitz baths, and analgesics are also a part of the postoperative regime. An adequate dietary supply of nutrients and supplements enhances wound healing and encourages rapid patient recovery.

The fourth most considerable point of postoperative wound management is educating the patients about maintaining good hygiene. After pilonidal sinus surgery, the navicular area should be kept clean.

The presence of co-morbidities like diabetes and hypertension, may hamper wound healing. The patients should be advised to continue with the medicines prescribed for these morbid conditions for a speedy recovery.

Take-Home Message
Wounds are reported to recover fast after minimally invasive procedures as the creation of the raw areas is very small. Timely and proper wound management, appropriate cleansing, and dressings can prevent the wound from becoming infected. During the patients' wound healing journey, the nurses and the treating surgeon must do their best to encourage, counsel, and adequately educate patients on wound care.

References

1. Britto EJ, Nezwek TA, Robins M. Wound dressings. In: StatPearls. Treasure Island, FL: StatPearls Publishing; 2022.
2. Al-Khamis A, McCallum I, King PM, Bruce J. Healing by primary versus secondary intention after surgical treatment for pilonidal sinus. Cochrane Database Syst Rev. 2010;2010(1):CD006213. https://doi.org/10.1002/14651858.CD006213.pub3.
3. Guo S, Dipietro LA. Factors affecting wound healing. J Dent Res. 2010;89(3):219–29. https://doi.org/10.1177/0022034509359125.
4. Gosain A, DiPietro LA. Aging and wound healing. World J Surg. 2004;28:321–6.
5. Mooventhan A, Nivethitha L. Scientific evidence-based effects of hydrotherapy on various systems of the body. N Am J Med Sci. 2014;6(5):199–209. https://doi.org/10.4103/1947-2714.132935.
6. McConnell EA. Giving your patient a Sitz bath. Nursing. 1993;23(12):14. https://doi.org/10.1097/00152193-199312000-00007.
7. LaFoy J, Geden EA. Postepisiotomy pain: warm versus cold Sitz bath. J Obstet Gynecol Neonatal Nurs. 1989;18(5):399–403. https://doi.org/10.1111/j.1552-6909.1989.tb00493.x.
8. Tejirian T, Abbas MA. Sitz bath: where is the evidence? Scientific basis of a common practice. Dis Colon Rectum. 2005;48(12):2336–40.
9. Shafik A. Role of warm-water bath in anorectal conditions. The "thermosphincteric reflex". J Clin Gastroenterol. 1993;16(4):304–8. https://doi.org/10.1097/00004836-199306000-00007.
10. Hsu KF, Chia JS, Jao SW, Wu CC, Yang HY, Mai CM, et al. Comparison of clinical effects between warm water spray and Sitz bath in the post-hemorrhoidectomy period. J Gastrointest Surg. 2009;13(7):1274–8.
11. Löfmark S, Edlund C, Nord CE. Metronidazole is still the drug of choice for the treatment of anaerobic infections. Clin Infect Dis. 2010;50(Suppl. S1):S16–23.
12. Nicholson TJ, Armstrong D. Topical metronidazole (10 percent) decrease post hemorrhoidectomy pain and improves healing. Dis Colon Rectum. 2004;47:711–6.
13. Gupta PJ, Heda PS, Kalaskar S, Tamaskar VP. Topical sucralfate decreases pain after hemorrhoidectomy and improves healing: a randomized, blinded, controlled study. Dis Colon Rectum. 2008;51(2):231–4. https://doi.org/10.1007/s10350-007-9092-4.
14. Alvandipour M, Ala S, Tavakoli H, Charati JY, Shiva A. Efficacy of 10% sucralfate ointment after anal fistulotomy: a prospective, double-blind, randomized, placebo-controlled trial. Int J Surg. 2016;36(Part A):13–7. https://doi.org/10.1016/j.ijsu.2016.10.017.
15. Electronic Medicines Compendium. Lidocaine 1% w/v solution for injection. Monograph. https://www.medicines.org.uk/emc/landing#gref.
16. Perrotti P, Bove A, Antropoli C, et al. Topical nifedipine with lidocaine ointment vs. active control for treatment of chronic anal fissure: results of a prospective, randomized, double-blind study. Dis Colon Rectum. 2002;45:1468–75.
17. Scaldaferri F, Ingravalle F, Zinicola T, Holleran G, Gasbarrini A. Medical therapy of hemorrhoidal disease. In: Ratto C, Parello A, Litta F, editors. Hemorrhoids, Coloproctology, vol. 2. Cham: Springer; 2018. p. 49–72. https://doi.org/10.1007/978-3-319-53357-5_6.
18. Patel HD, Bhedi AN, Chauhan AP, Joshi RM. Calcium dobesilate in symptomatic treatment of hemorrhoidal disease: an interventional study. Nat J Med Res. 2013;3:42–4.
19. Katsinelos P, Kountouras J, Paroutoglou G, Beltsis A, Chatzimavroudis G, Zavos C, Katsinelos T, Papaziogas B. Aggressive treatment of acute anal fissure with 0.5% nifedipine ointment prevents its evolution to chronicity. World J Gastroenterol. 2006;12(38):6203–6. https://doi.org/10.3748/wjg.v12.i38.6203.
20. Liu LW. Chronic constipation: current treatment options. Can J Gastroenterol. 2011;25(Suppl. B):22B–8B.

21. Leung L, Riutta T, Kotecha J, Rosser W. Chronic constipation: an evidence-based review. J Am Board Fam Med. 2011;24(4):436–51.

22. Bashir A, Sizar O. Laxatives. In: StatPearls. Treasure Island, FL: StatPearls Publishing; 2020.

23. Barr JE. Principles of wound cleansing. Ostomy Wound Manage. 1995;41:15S–21S.

24. Cunliffe PJ, Fawcett TN. Wound cleansing: the evidence for the techniques and solutions used. Prof Nurse. 2002;18:95–9.

25. Ovington LG. Battling bacteria in wound care. Home Healthc Nurse. 2001;19:622–30.

26. Beam JW. Wound cleansing: water or saline? J Athl Train. 2006;41(2):196–7.

27. Harris C, Sibbald RG, Mufti A, Somayaji R. Pilonidal sinus disease: 10 steps to optimize care. Adv Skin Wound Care. 2016;29(10):469–78. https://doi.org/10.1097/01.ASW.0000491324.29246.96.

28. Scholander PF. Oxygen transport through hemoglobin solutions. Science. 1960;131:585–90.

29. Sen C. Wound healing essentials: let there be oxygen. Wound Repair Regen. 2009;17(1):1–18.

30. Elg F, Hunt S. Hemoglobin spray as adjunct therapy in complex wounds: Meta-analysis versus standard care alone in pooled data by wound type across three retrospective cohort controlled evaluations. SAGE Open Med. 2018;6:2050312118784313. https://doi.org/10.1177/2050312118784313.

31. Hunt SD, Elg F. Clinical effectiveness of hemoglobin spray (Granulox®) as adjunctive therapy in the treatment of chronic diabetic foot ulcers. Diabetic Foot Ankle. 2016;7:33101. https://doi.org/10.3402/dfa.v7.33101.

32. Castilla DM, Liu ZJ, Velazquez OC. Oxygen: implications for wound healing. Adv Wound Care. 2012;1(6):225–30. https://doi.org/10.1089/wound.2011.0319.

33. John T. Human amniotic membrane transplantation: past, present, and future. Ophthalmol Clin N Am. 2003;16(1):43–65.

34. Hawkins B. The use of micronized dehydrated human amnion/chorion membrane allograft for the treatment of diabetic foot ulcers: a case series. Wounds. 2016;28(5):152–7.

35. Odet S, Louvrier A, Meyer C, Nicolas FJ, Hofman N, Chatelain B, et al. Surgical application of human amniotic membrane and amnion-chorion membrane in the oral cavity and efficacy evaluation: corollary with ophthalmological and wound healing experiences. Front Bioeng Biotechnol. 2021;9:443.

36. Chindera K, Mahato M, Sharma AK, Horsley H, Kloc-Muniak K, Kamaruzzaman NF, Kumar S, McFarlane A, Stach J, Bentin T, Good L. The antimicrobial polymer PHMB enters cells and selectively condenses bacterial chromosomes. Sci Rep. 2016;6:23121. https://doi.org/10.1038/srep23121

37. Bishop A. Wound assessment and dressing selection: an overview. Br J Nurs. 2021;30(5):S12–20.

38. Atiyeh BS, Dibo SA, Hayek SN. Wound cleansing, topical antiseptics, and wound healing. Int Wound J. 2009;6(6):420–30. https://doi.org/10.1111/j.1742-481X.2009.00639.x.

39. Main RC. Should chlorhexidine gluconate be used in wound cleansing? J Wound Care. 2008;17(3):112–4.

40. Yang W, Shen C, Ji Q, An H, Wang J, Liu Q, Zhang Z. Food storage material silver nanoparticles interfere with DNA replication fidelity and bind with DNA. Nanotechnology. 2009;20(8):085102.

41. Lansdown AB. Silver I: its antibacterial properties and mechanism of action. J Wound Care. 2002;11(4):125–30.

42. Feyzi KURT. The use of silver nitrate in pilonidal sinus patients. Chirurgia. 2021;34(4):158–61.

Hemorrhoids

3rd Degree Hemorrhoids—https://goo.by/D4i0F

4th Degree Haemorrhoids (Failure of Inj. Hylase)—https://goo.by/0Q6dF

4th Degree hemorrhoids Prolapsed and Thrombosed Piles—https://goo.by/fF9cm

Sclerotherapy for 1st Degree Hemorrhoids—https://goo.by/KvqHH

Local and Digital Rectal Examination (DRE)—https://goo.by/49hYj

K. Gupta, *Lasers in Proctology*, https://doi.org/10.1007/978-981-19-5825-0

Fistula in Ano

Two internal openings with two external openings (Distal Coring Proximal Fistulotomy (DCPF)—https://goo.by/RVjiO

Complex Fistula in Ano (Penoscrotal Junction)—https://goo.by/wwptl

Intersphincteric tract without External opening with Horseshoe intersphincteric tract (Type A4)—https://goo.by/eqF3P

© The Editor(s) (if applicable) and The Author(s), under exclusive license to Springer Nature Singapore Pte Ltd. 2022
K. Gupta, *Lasers in Proctology*, https://doi.org/10.1007/978-981-19-5825-0

Pilonidal Sinus

Video Assisted Laser Ablation of Pilonidal Sinus (VALAPS)—https://goo.by/HWrNO

Sinus Laser Treatment (SiLaT)—https://goo.by/4FoD8

Fissure in Ano

Fissure in Ano—https://goo.by/7Oecy
  Fissure in Ano with Skin Tag—https://goo.by/
va4lR

K. Gupta, *Lasers in Proctology*, https://doi.org/10.1007/978-981-19-5825-0